FRCR PART

FRCR PART 2A

Single Best Answer (SBA) Questions

Authors

Dr Tristan Barrett, Dr Nadeem Shaida,
Dr Owen Thomas, Dr Ashley Shaw

Addenbrooke's Hospital, Cambridge, UK

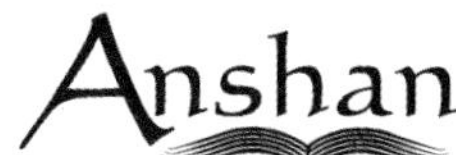

First published in 2010 by

Anshan Ltd
11a Little Mount Sion
Tunbridge Wells
Kent. TN1 1YS

Tel: +44 (0) 1892 557767
Fax: +44 (0) 1892 530358
E-mail: info@anshan.co.uk
www.anshan.co.uk

ISBN: 978 1848290 419

British Library Cataloguing in Publication Data
A catalogue record for this book is available from the British Library

Copy Editor: Andrew White
Cover Design: Terry Griffiths

Typeset by Replika Press Pvt Ltd, India

Preface

In March 2009, the Royal College of Radiologists confirmed that the long anticipated change in format of the written final FRCR Part 2A examinations was to come into effect from the autumn 2009 sitting. The previous negatively marked true-false MCQs were to be replaced by 'single best answer' (SBA) questions. The SBA format comprises a 'stem' question and 5 'options' (a) – (e) to choose from, only one of which represents the best answer to the question posed in the stem. Each of the 6 modules will consist of 75 stem questions; negative marking is to be discontinued.

Introduction

Single Best Answer questions, also known as 'One Best Answer', or 'Best of Five' questions have recently been adopted for various undergraduate and postgraduate medical examinations in multiple specialities in both the USA and the UK. They potentially offer many advantages over the previously used format of negatively marked true-false MCQs. A major criticism of the old style MCQ format relates to concerns that technique alone can get the 'exam-wise' candidate through the exam. Also, in order to avoid 'absolute' terms (always/never), the writer may use ambiguous terms such as 'commonly', 'usually', or 'frequently' which can be confusing; alternatively, in order to avoid ambiguity, the candidate may be asked to recall an isolated fact. SBA questions are designed to test the application of knowledge to help avoid such problems, and they are additionally thought to be fairer to candidates for whom English is not their first language. Candidates will require longer to complete SBA style questions due to the time taken to read and assess the stem; this has been reflected in the fact that the RCR has increased the allotted time for each examination to 2 hours, with the modules now taking place over 3, rather than 2 days.

The SBA question is composed of 3 parts: the stem, the lead in, and the options, and has 1 correct answer with 4 distracters. The ideal question has a long stem with a concise lead-in and short options. The stem typically comprises a clinical vignette and may consist of history, examination findings, pathological data or initial radiological findings. The vignette should present data which would be relevant and available to a practicing radiologist such as a clinician asking for advice on how to investigate a patient, or the details entered on a request card. Ideally, the stronger candidates would be able to answer the stem directly before even looking at the 5 options. The options should be continuous (*i.e.* all diagnoses, or all investigations), and should all grammatically follow the stem. The incorrect options should be plausible, and in some cases may not be completely wrong, but given the information stated in the stem, should be unequivocally 'less correct' than the intended answer. If couplets, or triplets are listed in the options, the correct answer should not be apparent due to its 'over representation' above other answers within the options. Additionally, the correct answer should not differ significantly in length or detail in comparison to the distracters.

We have extensively researched and cross-checked the questions, and relevant topics have been drawn from major radiology textbooks, as well as current radiological journals such as *Clinical Radiology* and *Radiographics*, and also from the 'Radiology Integrated Training Initiative' (RITI) website, an initiative of the Royal College of Radiologists. We have produced 750 'stem' questions covering all 6 modules and divided them into 2 sections. The first section consists of 50 questions per module and provides an overview; the second section consists of 75 stem questions per module and is in the format of a 'mock' examination. Readers can use this to test themselves against the clock and under examination conditions, in order to hone their technique prior to sitting the examination. Answers are given with detailed explanations and references are provided, which can also be used for further reading as appropriate.

References and further reading: Clin Rad (2008); 63(5): 506–10, and Case SM & Swanson DB, Constructing Written Test Questions for the Basic and Clinical Sciences (2008).

Contents

Abbreviation

Abbreviation	Full
α1AT	α1-antitrypsin deficiency
α-FP	α-Fetoprotein
β-HCG	β-Human chorionic gonadotropin
A&E	Accident & Emergency
AAA	Abdominal aortic aneurysm
AAST	American Association for the Surgery of Trauma
ABC	Aneurysmal bone cyst
ABPA	Allergic bronchopulmonary aspergillosis
AC	Acromio-clavicular
ACTH	Adrenocorticotropic hormone
ADC	Apparent diffusion co-efficient
ADPKD	Autosomal dominant polycystic kidney disease
AF	Atrial fibrillation
AIDS	Acquired immuno-deficiency syndrome
AIIS	Anterior inferior iliac spine
ALP	Alkaline phosphatase
ALT	Alanine aminotransferase
AP	Antero-posterior
ARDS	Adult respiratory distress syndrome
ARPKD	Autosomal recessive polycystic kidney disease
ASD	Atrial septal defect
ASIS	Anterior superior iliac spine
AVF	Arteriovenous fistula
AVM	Arteriovenous malformation
AVN	Avascular necrosis
AXR	Abdominal x-ray
BAC	Bronchoalveolar cell carcinoma
BMT	Bone marrow transplant
BP	Blood pressure
BPD	Bronchopulmonary dysplasia
CADASIL	Cerebral autosomal dominant arteriopathy with subcortical infarcts and leukoencephalopathy
CAF	Coronary artery fistula
CBD	Common bile duct
CBF	Cerebral blood flow
CBV	Cerebral blood volume
CC	Coraco-clavicular

CEA	Carcinoembryogenic antigen
CE-CT	Contrast-enhanced computed tomography
CF	Cystic fibrosis
CFA	Common femoral artery
CFV	Common femoral vein
CHD	Congenital heart disease
CNS	Central nervous system
COPD	Chronic obstructive pulmonary disease
CPA	Cerebello-pontine angle
CRL	Crown-rump length
CSF	Cerebro-spinal fluid
CT	Computed tomography
CTKUB	Computed tomography kidneys ureter bladder
CTPA	Computed tomography pulmonary angiography
CVA	Cerebro-vascular accident (stroke)
CXR	Chest x-ray
D+C	Dilation and curettage
DDH	Developmental dysplasia of the hip
DJJ	Duodeno-jejunal junction
DMSA	Dimercaptosuccinic acid
DNET	Dysembryoplastic neuroepithelial tumour
DRE	Digital rectal examination
DSA	Digital subtraction angiography
DVT	Deep vein thrombosis
DWI	Diffusion weighted imaging
EAA	Extrinsic allergic alveolitis
EAS	External anal sphincter
EBV	Epstein-Barr virus
ECA	External carotid artery
ECG	Electro-cardiogram
EDH	Extra-dural haematoma
EG	Eosinophillic granuloma
EIA	External iliac artery
ER	Estrogen receptor
ESM	Ejection systolic murmur
EUS	Endoscopic ultrasound
EVAR	Endovascular aneurysm repair
FAST	Focused assessment with sonography for trauma
FDG	Fluoro-deoxy-glucose
FEV-1	Forced expiratory volume in 1 second
FIGO	Federation-International of Gynaecology and Obstetrics
FNA	Fine needle aspiration
FOV	Field of view

GCS	Glasgow coma scale
GCT	Giant cell tumour
GFR	Glomerular filtration rate
GI	Gastrointestinal
GIST	Gastrointestinal stromal tumour
HIDA	Hepatobiliary iminodiacetic acid
HIV	Human immunodeficiency virus
HMD	Hyaline Membrane Disease
HMPAO	Hexamethylpropyleneamine oxime
HRCT	High resolution computed tomography
HRT	Hormone replacement therapy
HSG	Hysterosalpingogram
HSV	Herpes Simplex virus
HU	Hounsfield units
HyCoSy	Hysterosalpingo contrast sonography
i.v.	Intravenous
IAS	Internal anal sphincter
ICA	Internal carotid artery
IIA	Internal iliac artery
IJV	Internal jugular vein
IMA	Inferior mesenteric artery
IMV	Inferior mesenteric vein
In	Indium
IPF	Idiopathic pulmonary fibrosis
IPMN	Intraductal papillary mucinous neoplasm
IUCD	Intrauterine contraceptive device
IVC	Inferior vena cava
IVU	Intravenous urogram
JCA	Juvenile chronic arthritis
KUB	Kidneys ureter bladder x-ray
LA	Left atrium
LAM	Lymphangioleiomyomatosis
LAO	Left anterior oblique
LC	Lymphangiitis Carcinomatosis
LCA	Left coronary artery
LCH	Langerhans cell histiocytosis
LIP	Lymphocytic interstitial pneumonia
LLL	Left lower lobe
LMP	Last menstrual period
LN	Lymph node
LUL	Left upper lobe
LV	Left ventricle
MALT	Mucosa-associated lymphoid tissue

MDP	Methyl diphosphonate
MELAS	Mitochondrial encephalopathy lactic acidosis with stroke-like episodes
MIBG	Meta-iodobenzylguanidine
MRA	Magnetic resonance angiography
MRCP	Magnetic resonance cholangiopancreatogram
MRI	Magnetic resonance imaging
MS	Multiple sclerosis
MTT	Mean transit time
MUGA	Multi-gated acquisition
NAI	Non accidental injury
NASH	Non alcoholic steatohepatitis
NEC	Necrotizing enterocolitis
NF	Neurofibromatosis
NHL	Non-Hodgkin's lymphoma
NICE	National institute for clinical excellence
NRH	Nodular regenerative hyperplasia
NSAID	Non-steroidal anti-inflammatory drug
NSIP	Non-specific interstitial pneumonia
OA	Osteoarthritis
OGD	Oesophogastroduodenoscopy
OI	Osteogenesis imperfecta
PA	Pulmonary artery
PAN	Polyarteritis nodosa
PAPVC	Partial anomalous pulmonary venous connection
PD	Protein density weighted
PE	Pulmonary embolus
PET	Positron emission tomography
PHT	Pulmonary Hypertension
PICC	Peripherally inserted central catheter
PID	Pelvic inflammatory disease
PIE	Pulmonary interstitial emphysema
PML	Progressive multifocal leukoencephalopathy
PPH	Primary pulmonary hypertension
PPV	Positive predictive value
PSA	Prostate specific antigen
PUJ	Pelvi-ureteric junction
PUO	Pyrexia of unknown origin
PV	Per vagina
PVL	Periventricular leukomalacia
PVNS	Pigmented villonodular synovitis
RA	Right atrium
RAO	Right anterior oblique

RAS	Renal artery stenosis
RCA	Right coronary artery
RCR	Royal College of Radiologists
RDS	Respiratory distress syndrome
RECIST	Response evaluation criteria in solid tumours
RhA	Rheumatoid arthritis
RHV	Right hepatic vein
RIF	Right iliac fossa
RLL	Right lower lobe
RML	Right middle lobe
RTA	Road traffic accident
rt-PA	Recombinant-tissue plasminogen activator
RUL	Right upper lobe
RUQ	Right upper quadrant
RVH	Right ventricular hypertrophy
SAH	Subarachnoid haemorrhage
SBO	Small bowel obstruction
SCA	Subclavian artery
SCC	Squamous cell carcinoma
SCD	Sickle cell disease
SDH	Sub dural haematoma
SFV	Superficial femoral vein
SLE	Systemic lupus erythematosus
SMA	Superior mesenteric artery
SMV	Superior mesenteric vein
SNR	Signal-to-noise ratio
SPECT	Single photon emission computed tomography
STIR	Short tau inversion recovery
SUFE	Slipped upper femoral epiphysis
SUV	Standardised uptake value
SVC	Superior vena cava
SVCO	Superior vena caval obstruction
T_1W	T_1-weighted imaging
T_2W	T_2-weighted imaging
TAPVC	Total anomalous pulmonary venous connection
TB	Tuberculosis
TCC	Transitional cell carcinoma
THR	Total hip replacement
TIPS	Transjugular intrahepatic portosystemic shunt
TOF	Tracheo-oesophageal fistula
TTN	Transient tachypnoea of the newborn
UAC	Umbilical artery catheter
UFE	Uterine fibroid embolisation

UIP	Usual interstitial pneumonia
US	Ultrasound
UTI	Urinary tract infection
UVC	Umbilical vein catheter
VACTERL	Vertebral/anal/cardiovascular/tracheal/esophageal/renal/limb anomalies
VAE	Venous air embolism
VMA	Vanillymandelic acid
VSD	Ventricular septal defect
WCC	White cell count
WG	Wegener's granulomatosis

About the authors

Tristan Barrett is currently a radiology registrar at Addenbrooke's Hospital, Cambridge. He qualified in 2002, has two years research experience at National Institutes for Health, Bethesda, USA, and gained MRCP membership in 2005.

Nadeem Shaida is currently a radiology registrar at Addenbrooke's Hospital, Cambridge, having graduated from St. Bartholomew's and the Royal London School of Medicine in 2000. His clinical interests include interventional and oncological radiology.

Owen Thomas is currently a radiology registrar/academic clinical fellow at Addenbrooke's Hospital, Cambridge. He obtained a DPhil before graduating from Oxford University Medical School in 2005. He will sub-specialise in neuroradiology.

Ashley Shaw is a consultant radiologist at Addenbrooke's Hospital, Cambridge, having been appointed in 2004, after training in radiology at King's College Hospital, London. He has clinical and research interests including oncology, transplantation and cross-sectional imaging.

Section 1:
Practice SBAs

Section 1
Practice SBAs

Cardiothoracic and Vascular Practice SBA Questions

1 **A 42 year old fit and well male has a CXR for emigration purposes. There is a rounded opacity in the right mediastinum. Subsequent CT chest reveals a 4.5 cm nodal mass with central calcification and marked enhancement following contrast administration. There are no focal lung lesions.**

Which of the following is the most likely diagnosis?

(a) Castleman's disease
(b) Colorectal cancer metastasis
(c) Langerhan's cell histiocystosis
(d) Non-Hodgkins lymphoma
(e) Silicosis

2 **A 54 year old woman with a 20 pack per year smoking history presents with worsening chronic dyspnoea. CXR shows prominence of the central pulmonary vasculature. Contrast enhanced CT is performed.**

Which of the following features would not support a diagnosis of pulmonary arterial hypertension?

(a) The patient's demographics
(b) Mosaic attenuation of the lung parenchyma
(c) Bowing of the interventricular septum convex to the right
(d) Pruning of peripheral pulmonary arteries
(e) Bronchial arteries measuring up to 4 mm in diameter

3 **A CXR is requested in a 52 year old man with chronic dyspnoea. The CXR shows bi-apical volume loss and reticulonodular changes within both upper zones.**

Which of the following is the most likely underlying aetiology?

(a) α1-anti-trypsin deficiency
(b) Bleomycin toxicity
(c) Silicosis
(d) Systemic sclerosis
(e) Usual interstitial pneumonitis

4 **A 25 year old woman presents with an acute seizure. CT shows a 2 cm ring enhancing lesion in the frontal lobe with surrounding oedema. CXR shows 3 opacities measuring between 1–3 cm in size, projected over the left lower zone. Contrast enhanced CT shows these lesions to be round, well defined and containing linear structures radiating away from the lesions.**

What is the likeliest diagnosis?

(a) Lymphangioleiomyomatosis
(b) Takayasu's arteritis
(c) Sarcoidosis
(d) Osler–Weber–Rendu syndrome
(e) Wegener's granulomatosis

5 **A 24 year old asymptomatic man has a CXR for insurance purposes. The report describes a solitary 2 cm pulmonary nodule. A subsequent CT is arranged.**

Which of the following features favour a diagnosis of carcinoid over hamartoma?

(a) Avid 18FDG-PET uptake
(b) Calcification
(c) Central location
(d) Hounsfield value of -30
(e) Solitary lesion

6 **A 38 year old non-smoker presents with pleuritic chest pain, shortness of breath and a raised D-Dimer. A CT pulmonary angiogram is performed which shows no pulmonary emboli. There is a solitary 3 mm, well circumscribed nodule in the right upper lobe.**

What follow-up should you recommend?

(a) No follow-up
(b) CT at 6–12 months
(c) CT at 3, 9, and 24 months
(d) CT 6-12 at months, then 18-24 months
(e) PET-CT or biopsy of nodule

7 **A 32 year old male patient has a routine CXR for insurance purposes. The film is well centred, the right heart border is indistinct and appears rotated. The lung parenchyma and vasculature appear normal.**

What is the most likely cause?
(a) Absent left pericardium
(b) Pectus excavatum
(c) Poor patient positioning
(d) Pulmonary artery enlargement
(e) Situs solitus

8 **In the staging of pleural mesothelioma, which of the following constitutes T4 disease?**

(a) Invasion of a rib
(b) Invasion of the endothoracic fascia
(c) Invasion of mediastinal fat
(d) Invasion of the soft tissue of the chest wall
(e) Non-transmural invasion of the pericardium

9 **A CXR is performed and shows a unilateral right-sided pleural effusion.**

Which of the following extra-pulmonary conditions is most likely to produce these appearances?
(a) Boerhaarve's syndrome
(b) Gastric neoplasm
(c) Stanford type B aortic dissection
(d) Transection of the proximal thoracic duct
(e) Traumatic aortic rupture

10 A 46 year old man presents to an A&E department with shortness of breath. The CXR shows a diffuse opacity in the RUL. On a previous film, taken 3 months ago, he had a similar appearance in the LUL which cleared on a CXR taken 10 days later; there was a similar episode a year prior to this with an opacity in the middle lobe, which subsequently cleared.

Which of the following conditions is the least likely diagnosis?

(a) Chronic eosinophilic pneumonia
(b) Churg-Strauss syndrome
(c) Extrinsic allergic alveolitis
(d) Goodpasture's syndrome
(e) Loeffler's syndrome

11 Which of the following sequelae of intravenous contrast medium is not dose dependent?

(a) Anaphylactoid reaction
(b) Bradycardia
(c) Nausea & vomiting
(d) Nephropathy
(e) Metallic taste

12 A 27 year old man under investigation for suspected liver disease has his venous pressures measured and is found to have a hepatic venous wedge gradient of 3 mmHg.

What does this indicate?

(a) There is no liver disease
(b) Pre-sinusoidal cause of portal venous hypertension
(c) Sinusoidal cause of portal venous hypertension
(d) Post-sinusoidal cause of portal venous hypertension
(e) There is insufficient data to draw a conclusion

13 When optimising a CT study of the aorta, which of the following would not improve arterial enhancement?

(a) Increasing the injection flow rate
(b) Increasing the Iodine concentration
(c) Increasing the duration of the injection
(d) Increasing the cardiac output
(e) Increasing the volume of contrast medium

14 A 76 year old man presents with central chest pain. He is haemodynamically stable and undergoes a thoracic CT study which demonstrates a hyperdense crescent in the wall of the descending thoracic aorta on the unenhanced study, which does not change following the administration of i.v. contrast medium.

What is the most likely diagnosis?

(a) Aortic dissection
(b) Atherosclerosis
(c) Intramural haematoma
(d) Vasculitis
(e) Mediastinal fibrosis

15 A 67 year old patient with cardiac risk factors presents with left calf claudication on walking 30 yards. An MR angiogram is performed and shows a focal stenosis of the right popliteal artery. The vascular surgeons discuss further management.

What is the best approach for subsequent catheter angiography?

(a) Antegrade, left common femoral artery
(b) Antegrade, right common femoral artery
(c) Retrograde, left common femoral artery
(d) Retrograde, left popliteal artery
(e) Retrograde, right common femoral artery

16 Regarding congenital abnormality of the IVC.

Which of the following is most likely to be associated with azygous continuation of the IVC?

(a) Asplenia
(b) Total anomalous pulmonary venous connection (TAPVC)
(c) Bilateral bi-lobed lungs
(d) Right isomerisation
(e) Eparterial bronchi

17 You are asked to review a follow-up CT for a patient with a metastatic carcinoma in a clinical trial. The initial CT showed 2 pulmonary lesions, measuring 6 and 4 cm respectively. The current CT shows 3 lesions, each measuring 2 cm.

How should you classify the response?

(a) Complete response
(b) Mixed response
(c) Partial response
(d) Stable disease
(e) Progressive disease

18 Which of the following is not a feature of idiopathic pulmonary fibrosis at CT?

(a) Ground glass opacification
(b) Tractional dilatation of the airways
(c) Honeycombing
(d) Basal predominance
(e) Subpleural distribution

19 A 29 year old active man presents with slowly progressive intermittent unilateral claudication brought on by exercise or prolonged standing. He has never smoked and has no relevant family history. On examination, plantar flexion against resistance reproduces the symptoms.

What is the likely diagnosis?

(a) Atherosclerosis
(b) Buerger's disease
(c) Cystic adventitial disease of the popliteal artery
(d) Popliteal artery entrapment syndrome
(e) Ruptured Achilles tendon

20 With regards to the anatomy seen on a normal plain chest radiograph, which of the following is incorrect?

(a) The anterior junctional line is formed by the apposition of the visceral and parietal pleura of the anteromedial aspect of the lungs, separated by mediastinal fat
(b) The anterior junctional line extends more cranially than the posterior junctional line
(c) The right paratracheal stripe measures up to 4 mm
(d) The left paratracheal stripe is seen less commonly than the right paratracheal stripe
(e) The left paraspinal line is seen more commonly than the right paraspinal line

21 A 56 year old smoker without pre-existing lung disease is found to have a suspicious peripheral 2cm mass in the middle lobe.

Which of the following statements is false with regards to CT guided percutaneous biopsy of this mass?
(a) The patient should be consented for a risk of pneumothorax of 40%
(b) Oxygen saturation during the procedure is mandatory
(c) If uncomplicated, biopsy could be performed as a day case
(d) The patient should be encouraged to breath hold during imaging
(e) The horizontal fissure should not be traversed if possible

22 Regarding CTPA for the investigation of pulmonary emboli.

Which of the following is not a cause of a false-positive CTPA result?
(a) Hilar lymphadenopathy
(b) Low signal-to-noise ratio
(c) Narrow windowing
(d) Respiratory artefact
(e) SVC obstruction

23 An 18 year old man presents with a long history of recurrent pneumonias. CXR shows a 6 cm right lower lobe cystic lesion with an air/ fluid level within it. Contrast enhanced CT shows a single lesion containing fluid of water density along with higher attenuation material within it. A single aberrant vessel arising from the distal thoracic aorta is seen to enter the lesion. Angiography confirms this vessel and also demonstrates venous drainage via the pulmonary veins into the left atrium

What is the likeliest diagnosis?

(a) Intralobar sequestration
(b) Extralobar sequestration
(c) Lateral thoracic meningocoele
(d) Extramedullary haematopoiesis
(e) Pulmonary abscess

24 A 20 year old male smoker presents with a history of recurrent spontaneous pneumothoraces. CXR and subsequent CT show bilateral upper zone fine reticulonodular change with some larger discrete upper thin-walled cysts and increased lung volumes.

What is the likeliest diagnosis?

(a) Sarcoidosis
(b) Non-specific interstitial pneumonitis
(c) Usual interstitial pneumonitis
(d) Langerhans cell histiocytosis
(e) Lymphangiomyomatosis

25 Regarding the primary cardiac tumour myxoma, which of the following statements is true?

(a) 40% occur in the right atrium
(b) Enlargement of the atrial appendage may be seen on CXR
(c) The majority are sessile
(d) Most tumours arise from the septum
(e) It typically presents in teenage years

26 A 66 year old man presents with right thigh claudication on walking 20 yards. He is referred for an angiogram with a view to possible angioplasty. The angiogram demonstrates a 3 cm focal stenosis of the right external iliac artery with no other significant disease seen.

What sized balloon would be appropriate for attempted angioplasty?

(a) 3 mm
(b) 5 mm
(c) 7 mm
(d) 10 mm
(e) 13 mm

27 A 46 year old man with a dry cough is referred for a CT of the thorax. This demonstrates multiple pulmonary nodules, each less than 4 mm in diameter, in a perilymphatic and subpleural distribution.

What is the most likely diagnosis?

(a) Sarcoidosis
(b) Metastases
(c) Tuberculosis
(d) Varicella pneumonia
(e) Extrinsic allergic alveolitis

28 Which of the following respiratory conditions is not associated with cigarette smoking?

(a) Idiopathic pulmonary fibrosis
(b) Langerhan's cell histiocytosis
(c) Extrinsic allergic alveolitis
(d) Desquamative interstitial pneumonitis
(e) Respiratory bronchiolitis-interstitial lung disease

29 The International Labour Office (ILO) 1980 International Classification of Radiographs pertains to which of the following conditions?

(a) Pneumoconiosis
(b) Sarcoidosis
(c) Extrinsic allergic alveolitis
(d) Hypersensitivity pneumonitis
(e) Asbestos-related lung disease

30 With regard to the thymus, which of the following statements is true?

(a) 30–40% of patients with myasthenia gravis have a thymoma
(b) 10% of patients with a thymoma have myasthenia gravis
(c) Thymoma usually presents before the age of 40
(d) Cyst formation in the thymus is a feature of malignant degeneration
(e) The average age of thymoma diagnosis is less in patients with associated myasthenia gravis

31 A 68 year old retired shipbuilder presents with shortness of breath. CXR shows a round 4 cm subpleural mass and a CT is performed.

Which of the following CT signs is not a feature of folded lung?

(a) Air bronchograms
(b) Interval growth
(c) Adjacent pleural thickening
(d) Cavitation
(e) Enhancement following intravenous contrast medium

32 With regard to emphysema, which of the following statements is not true?

(a) It is clinically evident in 15% of smokers
(b) Panacinar emphysema has a predilection for the lower lobes
(c) The chest radiograph has a high sensitivity for diagnosing emphysema
(d) Heterogeneous involvement of the lungs improves outcome following volume reduction surgery
(e) Panacinar emphysema is associated with bronchiectasis

33 A 55 year old man presents with chest pain radiating to the back, the arm pulses are unequal, but the patient is haemodynamically stable. CXR shows a widened mediastinum, and non-contrast CT demonstrates crescentic high attenuation material along the outer wall of the distal descending thoracic aorta.

Which of the following sub-classifications most accurately describes this dissection?

(a) Stanford A and DeBakey I
(b) Stanford A and DeBakey II
(c) Stanford B and DeBakey I
(d) Stanford B and DeBakey II
(e) Stanford B and DeBakey III

34 According to the British Thoracic Society guidelines, what distance between the lung edge and the chest wall constitutes a 'large' pneumothorax?

(a) >1 cm
(b) >2 cm
(c) >3 cm
(d) >4 cm
(e) >5 cm

35 A 20 year old woman undergoes a CXR as part of an occupational assessment. She is found to have an abnormal lesion in the right cardiophrenic space and subsequently undergoes CT examination which shows an anterior mass predominantly composed of fat with fine higher attenuation linear structures within it. The lesion also contains some round, well defined gas containing areas.

What is the likeliest diagnosis?

(a) Liposarcoma
(b) Pericardial fat necrosis
(c) Thymolipoma
(d) Diaphragmatic hernia
(e) Teratoma

36 A patient undergoes myocardial perfusion imaging and you are shown the standard short axis view.

Which part of the myocardium is uppermost as you look at it?

(a) Anterior wall
(b) Interventricular septum
(c) Posterior wall
(d) Inferior wall
(e) Lateral wall

37 With regard to cardiac CT imaging, which of the following statements is true?

(a) Prospective gating enables wall motion to be evaluated
(b) Retrospective gating reduces dose in cardiac imaging
(c) The coronary arteries are best evaluated during systole
(d) Ejection fraction evaluation requires retrospective gating
(e) Pacemakers are a contraindication to cardiac CT

38 A 40 year old woman presents haemoptysis. CXR shows multiple cavitating lesions in both lungs. Needle biopsy confirms the lesions are metastatic.

Which of the following is the least likely cause?
(a) Squamous cell carcinoma of the larynx
(b) Adenocarcinoma of the cervix
(c) Transitional cell carcinoma of the bladder
(d) Adenocarcinoma of the colon
(e) Giant cell tumour of the distal femur

39 A previously healthy 24 year old man presents following an RTA with pelvic and lower limb fractures. 3 days after admission he becomes progressively breathless and has a headache. Examination shows a petechial rash. CXR is normal; V/Q imaging demonstrates multiple peripheral subsegmental defects.

What is the most likely diagnosis?
(a) Pulmonary embolism
(b) Pneumocystis infection
(c) Acute interstitial pneumonitis
(d) Fat embolism
(e) Pulmonary contusions

40 A CT-angiogram in a 67 year old man shows a focal 1 cm popliteal occlusion with reconstitution and 3-vessel run-off. Initial sub-intimal angioplasty is successful, but acute thrombosis forms in the peroneal trunk late in the procedure. Thrombolysis with rt-PA is considered.

Which of the following factors would be an absolute contra-indication to thrombolysis?
(a) CVA 3 months ago
(b) Irreversible ischaemia
(c) Major abdominal surgery 4 weeks ago
(d) Primary cerebral tumour
(e) Recent warfarin use

41 Which of the following CT features indicates post-primary rather than primary pulmonary tuberculosis?

(a) Miliary nodules
(b) Bronchiectasis
(c) Cavitation
(d) Tree-in-bud opacification
(e) Lymphadenopathy

42 Following a prolonged angioplasty procedure is noted to have a swelling at the CFA puncture site. US confirms a 4 cm pseudoaneurysm. The patient is haemodynamically stable.

What is the most appropriate immediate treatment?
(a) Conservative management
(b) Manual compression
(c) Stent-graft placement
(d) Surgical repair
(e) US-guided thrombin injection

43 With respect to Mycoplasma pneumoniae infection, which of the following statements is not true?

(a) It is the commonest non-bacterial cause of pneumonia
(b) It usually affects previously healthy individuals
(c) It usually affects the upper lobes
(d) Cavitation is not a feature
(e) Radiographic resolution may take up to 2 months

44 A 32 year old lady, 27 weeks pregnant, is referred for a CT pulmonary angiogram.

Which of the following technique modifications would not be appropriate?
(a) Reduced tube current
(b) Reduced tube voltage
(c) Reduced z-axis
(d) Reduced pitch
(e) Increased collimation thickness

45 A previously healthy 32 year old man presents to A&E with progressive breathlessness. He has a 3-day history of a flu-like illness. Initial chest radiography demonstrates patchy bilateral consolidation. Over the next few days he develops fulminant respiratory failure. A CT performed 1 week after the onset of symptoms demonstrates areas of consolidation and ground glass opacification; in addition, tractional dilatation of the airways is evident on a CT performed at 2 weeks.

What is the most likely diagnosis?

(a) Desquamative interstitial pneumonia
(b) Pneumocystis infection
(c) Lymphoid interstitial pneumonia
(d) Accelerated-phase usual interstitial pneumonia
(e) Acute interstitial pneumonia

46 Which of the following is not a recognised indication for a transjugular intrahepatic porto-systemic shunt (TIPS) procedure?

(a) Budd-Chiari syndrome
(b) Hepatic encephalopathy
(c) Hepato-pulmonary syndrome
(d) Refractory ascites
(e) Uncontrolled variceal bleed

47 With regard to ventilation/perfusion (V/Q) studies, which of the following statements is not true?

(a) Ventilation should be performed with the patient upright
(b) A low probability study is associated with a PE in around 10% of cases
(c) Perfusion images should be acquired with the patient upright
(d) A high probability study is associated with no PE in around 10% of cases
(e) Technetium agents have better imaging characteristics than Krypton for the ventilation phase

48 The ITU team wish to discuss a chest radiograph on one of their patients.

Which of the following features suggest ARDS over cardiogenic pulmonary oedema?

(a) Ratio of arterial oxygenation to inspired oxygen fraction 300 mmHg
(b) Bilateral pulmonary infiltrates
(c) Pulmonary arterial wedge pressure 20 mmHg
(d) Heart size 15 cm
(e) Bilateral pleural effusions

49 A 53 year old man presents with abdominal pain. A post-contrast abdominal CT examination is performed in the portal phase which reveals an enlarged aorta with an eccentric thrombosed channel, extending over 8 cm.

Which of the following features makes a thrombosed aneurysm more likely than a chronic dissection?

(a) Involvement of the SMA
(b) Small aortic lumen
(c) Mural calcification displaced outwards
(d) Thrombus extending over 6 cm cranio-caudally
(e) Total aortic diameter > 5 cm

50 A 56 year old man undergoes single lung transplantation for sarcoid-related lung disease. At day 10 post-operatively he becomes increasingly dyspnoeic. The CXR shows increased consolidation within the graft lung.

What is the most likely cause for these appearances?

(a) Acute rejection
(b) Aspergillus infection
(c) Cytomegalovirus infection
(d) Post-transplant lymphoproliferative disorder
(e) Recurrent sarcoidosis18

Cardiothoracic and Vascular Practice SBA Answers

1 (a)
Castleman's disease is a low-grade B-cell lymphoid proliferation of unknown aetiology. It can be localised or multicentric (multiple LNs, typically with systemic symptoms, with a poorer prognosis). The nodes may be as large as 16 cm, classically enhance avidly, and may have central calcification. Resection is curative in 90% of patients with the localised form. Metastases from vascular tumours may also produce similar findings (*e.g.* melanoma, RCC, papillary thyroid cancer). NHL can have similar features, but untreated lymphoma is not expected to produce calcified lymph nodes. The acute disseminated form of LCH can be associated with lymphadenopathy, but this is usually generalised, the patient would be expected to be systemically unwell, and these nodes do not typically calcify.

Ref: Parker MS, et al. (2007). Clin Rad; 62(7): 707–10

2 (c)
There are multiple causes of pulmonary arterial hypertension which can broadly be divided into vascular, lung and cardiac causes along with idiopathic PAH. Signs include enlargement of the main PA (greater than 2.9 cm), a PA to corresponding aorta ratio of > 1 and signs of right ventricular strain which would eventually cause bowing of the interventricular system convex to the left.

Ref: Clin Rad (2009); 64 (8): 751–60.

3 (c)
Causes of interstitial lung disease which predominantly affects the upper lobes include TB, silicosis, sarcoid, prior radiation therapy, ankylosing spondylitis, chronic EAA, histoplasmosis, and PCP in patients who have received aerosol pentamidine prophylaxis. The typical distribution of UIP is peripheral and basal, the other conditions predominantly affect the lower zones.

Ref: Radiology Review Manual, 6th Ed, p. 416–7.

4 (d)
Also known as hereditary haemorrhagic telengiectasia, it is a group of inherited disorders that result in a number of systemic fibrovascular disorders affecting mucus membranes, skin, brain and lung. It is associated with the presence of multiple pulmonary arterio-venous fistulae. These can act as a right to left shunt and embolic sequelae in the brain can be the presenting symptom.

Ref: Radiology Review Manual, 6th Ed, p. 521.

5 (c)
Pulmonary carcinoids represent < 4% of all lung tumours and approximately 15% of all carcinoid tumours within the body. They can be typical (type 1; local tumour; 90%) or atypical (type 2; metastasises to local LNs, rarely to liver), 80% are centrally located. They rarely cause carcinoid syndrome, often enhance strongly, 1/3 contain calcification, and they typically have no uptake at PET. Hamartomas are well circumscribed solitary nodules; 90% are peripheral. They are benign tumours composed of cartilage, connective tissue, muscle, fat, and bone. Fat attenuation at CT is described as pathognomonic, 'popcorn' calcification is also diagnostic but is seen in only 20%.

Ref: Primer of Diagnostic Imaging, 4th Ed. p. 31–2.

6 (a)
The Fleischner society guidelines were published in 2005 and relate to the management of incidentally detected new lung nodules. They do not aply to patients < 35 yrs (as the risk of lung cancer is minimal below this age), with underlying malignancy, or with unexplained fever. Low risk patients are defined as having a minimal or absent history of smoking and of other known risk factors (*e.g.* family history, asbestos/ radon exposure). NB non or partly solid (*e.g.* ground-glass nodules) may require longer follow-up to rule out adenocarcinoma.

Size (mm)	Low risk patients	High risk patients
≤ 4	No follow-up	Follow-up 12 months. If no change, no further imaging
4–6	Follow-up 12 months. If no change, no further imaging	Follow-up 6–12 months, then 18–24 months if no change
6–8	Follow-up 6–12 months, then	Follow-up at 3, 9, and 24
months		
	18–24 months if no change	if no change
> 8	Follow-up at 3, 9, and 24 months. Consider dynamic CT/PET/biopsy	Same as for low risk patients

Ref: MacMahon H, et al. (2005). Radiology; 237(2): 395–400.

7 (a)

Congenital absence of the pericardium may be partial (91%) or total (9%). Large defects can cause strangulation and have the appearance of the large cardiac silhouette seen in pericardial effusions, small defects are usually asymptomatic. Partial defects are more common on the left (complete left-sided absence 35%, foraminal defect left side 35%). In complete left-sided absence, the heart is shifted to the left and rotated, the PA view of the heart mimics an RAO view and the heart is separated from the sternum on the lateral view. In foraminal left-sided defects, there may only be prominence of the left atrial appendage (appears as left hilar mass, may mimic left PA enlargement). They are associated with bronchogenic cysts (30%), VSD, PDAs, CDHs and mitral stenosis.

Ref: Primer of Diagnostic Imaging, 4th Ed, p. 150 & Radiology Review Manual, 6th Ed, p. 648–9.

8 (a)

The remaining scenarios constitute T3 disease.
Ref: TNM Atlas, 5th Ed, p. 169–176.

9 (d)
Unilateral right-sided pleural effusions are associated with congestive cardiac failure and proximal thoracic duct transaction and, rarely pancreatitis (which can be unilateral left (68%), unilateral right (10%) or bilateral, in 22%). Unilateral left-sided pleural effusions include those mentioned and transection of the distal thoracic duct. The vast majority of traumatic aortic transections occur at the isthmus, distal to the left SCA origin, thus result in left-sided pleural effusions.

Ref: Radiology Review Manual, 6th Ed, p. 439.

10 (a)
Loeffler's syndrome is also known as transient pulmonary eosinophillia. Churg-Strauss syndrome (allergic angiitis granulomatosis) classically presents with fleeting pulmonary opacities. Causes of pulmonary haemorrhage/vasculitis can also give this appearance (*e.g.* Wegener's granulomatosis or Goodpasture's syndrome). EAA can occur following exposure to the relevant trigger, which subsequently resolves on its removal. Chronic eosinophilic pneumonia typically has a peripheral distribution (the 'photographic negative' of pulmonary oedema) and appearances typically remain unchanged for weeks or months.

Ref: Radiology Review Manual, 6th Ed, p. 483 & 493–4.

11 (a)
Anaphylactoid reactions mimic anaphylactic reactions but do not involve IgE and are not true hypersensitivity reactions. They may occur with as little as 1 ml of contrast medium and do not require pre-sensitisation; patients may not have the same reaction after a second exposure. The remaining features are dose-dependent reactions to intravenous contrast medium.

Ref: R-ITI. 3_034. Common Clinical Problems: Managing Abdominal Radiological Emergencies.

12 (e)
These are normal physiological measurements (1–4 mmHg), but may be seen in normal patients, extrahepatic portal hypertension and some cases of pre-sinusoidal portal hypertension. Elevation in sinusoidal disease is seen and correlates with Child score and risk of oesophageal variceal haemorrhage.

Ref: Am J Physiol. 1997; 272: 2826–32

13 (d)
Cardiac output is inversely proportional to arterial opacification. The other 4 techniques are used to increase arterial opacification. Rates above 8 ml/s offer no incremental value, whilst matching dose to body weight will give more uniform enhancement across a patient group.

Ref: Radiologic Clinics of North America (2009); 47(1): 13–26

14 (c)
This results from the rupture of the vasa vasorum and haemorrhage in to the arterial media. It is associated with hypertension (50%, is more common in men (60%) and presents in the same manner as aortic dissection, with most (> 90%) cases non-traumatic. It has a mortality rate of around 20%.

Ref: Radiographics (2009); 29: 791–804.

15 (b)
The likely location and extent of the lesion is known. As intervention is likely, the antegrade ('down the leg') approach should be adopted on the symptomatic side. A diagnostic run should be performed to confirm disease extent as MR can over-estimate it, alternatively there may have been disease progression depending on the elapsed time-interval.

16 (c)
Azygous continuation of the IVC is congenital absence of the hepatic segment of the IVC with continuation to the right atrium occurring via the azygous or hemi-azygous veins, prevalence = 0.6%. It is often associated with polysplenia syndrome (left isomerisation) and only rarely with asplenia syndrome (right isomerisation). Polysplenia syndrome is associated with bilateral bi-lobed lungs, partial anomalous pulmonary venous connection (PAPVC), persistent left SVC, situs ambiguous, hyparterial bronchi, atrial septal defects (ASD) and double outlet right ventricle (DORV).

Ref: Radiology Review Manual, 6th Ed, p. 626 & Primer of Diagnostic Imaging, 4th Ed, p. 140.

17 (e)
The development of any new lesion, or an increase in the overall size of lesions by 20% or more, indicates progressive disease. There is no 'mixed response' category in the RECIST system.

Ref: European Journal of Cancer (2009); 45: 228–247.

18 (a)
Answers (b) – (e) are the classical features of IPF on CT. Ground glass opacification is not a significant feature of IPF. IPF is more common in smokers and, as such, may co-exist with emphysema which may preserve total lung volumes. Irrespective of smoking history, the incidence of bronchogenic carcinoma is increased 7x in IPF.

Ref: R-ITI 1b_016. Idiopathic interstitial pneumonias

19 (d)
PAES is most common in young active male patients (60% are < 30 yrs) and must be considered in an individual of this demographic who develops calf claudication on exercise. It is bilateral in up to 67% and usually results from an anomalous course of the medial head of gastrocnemius which causes compression of the popliteal artery. It can rarely be caused by a fibrous band, or muscle hypertrophy in athletes. Surgical release of the muscle or tendon is the optimal treatment, there is no role for angioplasty/ stenting.

Ref: Radiographics (2004); 24: 467–79.

20 (b)
The posterior junctional line is formed by the junction between the lungs posterior to the oesophagus and anterior to the 3rd – 5th thoracic vertebrae. It appears as a straight or mildly leftward convex line seen projected over the trachea. Unlike the anterior junctional line, it can extend above the clavicles.

Ref: RadioGraphics (2007); 27: 33–48.

21 (a)
The risk of pneumothorax is 15–20%, depending on location and the presence of bullae. Only 2–5% require formal drainage. The patient should be warned that minor haemoptysis can occur. If multiple passes are required a co-axial system is usually employed. The patient is usually asked to hold their breath during inspiration in an attempt to reduce the degree of movement of the lesion between scans.

Ref: Interventional Radiology: A Survival Guide, 2nd Ed, p. 313.

22 (c)
If a technically adequate study is performed CTPA is > 90% sensitive and specific for large, central PEs. False-positive results may occur if there is increased noise (hence reduced SNR), particularly in larger patients or if patients are too unwell to lift their arms above their head. Others include SVC obstruction (due to partial opacification of the vessels), hyperdynamic circulation, lymphadenopathy, and respiration/motion (due to partial voluming). Narrow windowing produces 'brighter' contrast thus filling defects may be obscured, resulting in a false *negative* result. Emboli can be detected within the proximal arteries of ≤ 5th/6th generation, sub-segmental emboli are usually undetectable (thus effectively produce a false negative result).

Ref: Radiology Review Manual, 6th Ed, p. 524–5.

23 (a)
Intralobar sequestration is congenital malformation involving a lesion enclosed within the visceral pleura of the affected pulmonary lobe but has no connection with the tracheobronchial tree. It is more common than extralobar sequestration and can present in adulthood. Venous drainage of the lesion is *via* the pulmonary as opposed to the systemic veins as seen in extralobar sequestration. CT shows single or multiple cystic lesions filled with a combination of fluid, pus and mucus.

Ref: Radiology Review Manual, 6th Ed, p. 479.

24 (d)
Pulmonary LCH is a rare condition affecting young male smokers, characterised by bilateral upper and mid zone changes starting with nodules (which may cavitate) and progressing through the spectrum of reticular change finishing with true fibrosis. It results in increased lung volumes in up to a third of patients.

Ref: Radiology Review Manual, 6th Ed, p. 504.

25 (d)
Myxoma is the most common primary cardiac tumour in adults. 90% of patients are between 30–60 years at presentation. The majority occur in the left atrium (80%), with 75% of these arising from the interatrial septum near the fossa ovalis. They are typically villous, pedunculated tumours, with only 25% seen as a sessile mass; the average size at presentation is 6 cm. Patients present with constitutional symptoms such as fever, weight loss, or syncope. Myxomas may also produce anaemia, emboli, and obstruction of the mitral valve, which can lead to pulmonary venous hypertension and pulmonary oedema. There is enlargement of the left atrium, but not of the atrial appendage.

Ref: Radiology Review Manual, 6th Ed, p. 646–7.

26 (c)
The more distal the occlusion, the smaller the balloon required for angioplasty, if the balloon is too big there is an increased risk of arterial rupture; if it's too small there is a reduced probability of success. Appropriate balloon sizes include: popliteal artery 3–4 mm, SFA or renal artery 4–6 mm, EIA 6–8 mm, and common iliac 8–10 mm.

Ref: Primer of Diagnostic Imaging, 4th Ed. p. 671.

27 (a)
This is the typical distribution of pulmonary sarcoid nodules. TB, varicella pneumonia, and metastatic disease are randomly distributed. EAA nodules are typically centrilobular.

Ref: Imaging of diseases of the chest, 3rd edn. p 637–655.

28 (c)
Smoking appears to have a somewhat protective effect in EAA, with the vast majority of patients being non-smokers. This may be due to peripheral airway constriction. The remaining conditions are associated with smoking, although curiously smokers with IPF appear to have better survival than non-smokers.

Ref: Clinical Radiology (2003); 58: 259–68.

29 (a)
This is the system most widely used to code pneumoconioses by comparing against a standardised set of chest radiographs for nodule size, shape and extent. This semi-quantitive measure enables international epidemiological studies to be carried out.

Ref: R-ITI. 1b_015. Pneumoconiosis.

30 (e)
Thymoma typically presents around 50 years of age and is associated with myasthenia gravis; the percentages values for (a) and (b) are reversed. Thymic cysts are benign and may be congenital or acquired, particularly after mediastinal radiotherapy.

Ref: R-ITI 1b_073-Anterior mediastinal masses.

31 (d)
Rounded atelectasis is the end result of an exudative pleural effusion; fibrous strands cause invagination of the pleura as the fluid resolves. Hence the 'mass' has a smooth margin except where the bronchi and vessels enter - often seen pulled in to the mass and described as a 'comet-tail' or 'crow's-foot' appearance.

Ref: Imaging of diseases of the chest, 3rd Ed, p. 97–98.

32 (c)
The chest radiograph has a low sensitivity, but high specificity, for diagnosing emphysema. Centrilobular and panacinar emphysema predominantly affect the upper and lower lobes respectivately, the latter being associated with bronchiectasis in 40% of cases. Centrilobular emphysema is the result of pollutants, notably smoking, whilst α1-antitrypsin deficiency is the commonest cause of the panacinar type.

Ref: R-ITI 1b_038. Emphysema.

33 (e)
Thoracic aortic dissections are classified by either the DeBakey or Stanford systems. DeBakey has 3 sub-divisions: I involves ascending and descending aorta, II ascending only, III descending only. Stanford has 2 subdivisions: A: ascending +/– descending thoracic aorta, B: descending only (NOT ascending). Thus, Stanford A incorporates DeBakey types I and II, and Stanford B is equivalent to DeBakey III.

Ref: Radiology Review Manual, 6th Ed, p. 618–20.

34 (b)
Measuring the volume of a pneumothorax from the 2-D chest film is difficult, not least because the distance from the chest wall to the lung edge varies along its course. These authors estimate 2 cm to be a 50% pneumothorax, although earlier papers would estimate it at 20%.

Ref: Thorax (2003); 58(Suppl II): ii39–ii52.

35 (d)
In the adult, congenital diaphragmatic hernias are typically asymptomatic. The presence of gas within bowel loops is pathognomonic. Mesenteric vessels typically appear as linear opacities. If the lesion only contains omental fat, it can be difficult to differentiate from lipoma or liposarcoma.

Ref: RadioGraphics (2007); 27: 19–32.

36 (a)
The short axis view shows a circle of myocardium. The lateral wall is on your right, the septum on your left and the inferior wall at the bottom.

Ref: R-ITI 7c_005. Basics of radionuclide image interpretation in myocardial perfusion imaging.

37 (d)
Prospective gating images the heart during a short period of diastole and, whilst reducing dose, only images the arteries. Evaluation of cardiac function requires imaging throughout the cardiac cycle and retrospective gating, but this has a dose penalty. Dose may be reduced by modulating mAs during systole.

Ref: R-ITI 1a_006. Normal cardiac CT

38 (e)
The differential diagnosis for cavitating metastases also includes melanoma. Giant cell tumour metastases may calcify.

Ref: Radiology Review Manual, 6th Ed, p. 515.

39 (d)
In fat embolism the radiographic features often progress to diffuse opacification with clearing in 7–14 days; ARDS may develop. The mottled appearance at V/Q is quite different from that seen with large pulmonary emboli. Neurological features are generalised and may progress from irritability to seizures and coma.

Ref: Imaging of diseases of the chest, 3rd Ed, p. 976.

40 (d)
Absolute contra-indications include major trauma/ surgery/CPR within 2 weeks, CVA within 2 months, bleeding diathesis, pregnancy, primary or secondary cerebral malignancy and irreversible ischaemia (the acute event and normal pre-morbid imaging in this scenario makes this answer wrong in this instance). Relative contraindications include the other options given, along with cardiac emboli, age > 80 years, and a 'white' limb (surgery would be a better option in this case).

Ref: Interventional Radiology: A Survival Guide, 2nd Ed, p. 181–2.

41 (a)
The difference between primary and post-primary (reactivated) TB is in the degree of previous exposure the patient has had to TB. Most features are seen in both to some degree with the exception of miliary nodules.

Ref: R-ITI 1b_056 - Tuberculosis - basic patterns.

42 (e)
Femoral artery pseudoaneurysms occur in 0.2% of diagnostic and 8% of interventional procedures; compression of adjacent structures or rupture are potential complications. Risk factors include low puncture, larger catheter size, lengthy procedures, and peri-procedural anti-coagulation. Treatment can be conservative for small aneurysms < 2 cm. US-guided thrombin injection has replaced US-guided compression as the treatment of choice in uncomplicated cases due to greater success rate, reduced procedural time and better patient tolerance. Stent-grafts are more commonly used in larger diameter arteries and have a lower complication rate compared to surgery. Surgery is reserved for cases of rapid aneurysm expansion, rupture, infection, or failure of other treatments.

Ref: Clin Rad (2008); 62(12): 1310–16.

43 (c)
Mycoplasma pneumoniae infection has a predilection for the lower lobes, although isolated upper lobe infection is well recognised. A nodular interstitial pattern may also be seen, the frequency of this finding varies significantly between series, as does the prevalence of pleural effusion.

Ref: Imaging of diseases of the chest, 3rd edn. p 236.

44 (d)
If anything the pitch should be increased to reduce dose. Breast shields, abdominal shielding and increased collimation thickness should also be considered in an effort to reduce dose.

Ref: Radiographics (2009); 29: 639–54.

45 (e)
The clinical history and CT appearances are characteristic of AIP, formerly known as Hamann-Rich syndrome, which pathologically resembles ARDS.

Ref: Imaging of diseases of the chest, 3rd Ed, p. 534–5.

46 (b)
Refractory ascites and variceal bleeding uncontrolled by endoscopic and medical therapy account for 99% of TIPS cases. Other indications include hepatorenal syndrome, hepatopulmonary syndrome, hepatic hydrothorax and Budd-Chiari. Hepatic encephalopathy is a relative contra-indication to a TIPS procedure.

Ref: Clin Rad (2009); 64(7): 664–74.

47 (e)
Krypton has better imaging characteristics with a short half-life (13 secs) and better penetration (it is a gas). Technetium is widely used for its low cost and ready availability.

Ref: R-ITI 7l_001 Basic Pathology and Clinical Aspects.

48 (d)
ARDS is a response of the lung to injury which may be direct or indirect; radiological features are those of non-cardiogenic oedema which develops as a consequence but unlike simple oedema an interstitial fibrosis may develop. Mechanical ventilation is thought to contribute to this process. Pulmonary arterial wedge pressure 18 mmHg suggests raised left atrial pressures. The diagnosis of ARDS requires the ratio of arterial oxygenation to inspired oxygen to be < 200 mmHg.

Ref: R-ITI 1b_032 ARDS-Radiology and Cause.

49 (c)

A thrombosed aneurysm and thrombosed blood within the false lumen of a chronic dissection can have similar appearances. In thrombosed aneurysm the calcium is typically displaced outwards, thus appears to be pushed outside from the aortic lumen (in dissection any calcium, if present would be displaced medially, 'inside' the lumen), in addition there is likely to be extensive calcification seen elsewhere in the wall. Dissection usually extends over a longer (> 6 cm) cranio-caudal distance and, although the overall aortic size is normal in the acute phase, it can be very large (> 5 cm) in the chronic phase. The aortic lumen is likely to be normal or small in dissection, but is expected to be large with an aneurysm. Involved vessels are not a reliable guide, but an aneurysm tends to involve the lumbar branches, a dissection of the renal arteries and the SMA.

Ref: Primer of Diagnostic Imaging, 4th Ed, p. 687.

50. (a)

Acute rejection typically presents within the first 4 weeks, CXR may be normal, or show oedema, worsening consolidation, peribronchial thickening, new pleural effusions, or septal lines without evidence of LVF. Infection in the first 4 weeks of transplantation is almost invariably bacterial. Acute rejection is the only other condition common within the first month and is extremely common after 1 week. CMV, PTLD and Aspergillus infection typically occur more than 4 weeks post transplantation; recurrent disease would also be expected later, but is more common in sarcoid (35%) than other conditions (< 1%).

Ref: R-ITI 1b_059 Thoracic Imaging in Heart and Lung Transplantation.

Musculoskeletal and Trauma Practice SBA Questions

1 **A plain radiograph reveals a well-defined lucent lesion within the metaphysic and epiphysis of the distal femur. There is eccentric expansion and the cortex is thin but intact. It does not reach the articular surface. CT reveals fluid-fluid levels.**

Which of the following is the most likely cause?
(a) Giant cell tumour
(b) Aneurysmal bone cyst
(c) Enchondroma
(d) Non-ossifying fibroma
(e) Chondromyxoid fibroma

2 **A 35 year old man suffers a knee injury during a football match and presents with pain, swelling, knee locking and an inability to fully extend his knee. He undergoes an MRI examination.**

What is the most common site of injury?
(a) Anterior cruciate ligament
(b) Posterior cruciate ligament
(c) Anterior horn medial meniscus
(d) Posterior horn medial meniscus
(e) Anterior horn lateral meniscus

3 **A 78 year old woman has left hip pain following a fall. On examination the left hip is shortened and externally rotated. X-rays show a fracture of the left neck of femur.**

Which of the following fractures is at highest risk of avascular necrosis?
(a) Basi-cervical fracture
(b) Inter-trochanteric fracture
(c) Sub-capital fracture
(d) Sub-trochanteric fracture
(e) Trans-cervical fracture

4 A stress fracture in which of the following areas would be most indicative of a pseudofracture (Looser's zone) of osteomalacia?

(a) Axillary margin of the scapula
(b) Distal 1/3 ulna
(c) Greater trochanter of the femur
(d) Lateral femoral neck
(e) Proximal 1/3 radius

5 A CXR is performed in a patient with increasing shortness of breath. The lungs are clear, but there is a bilateral symmetrical absence of the lateral end of the clavicles.

Which is the least likely cause of these appearances?

(a) Cleidocranial dysplasia
(b) Eosinophilic granuloma
(c) Hyperparathyroidism
(d) Pyknodysostosis
(e) Rheumatoid arthritis

6 A 45 year old man has an acute episode of shortness of breath. A CXR is requested; this shows concave scalloping of the undersurface of the right 2nd and 3rd ribs, there is a slight scoliosis of the inferior aspect of the thoracic spine, but the lung parenchyma is clear.

Which of the following is the most likely cause of these appearances?

(a) Marfan's syndrome
(b) Neurofibromatosis Type I
(c) Rheumatoid arthritis
(d) SLE
(e) Scleroderma

7 **Which of the following forms of micromelic dwarfism is considered to be the most severe?**

(a) Diastrophic dysplasia
(b) Heterozygous achondroplasia
(c) Nievergelt syndrome
(d) Osteogenesis Imperfecta Type 1
(e) Thanatophoric dysplasia

8 **A 12 year old boy falls and sustains a fracture to the proximal phalanx of his right index finger which extends from the articular surface to the epiphyseal plate but not extending to the metaphysis.**

What is the Salter-Harris classification of this injury?
(a) I
(b) II
(c) III
(d) IV
(e) V

9 **A young man sustains blunt trauma to the chest. There is suspicion of a pneumothorax. A supine chest radiograph is available.**

On this radiograph, which of the following would be the least supportive of this diagnosis?
(a) Presence of the 'deep sulcus sign'
(b) A sharply outlined dome of the diaphragm
(c) A hyperlucent right upper abdominal quadrant
(d) A sharply defined anterior junctional line
(e) A poorly defined anterior cardiophrenic sulcus

10 **In the evaluation of a splenic injury following trauma, which of the following features favours pseudoaneurysm over active extravasation?**

(a) Less apparent on delayed imaging
(b) Layering
(c) Ill-defined
(d) Increased size on delayed imaging
(e) Jet of contrast medium

11 A 32 year old man presents with a painful elbow, having fallen off his bicycle. AP and lateral radiographs of the elbow are taken; an A&E doctor is unsure if an abnormality is present and phones to ask your advice.

Which of the following indicates an underlying abnormality?

(a) A visible anterior fat pad
(b) On the lateral view, a line drawn through the long axis of the proximal radius passes through the capitellum
(c) The posterior fat pad is not visible
(d) 'Hourglass' or 'figure 8' sign of the distal humerus on lateral film
(e) The anterior humeral line passes through the anterior third of the capitellum

12 A 27 year old undergoes a CXR as part of an occupational assessment. The CXR shows a solitary expansile right 5th posterior rib mass. CT confirms the mass is arising from the rib and that it shows no aggressive features.

What is the likeliest diagnosis?

(a) Exostosis of the rib
(b) Benign cortical defect
(c) Langerhans cell histiocytosis
(d) Fibrous dysplasia
(e) Osteoblastoma

13 A calcified mass is seen on a plain radiograph of a young man's femur. The mass appears to be centred within the soft tissues of the thigh and the calcification is more prominent on the periphery of the mass. There is a radiolucent zone separating the lesion from the underlying bone, the cortex of which appears unaffected.

Which of the following is the most likely diagnosis?

(a) Myositis ossificans
(b) Parosteal osteosarcoma
(c) Juxtacortical chondroma
(d) Osteochondroma
(e) Rhabdomyosarcoma

14 **A patient presents with painful swelling of the limbs and joints, particularly the knees, ankles, wrists and elbows. Digital clubbing and joint effusions are noted. Plain radiographs show marked bilateral, smooth periosteal reactions affecting the radius, ulna, tibia and fibula.**

Which one of the following diseases is not associated with the most likely unifying condition?

(a) Gaucher's disease
(b) Carcinoma of the bronchus
(c) Undifferentiated nasopharyngeal carcinoma
(d) Pleural fibroma
(e) Ulcerative colitis

15 **A lady suffers from long-standing rheumatoid arthritis. She is noted to have splenomegaly on a clinic visit. A diagnosis of Felty's syndrome is suspected clinically.**

Which of the following is not a recognised feature of Felty's syndrome?

(a) Ulceration
(b) Neutropaenia
(c) Skin pigmentation
(d) Weight loss
(e) Low titres of rheumatoid factor

16 **A patient presents with back pain. He is found to be HLA-B27 positive and a diagnosis of ankylosing spondylitis is suspected. Plain films of the spine are requested.**

Which of the following would be the least supportive of this diagnosis?

(a) Calcification of the anterior longitudinal ligament
(b) Osteitis
(c) Syndesmophytes
(d) Sclerosis of the costotransverse joints
(e) Ankylosis of the costovertebral joints

17 You are asked to review a series of plain films of the cervical spine of an adult patient.

Which of the following is abnormal?

(a) On the lateral view, the distance between the anterior arch of C1 and the anterior aspect of the odontoid peg is 2 mm
(b) On the lateral view, the soft tissues anterior to C2 are 9 mm thick
(c) Harris' white ring is incomplete in its inferior aspect
(d) On the lateral view, the C4-5 interspinous distance is 30% greater than the C5-6 interspinous distance
(e) On the lateral view, the soft tissues anterior to C6 are 20 mm thick

18 A pregnant lady suffers from sudden, spontaneous hip pain, worsened by weight bearing. The range of movement is relatively well preserved. Plain radiographs and an MR examination are performed.

Which of the following would be more suggestive of avascular necrosis rather than transient osteoporosis of the hip?

(a) Acetabular oedema on MR imaging
(b) A 'double line' sign on MR imaging
(c) Osteoporosis on plain radiographs
(d) Increased uptake in the femoral head on ^{99m}Tc-MDP imaging
(e) Preservation of the articular cartilage on MR imaging

19 An 8 year old child presents with a limp. Which of the following would favour a diagnosis of bacterial infection over Perthe's disease?

(a) A smaller femoral epiphysis than on the contralateral side
(b) Joint space widening
(c) Destruction of the articular cortex
(d) Alteration of the periarticular soft tissue outline
(e) Localised bone demineralization

20 A young man is involved in an RTA and arrives in hospital with a markedly reduced GCS. Anterior tilt of the odontoid peg is noted and an oblique fracture line is seen through the upper portion of the dens.

Which type of odontoid fracture is this?

(a) Type I
(b) Type II
(c) Type III
(d) Type IV
(e) Type V

21 Following penetrating abdominal trauma, which organ is most frequently injured?

(a) Liver
(b) Pancreas
(c) Spleen
(d) Kidney
(e) Small bowel

22 With regards to the Ottawa rules for plain radiographs of the foot and ankle, which of the following is incorrect?

(a) An ankle X-ray is indicated if the patient cannot weight bear at the time of injury
(b) An ankle X-ray is indicated if there is pain in the malleolar zone and bony tenderness over the base of the 5th metatarsal
(c) A foot X-ray is indicated if there is pain in the midfoot zone and bony tenderness over the navicular
(d) An ankle X-ray is indicated if the patient cannot weight bear in the department
(e) An ankle X-ray is indicated if there is pain in the malleolar zone and bony tenderness over the posterior edge of the lateral malleolus

23 A 7 year old boy is brought to the GP by his parents, having noticed soft, blue-coloured growths on his right hand. The hand X-ray reveals multiple enchondromas.

Which of the following features would confirm Mafucci's syndrome as the diagnosis rather than Ollier's disease?

(a) A first degree relative also affected
(b) Bilateral, predominantly symmetrical disease
(c) A discrepancy in arm length
(d) Sarcomatous degeneration
(e) Soft tissue haemangiomas

24 A 32 year old man falls on his outstretched right wrist whilst playing football. Wrist X-ray reveals a displaced, oblique intra-articular fracture of the dorsal lip of the distal radius.

What is the fracture type described?

(a) Barton's
(b) Chauffeur's
(c) Colles'
(d) Smith's
(e) Salter Harris Type II

25 A 32 year old presents with acute abdominal pain. An AXR demonstrates calcification in the LUQ, with loops of bowel in this region, central depressions in the superior and inferior endplates of L3 and L4, and a mixed lysis/sclerosis appearance to the superior aspect of the left femoral head.

What is the likely unifying diagnosis?

(a) Achondroplasia
(b) Hyperparathyroidism
(c) Lymphoma
(d) Renal osteodystrophy
(e) Sickle cell disease

26 Which of the following statements regarding blunt thoracic trauma is not true?

(a) Pericardial injuries are usually left sided
(b) The tricuspid valve is the most commonly injured valve
(c) Cardiac herniation through the pericardium may result in cardiac dysfunction
(d) The right ventricle is injured more frequently than the left
(e) Blunt cardiac injuries are most commonly the result of road traffic accidents

27 Axial MR imaging of the ankle is performed. You are asked to review a single image at the level of the tibio-talar joint. You note a tendon which is swollen and contains unusually high signal, located immediately posterior to the tendon of tibialis posterior.

What is the likely diagnosis?
(a) Tendonitis of extensor hallucis longus
(b) Tendonitis of extensor digitorum longus
(c) Tendonitis of flexor hallucis longus
(d) Tendonitis of flexor digitorum longus
(e) Tendonitis of tibialis anterior

28 A 14 year old boy is referred for a CT following blunt abdominal trauma. This demonstrates a transection of the distal pancreas with free fluid in the peri-pancreatic space.

According to the American Association for the Surgery of Trauma (AAST), what grade is this injury?
(a) Grade I
(b) Grade II
(c) Grade III
(d) Grade IV
(e) Grade V

29 A man suffers a supination-abduction ankle injury. Plain films reveal an oblique fibular fracture through the tibiofibular syndesmosis.

Which Weber category does this represent?

(a) A
(b) B
(c) C
(d) D
(e) E

30 You are asked to review a hand x-ray of a 6 year old boy. The request simply states "Please assess bone age", there are no prior films available for comparison. There is osteopaenia and mild expansion of the medullary cavities of all the metacarpals and phalanges. There is additional atrophy of the trabeculae and cortical thinning.

What is the likely diagnosis?

(a) Engelmann's disease
(b) Hurler's syndrome
(c) Ollier's disease
(d) Pseudo-pseudohyperparathyroidism
(e) Thalassaemia

31 Plain radiographs are taken of a 9 year old's elbow. Five ossification centres are seen.

Which of the visible ossification centres would have been last to appear?

(a) Radial head
(b) Lateral epicondyle
(c) Medial epicondyle
(d) Olecranon
(e) Trochlear

32 Regarding idiopathic scoliosis.

Which of the following statements is true?

(a) Adolescent idiopathic scoliosis is the commonest form
(b) It affects males more than females
(c) There is a worse prognosis with lumbar scoliosis
(d) Scaphocephaly is associated with infantile idiopathic scoliosis
(e) Subtle neurological abnormalities can be expected

33 A patient has injured his knee and is unable to weight bear. AP and lateral radiographs are taken.

Which of the following is an abnormal finding?

(a) On the lateral view, the distance from the lower pole of the patella to the tibial tubercle is 1.5 times the length of the patella
(b) There is irregularity of the tibial tubercle
(c) On the AP view, a perpendicular line drawn from the lateral margin of the femoral condyle has 3 mm of the lateral margin of the tibal condyle outside of it
(d) There is a corticated, calcified body in the lateral head of the gastrocnemius muscle
(e) There is a multipartite patella

34 A patient presents with foot and ankle tenderness after a sports injury. Plain radiographs of the ankle and foot are taken.

Which of the following is an abnormal finding?

(a) Bohler's angle is 31 degrees
(b) On an AP view of the midfoot, the medial margin of the second metatarsal aligns with the medial margin of the intermediate cuneiform
(c) On an AP view of the midfoot, the medial margin of the third metatarsal aligns with the medial margin of the lateral cuneiform
(d) The width of the space between the distal tibia and fibula at a point 1 cm from the articular surface is 8 mm
(e) On the AP view of the midfoot, there is a lucent line through the base of the 5th metatarsal which runs parallel to the metatarsal shaft

35 A 50 year old man presents with knee pain. Plain radiographs show an 8 cm lytic lesion within the distal femoral metaphysis with endosteal scalloping and cortical thickening. CT shows matrix mineralisation.

Which of the following features does not favour a diagnosis of chondrosarcoma over enchondroma?

(a) The patient's age
(b) The patient's sex
(c) The lesion size
(d) The lesion site
(e) The CT findings

36 A patient has injured his right shoulder. An AP view demonstrates an acromio-clavicular distance of 12 mm and a coraco-clavicular distance of 10 mm. The clavicle is not otherwise grossly displaced.

What is the grade of the acromio-clavicular joint injury?

(a) Grade I
(b) Grade II
(c) Grade III
(d) Grade IV
(e) Grade V

37 An MRI examination of the lumbar spine demonstrates endplates with reduced signal intensity on T1W and increased signal intensity on T2W.

What is the most appropriate diagnosis?

(a) Normal
(b) Type I Modic change
(c) Type II Modic change
(d) Type III Modic change
(e) Type IV Modic change

38 A patient presents with tenderness in the anatomical snuffbox and a scaphoid series of plain radiographs are taken. There is a fracture across the proximal pole of the scaphoid.

Which of the following is incorrect?

(a) Compared to other scaphoid fractures, those across the proximal pole have the highest risk of avascular necrosis
(b) Most scaphoid fractures occur across the waist
(c) Most scaphoid fractures are not displaced
(d) Scaphoid waist fractures may take up to 2 years to heal
(e) A vertical oblique fracture is considered more stable compared to a transverse fracture

39 Regarding giant cell tumours, which of the following statements is true?

(a) GCT usually regresses during pregnancy
(b) It is a highly malignant lesion
(c) Surgical resection is usually curative
(d) The majority arise in the spine
(e) Vertebral body involvement is more common than the posterior elements

40 A patient presents with suspected transient patellar dislocation. MR imaging is performed.

Which of the following MR imaging features would be least expected in this condition?

(a) Disruption of the medial retinaculum
(b) Lateral patellar tilt
(c) Elevation of the vastus medialis obliquus muscle
(d) Bone contusion of the medial aspect of the medial femoral condyle
(e) Bone contusion of the inferomedial aspect of the patella

41 A patient with joint pain has plain radiographs of the hands and spine. The differential diagnosis is considered to be between psoriatic arthropathy and rheumatoid arthritis.

Which of the following features is more common in rheumatoid arthritis rather than psoriatic arthropathy?

(a) Phalangeal enthesophytes
(b) Involvement of the distal interphalangeal joints
(c) Fusiform soft tissue swelling of the digits
(d) Asymmetric joint involvement
(e) Involvement of the wrist joints

42 A patient with Paget's disease has a series of plain radiographs.

Which of the following is a feature of the active phase of the disease?

(a) Widened and coarsened trabeculation of the pelvic ring
(b) 'Cotton wool' skull
(c) 'Ivory vertebra'
(d) Osteoporosis circumscripta
(e) Splitting of the iliopectineal line

43 A CT is performed following major trauma. A Hangman's fracture is suspected.

Which of the following features would be unusual with this diagnosis?

(a) Avulsion of the anteroinferior corner of C2
(b) Posterior subluxation of C2 on C3
(c) Bilateral pars fracture of C2
(d) Prevertebral soft tissue swelling
(e) Disruption of the C1-C2 spinolaminar line

44 A 38 year old woman presents with a palpable lump in her thigh. Plain films show a lobulated ossified mass lying posterior to the femur with a connection to the cortex. The centre of the lesion is denser than the periphery. MRI shows a large associated soft tissue component.

What is the likeliest diagnosis?

(a) Myositis ossificans
(b) Osteochondroma
(c) Parosteal osteosarcoma
(d) Periosteal osteosarcoma
(e) Extraosseous osteosarcoma

45 An MR arthrogram of the shoulder is performed in a patient with a known history of shoulder dislocation.

Which of the following features would be more supportive of prior posterior, rather than anterior, glenohumeral dislocation?

(a) Hill-Sach's lesion
(b) Anterior labral tear
(c) Torn glenohumeral ligaments
(d) Posterior capsule stripping
(e) Bankart lesion

46 A child presents with bruising and a tibial fracture. The possibility of non accidental injury is raised.

Which of the following statements with regards to NAI is incorrect?

(a) Metaphyseal 'corner' fractures are the commonest fracture type
(b) Multiple fractures at different stages of healing is a highly specific sign
(c) Skull fractures are seen in 20% of cases
(d) Interhemispheric haemorrhage is the commonest site of intracranial haemorrhage
(e) Exuberant callus formation is a feature

47 A 40 year old man presents with heel pain. Lateral radiograph of the foot reveals a well defined 3 cm lesion located between the anterior and middle thirds of the calcaneus. The lesion is radiolucent with a thin rim of sclerosis and central calcification.

What is the likely diagnosis?

(a) Desmoplastic fibroma
(b) Giant cell tumour
(c) Intraosseous lipoma
(d) Osteoid osteoma
(e) Unicameral bone cyst

48 Regarding osteoblastomas, which of the following is true?

(a) An expansile appearance on plain film implies malignancy
(b) Matrix calcification is a common plain film feature
(c) They result in scoliosis more commonly than osteoid osteoma
(d) They rarely grow beyond 2 cm
(e) They usually present in the 6th–7th decades

49 The pelvic radiograph of a young woman reveals bilateral, symmetrical triangular areas of subchrondral sclerosis on the inferior aspect of the iliac side of the joint. The joint spaces are normal and the joint margin is well-defined. There is no evidence of bone or joint disease elsewhere.

What is the most likely diagnosis?

(a) Osteitis condensans ilii
(b) Infection
(c) Osteoarthritis
(d) Hyperparathyroidism
(e) Alkaptonuria

50 A 3 month old infant presents with tender, hard swellings over a number of bones. Radiographs reveal a cortical hyperostosis and marked, diffuse, symmetrical periosteal reaction of the clavicles, ribs and mandible.

Which of the following is the most likely diagnosis?

(a) Rickets
(b) Caffey's disease
(c) Hypothyroidism
(d) Scurvy
(e) Ulcerative colitis

Musculoskeletal and Trauma Practice SBA Answers

1 (b)
Of the conditions that typically cause lucent, eccentrically expanded lesions, only GCTs and ABCs have fluid-fluid levels on CT imaging. As GCTs do not reach the articular surface, this is most likely to be an ABC.

Ref: Aids to Radiological Differential Diagnosis, 4th Ed, p. 62.

2 (d)
The symptoms described are more consistent with those of a meniscal injury, rather than a ligamentous tear. Such tears are commonest in the posterior horn of the medial meniscus.

Ref: Radiology Review Manual 6th Ed, p. 117.

3 (c)
Proximal femoral fractures are divided in subcapsular and extracapsular. The joint capsule runs from the acetabulum to the inter-trochanteric line anteriorly and to the junction of the middle/distal third of the femoral neck posteriorly. Thus intracapsular fractures are those of the femoral neck: sub-capital, trans-cervical and basi-cervical fractures, and extracapsular include inter-trochanteric, sub-trochanteric and femoral shaft fractures. Intracapsular fractures are more susceptible to AVN because the main supply to the femoral head is from the circumflex femoral arteries, which enter *via* the capsule and are more likely to be disrupted by such fractures. Additional blood supply from the ligamentum teres artery *via* the acetabular fossa and the retinacular branches on the surface of the femoral neck, are usually insufficient to prevent AVN. Furthermore they may be compromised by the raised pressure secondary to blood within the joint capsule. The more proximal the subcapsular fracture, the greater the risk of vascular compromise, thus a sub-capital fracture has the greatest risk of AVN.

Ref: Orthop Clin North Am (2002); 33(1): 97–111, viii.

4 (a)
Pseudofractures (Looser's zones) are insufficiency stress fractures with poor healing due to mineral deficiency. These are classically associated with osteomalacia, but can also be due to Paget's disease, osteogenesis imperfecta, or fibrous dysplasia. The fractures are typically bilateral and symmetrical and are at right angles to the cortical margin. Other common locations include distal 1/3 radius, proximal 1/3 ulna, lesser trochanter, medial femoral neck, ischial tuberosity, clavicle, long bones of the feet and hands.

Ref: Radiology Review Manual, 6th Ed, p. 148.

5 (b)
Other causes include trauma, infection, metastases and myeloma (but these are less likely to be bilaterally symmetrical). EG is a cause of destruction of the medial end of the clavicle, which can also be caused by metastases, infection, lymphoma and rheumatoid arthritis.

Ref: Radiology Review Manual, 6th Ed, p. 19.

6 (b)
The other listed diagnoses would be expected to cause superior rib notching. Superior notching is typically caused by connective tissue disorders, inferior notching is typically of vascular origin due to enlarged collateral vessels: coarctation, interrupted aortic arch, subclavian stenosis (Takayasu's), or SVC obstruction with venous collaterals, or AVMs. Hyperparathyroidism and NF-I can cause superior or inferior rib notching, the latter diagnosis is further suggested by the presence of scoliosis.

Ref: Radiology Review Manual, 6th Ed, p. 18–9.

7 (e)
Thanatophoric dysplasia is the commonest type of lethal micromelic dwarfism. Features include clover-leaf skull (15%), limb bowing, narrow thorax, non-immune hydrops. Other lethal dwarfisms include camptomelic dysplasia, Ellis-van Creveld syndrome, Jeune's syndrome, achondrogenesis, hypophosphatasia, homozygous achondroplasia, OI Type 2, and chondrodysplasia punctata. Heterozygous achondroplasia, OI Types 1, 3 and 4, diastrophic dysplasia, and Nievergelt syndrome are non-lethal variants.

Ref: Primer of Diagnostic Imaging, 4th Ed, p. 883–5.

8 (c)
Type I (6–8%) is an epiphyseal slip. Type II (73–75%) extends through the physis separating a metaphyseal fragment. Type IV (10–12%) involves the metaphysic, physis and epiphysis. Type III (8–10%) is described. Type V (< 1%) is a crush injury with damage to the vascular supply to the epiphysis. Common sites include the distal radius (28%), hand phalanges (26%), and distal tibia (10%). The prognosis gets worse as the grade increases, with type V injuries particularly associated with subsequent growth disturbance. Lower extremity injuries are also associated with a worse prognosis than upper limb injuries.

Ref: Radiology Review Manual, 6th Ed, p. 84.

9 (e)
In the supine position, air may collect in the anterior cardiophrenic sulcus, which will therefore appear well defined against the inferior border of the heart.

Ref: The Chest X-ray: A Survival Guide, 1st Ed, p. 96.

10 (a)
Pseudoaneurysms are typically well-defined, rounded and may be seen to have a neck adjoining an adjacent vessel. They are more difficult to detect on delayed images and there is no change in the haematoma. Management may be by embolisation or surgery depending on the clinical condition of the patient.

Ref: Radiographics (2008); 28: 1603–16.

11 (e)
More than one third of the capitellum should lie anterior to the anterior humeral line – if not, a supracondylar fracture should be suspected. A visible posterior fat pad is always abnormal. Displacement of the anterior fat pat raises the possibility of a fracture. In a true lateral film the distal humerus appears to form an 'hourglass', loss of this or apparent asymmetry are indicators of a supracondylar fracture.

Ref: Accident and Emergency Radiology, 2nd Ed, p. 106.

12 (d)
Fibrous dysplasia is the commonest benign rib tumour. Second most common is osteochondroma/bony exostosis but this typically occurs at the costochondral junction. Other benign possibilities include GCT and aneurysmal bone cyst.

Ref: Radiology Review Manual, 6th Ed, p. 18.

13 (a)
Myositis ossificans is a form of heterotopic bone formation within skeletal muscle, usually resulting from blunt trauma. Although parosteal osteosarcoma can have similar appearances, myositis ossificans typically has denser calcification in the periphery; osteosarcoma shows the reverse phenomenon, with denser calcification centrally. Juxtacortical chondroma typically scallops the underlying cortex. An osteochondroma is continuous with the underlying bone.

Ref: Musculoskeletal Imaging: the Requisites, 3rd Ed, p. 524.

14 (a)
The patient is most likely to be suffering from hypertrophic osteoarthropathy. This is commonly secondary to disease within the chest but many extra-thoracic causes are also recognised. Possible thoracic causes include: Bronchogenic carcinoma, lymphoma, pulmonary metastasis, a benign tumour (*e.g.* pleural fibroma), and chronic inflammation/infection (*e.g.* an abscess, bronchiectasis). Extrathoracic causes include, amongst others: inflammatory bowel disease, whipple's disease, coeliac disease, cirrhosis, dysentery and undifferentiated nasopharyngeal carcinomas.

Ref: Aids to Radiological Differential Diagnosis, 4th Ed, p. 37.

15 (e)
Felty's syndrome is characterised by the combination of long-standing rheumatoid arthritis, splenomegaly and neutropaenia. Associated features include weight loss, leg ulceration, and brown skin pigmentation. Almost all have high titres of rheumatoid factor.

Ref: Musculoskeletal Imaging: the Requisites, 3rd Ed, p. 291.

16 (a)
Ossification of the posterior, rather than anterior longitudinal ligament is typical of ankylosing spondylitis.

Ref: Aids to Radiological Differential Diagnosis, 4th Ed, p. 383.

17 (b)
The distance between the anterior arch of C1 and the anterior aspect of the odontoid peg should be no more than 3 mm in an adult. On the lateral view, the maximum width of the prevertebral soft tissues is: 7 mm at C1-4, 22 mm at C5-7. Harris' ring is often incomplete in its inferior aspect. On the long AP view, no single interspinous distance should be more than 50% wider than the one immediately above or below it.

Ref: Accident and Emergency Radiology, 2nd Ed, p. 87.

18 (b)
Transient osteoporosis of the hip is a sudden, painful but self limiting condition, first described in patients in the third trimester of pregnancy, but seen most frequently in middle-aged men. Radiographs show diffuse ostepaenia 4–8 weeks after symptom onset. MR imaging demonstrates diffuse oedema, without focal defects: oedema localised to the subchondral surface or a 'double-line' sign suggest AVN. ^{99m}Tc-MDP imaging shows homogeneously increased uptake in the femoral head and neck.

Ref: Can J Surg (2003); 46(3): 187–192.

19 (c)
Articular cortex destruction is not seen in Perthe's disease, which classically demonstrates sclerosis of the femoral head along with the findings above in the early phase. Later changes include subchondral fractures, femoral head fragmentation, femoral neck cysts and loose body formation.

Ref: Radiology Review Manual, 6th Ed, p. 51.

20 (a)
Type I: a fracture through the upper portion of the dens. Type II: a transverse fracture through the junction of the dens and the body of the axis. Type III: a fracture through the body of the axis. There is no type IV nor V.

Ref: Neuroradiology: the requisites, 2nd Ed, p. 844.

21 (a)
The spleen accounts for 40% of organ injuries following blunt abdominal trauma, with the liver accounting for 20%. If penetrating trauma is taken in to account as well, the liver is the most commonly injured organ.

Ref: Radiographics (2007); 1: 109–125.

22 (b)
A foot x-ray is indicated with bony tenderness over the base of the 5th metatarsal (and midfoot pain).

Ref: JAMA (1994); 271(11): 271–82.

23 (e)
Both conditions describe multiple enchondromas affecting the hands and/or feet, and both tend to be unilateral; neither has a genetic component. Both conditions can lead to shortening of the involved arm/leg, resulting in length discrepancy. Malignant degeneration can be to osteosarcoma (young adults), or chondro/fibrosarcoma (older patients); it is more common in Mafucci's syndrome, but is still seen in 5–30% of cases of Ollier's disease. Maffucci's syndrome describes enchondromas with additional multiple soft tissue haemangiomas, if bilateral there is marked asymmetry.

Ref: Diagnostic Radiology, 5th Ed, p. 1037–8.

24 (a)
A Barton's fracture refers to an intra-articular fracture through the distal radius. The conventional Barton fracture involves the dorsal rim of the radius, the reverse Barton involves the volar rim. Salter-Harris fractures involve the growth plate before closure; the other types described are not intra-articular. Colles' and Smith's are fractures of the distal radius with dorsal and volar displacement of the distal fragments, respectively. A chauffeur fracture is a triangular fracture of the radial styloid process.

25 (e)
The described findings are of an H-shaped vertebrae (often better appreciated on lateral films), left femoral head AVN, and auto-infarction of the spleen. In SCD, the Hb deforms at low oxygen tension, and obstructs small blood vessels, leading to hypoxia/ anoxia (AVN), and splenic auto-infarction (on AXR: prominent bowel loops in the LUQ +/– calcification of the spleen). Other skeletal features include 'hair-on-end' appearance to the skull, secondary osteomyelitis (often due to *Salmonella*), and premature epiphyseal fusion. Cholelithiasis, cardiomegaly, PE, cerebral infarcts, and renal papillary necrosis are also associated.

Ref: Diagnostic Radiology, 5th Ed, p. 1773–6.

26 (b)
The aortic and mitral valves are more commonly affected.

Ref: Radiographics (2009); 28: 1555–70.

27 (d)
The flexor tendons occur in the order (from anterior to posterior): tibialis posterior, flexor digitorum longus, flexor hallucis longus – the mnemonic 'Tom, Dick, and Harry' aids memory.

Ref: Fundamentals of Skeletal Radiology, 3rd Ed, p. 209.

28 (c)
Grade I injury is a minor contusion/superficial laceration. Grade II injury is a major contusion/laceration without duct injury. Grade III injury is a distal transection/injury involving the duct. Grade IV injury is a proximal transection or injury involving the ampulla or bile duct. Grade V injury is massive disruption of the pancreatic head.

Ref: Radiographics (2009); 28: 1591–1601.

29 (b)
The Weber classification is based on the location of the distal fibular fracture relative to the tibiotalar joint. Type A is a transverse fracture distal to the ankle joint; type B is an oblique fracture at the level of the joint; type C is a fibular fracture proximal to the level of the joint. There is no type D or E.

Ref: Musculoskeletal Imaging: the Requisites, 3rd Ed, p. 253.

30 (e)
The earliest changes of thalassaemia can be seen in the small bones of the hand and feet. The appearances described are due to marrow hyperplasia secondary to anaemia. The changes are typically symmetrical with osteopaenia/osteoporosis, atrophy and coarsening of the trabeculae, widening of the medullary spaces, and thinning of the cortices.

Ref: Radiology Review Manual, 6th Ed, p. 168–70.

31 (d)
Although there can be some variation in the order, the usual sequence of appearance is shown below:

Approximate age at appearance (years)	Ossification centre
1	Capitellum
3	Radial head
4–5	Internal (medial) epicondyle
7–8	Trochlea
8–10	Olecranon
9–13	Lateral (external) epicondyle

Ref: Accident and Emergency Radiology, 2nd Ed, p. 100.

32 (a)
Scoliosis can be divided into three broad categories: congenital, idiopathic, and secondary. Idiopathic scoliosis is described as infantile (0–3 years), juvenile (4–10 years), adolescent (> 10 years), or adult onset. Adolescent idiopathic scoliosis accounts for 80% of cases, and rapid progression tends to occur during growth spurts. Prognosis is worse with a high thoracic scoliosis. Females are more commonly affected. The presence of neurological signs implies an underlying abnormality. Plagiocephaly is associated with infantile idiopathic scoliosis.

Ref: RITI 2_018 Painful scoliosis & 5_115 Scoliosis.

33 (a)
On the lateral view, the distance from the lower pole of the patella to the tibial tubercle should equal the length of the patella plus or minus 20%. If this rule is broken, a ruptured patellar ligament must be suspected. On the AP view a perpendicular line drawn from the lateral margin of the femoral condyle should have ≤ 5 mm of the lateral margin of the tibal condyle outside of it. The fabella is a common sesamoid bone within the lateral head of gastrocnemius.

Ref: Accident and Emergency Radiology, 2nd Ed, p. 214.

34 (d)
The width of the space between the distal tibia and fibula at a point 1 cm from the articular surface should be ≤ 6 mm. Bohler's angle is normally 30–40 degrees. In contradistinction to a fracture, the long axis of an unfused apophysis of the base of the 5th metatarsal runs parallel to the metatarsal shaft. On an AP view of the midfoot, the medial margin of the second metatarsal should align with the medial margin of the intermediate cuneiform. On an AP view of the midfoot, the medial margin of the third metatarsal aligns with the medial margin of the lateral cuneiform.

Ref: Accident and Emergency Radiology, 2nd Ed, p. 234.

35 (e)
Enchondromas present in a slightly younger age group and are more common in females. They typically affect the bones of the hands and feet and are usually less than 5 cm in size. Although both lesions show matrix mineralisation, this feature is slightly commoner in enchondromas. Other features to favour chondrosarcoma over enchondroma include presentation with a mass, cortical destruction and the presence of a soft tissue mass.

Ref: Radiology Review Manual 6th Ed, p. 59.

36 (b)

Grade	Features
I	Normal radiograph
II	AC distance > 8–10 mm; CC distance ≤ 13 mm
III	AC distance > 8–10 mm; CC distance > 13 mm
IV	Total dislocation, clavicle dislocated into trapezius
V	Total dislocation, clavicle dislocated into neck
VI	Total dislocation, clavicle dislocated inferiorly

Ref: Accident and Emergency Radiology, 2nd Ed, p. 87.

37 (b)
Modic degenerative changes are bone marrow and endplate changes adjacent to degenerative lumbar intervertebral discs; they are commonest at the L4-L5 and L5-S1 level. Modic II is more prevalent, but Modic I changes are more likely to be symptomatic. Type I changes have MRI appearances of fluid (low T1, high T2), type II changes have the characteristics of fat due to red marrow replacement (high T1 and T2), and type III changes are due to sclerosis (low on T1 and T2).

Ref: Radiology (2007); 245(1): 43–61.

38 (e)
Fractures across the proximal pole and waist both carry a high risk of subsequent AVN. 80% of fractures occur across the waist, compared to 10% for each of the poles. Transverse/horizontal oblique fractures are relatively stable compared to vertical oblique fractures.

Ref: Musculoskeletal Imaging: the Requisites, 3rd Ed, p. 144.

39 (e)
GCTs are usually benign lesions. Malignancy occurs in 5–10% of cases and is usually secondary to previous radiation therapy. The majority of spinal lesions arise within the sacrum. Vertebral involvement accounts for only 7% of cases: thoracic spine is the most common location, followed by cervical and lumbar regions. They typically increase in size during pregnancy, thought to be due to hormonal influences. GCTs tend to be locally aggressive and complete surgical resection is uncommon; adjuvant radiotherapy is often administered. Recurrence occurs in 40-60%, and is suggested on plain film by the presence of new areas of osseous destruction.

Ref: RITI 2_018 Painful scoliosis.

40 (d)
In transient patella dislocation, the patella dislocates laterally and then relocates. This causes impaction between the inferomedial aspect of the patella and the anterolateral aspect of the lateral femoral condyle, which results in bone contusions. In addition to the above signs, a haemarthrosis is also usually present.

Ref: Radiology Review Manual, 6th Ed, p. 69.

41 (e)
The wrists are more commonly involved in rheumatoid arthritis.

Ref: Musculoskeletal Imaging: the Requisites, 3rd Ed, p. 322.

42 (d)
The active phase is the osteolytic phase, also known as the 'hot' phase. Typical lesions include osteoporosis circumscripta of the skull (especially frontal and occipital bones) and well-defined, 'flame-shaped' radiolucencies of the long bones.

Ref: Aids to Radiological Differential Diagnosis, 4th Ed, p. 590.

43 (b)
The Hangman's fracture is a traumatic bilateral neural arch fracture, most commonly of the pars, resulting from hyperextension. When subluxation occurs, it is more commonly an anterior, rather than posterior subluxation of C2 on C3.

Ref: Musculoskeletal Imaging: the Requisites, 3rd Ed, p. 170.

44 (c)
Parosteal osteosarcomas have the best prognosis of all osteosarcomas. If no stalk can be clearly identified they can be distinguished from myositis ossificans by the relative density of the centre of the ossified part of the lesion.

Ref: Radiology Review Manual, 6th Ed, p. 143.

45 (d)
Posterior dislocations produce posterior, rather than anterior, capsule stripping. Other evidence of a prior posterior dislocation include: a reverse Bankart lesion, a reverse Hill-Sach's lesions, or a posterior labral tear.

Ref: Musculoskeletal Imaging: the Requisites, 3rd Ed, p. 99.

46 (a)
Metaphyseal corner fractures are relatively specific for NAI, however overall they are less common than diaphyseal fractures. Subdural haemorrhage with an interhemispheric location is the commonest type of intracranial haemorrhage.

Ref: Radiology Review Manual, 6th Ed, p. 52.

47 (c)
Intraosseous lipomas are rare bone tumours; they are often asymptomatic and present incidental, but can be associated with pain. The commonest locations are within the proximal femur (Ward's triangle) and in the area of the calcaneus described. In these areas there is a relative paucity of trabecular bone and it is thought that this leads to an 'overshoot' phenomenon during the transition of haematopoietic to fatty marrow, with the resultant formation of the lipoma. Central or ring calcification in a lucent lesion in this location of the calcaneus is said to be pathognomonic of an intraosseous lipoma and allows its distinction from a UBC. If clinical doubt persists MR imaging can be used for further clarification and to confirm the presence of fat.

Ref: Radiographics (2004); 24: 1433–1466.

48 (b)
Osteoblastomas are uncommon primary bone tumours (< 1%). 90% occur in 2nd – 3rd decades, although cases have been documented up to 72 years. They are histologically similar to osteoid osteoma but less well organised and by definition larger (> 2 cm). The majority (30–40%) of cases occur in the spine, with a slight predominance for the posterior elements (55%). An expansile lesion in osteoblastoma is not typically associated with malignancy. Scoliosis can occur in both and is typically painful, but occurs more commonly in osteoid osteoma, where the scoliosis results from muscle spasm secondary to the inflammatory mediators produced. Osteoblastomas are not radiosensitive and surgical excision is performed in most cases, however, recurrence is seen in up to 50%.

Ref: RITI 2_018 Painful scoliosis.

49 (a)
Osteitis condensans ilii produces this radiographic appearance, typically in young multiparous women. Possible differential diagnoses include: ankylosing spondylitis, rheumatoid arthritis (both would be associated with joint space changes) and Paget's disease.

Ref: Aids to Radiological Differential Diagnosis, 4th Ed, p. 101.

50 (b)
The appearances are typical of Caffey's disease, also known as infantile cortical hyperostosis. Scurvy and rickets are unlikely to produce this picture in those < 6 months old.

Ref: Aids to Radiological Differential Diagnosis, 4th Ed, p. 38.

Gastro-intestinal Practice SBA Questions

1 **A 42 year old man presents with severe central abdominal pain and a raised serum amylase. 4 days later, extremely ill, the patient undergoes a CT of the abdomen which demonstrates that only the head and uncinate process of the pancreas are enhancing and there is extensive free fluid in the peri-pancreatic tissues.**

How would you interpret these findings?
(a) Acute pancreatitis
(b) Acute pancreatitis with necrosis
(c) Acute pancreatitis with infected necrosis
(d) Acute pancreatitis with abscess
(e) Acute pancreatitis with pseudocyst formation

2 **A patient with proven Hodgkin lymphoma is referred for a staging PET-CT. This shows a solitary focal lung lesion with cervical and mediastinal lymph node enlargement. All of these lesions are PET positive with no other sites of disease.**

What stage is this disease?
(a) I
(b) II
(c) IIE
(d) III
(e) IV

3 **A 47 year old patient is referred for an abdominal US. In the spleen, several rounded, thin-walled hypoechoic lesions are seen in a subcapsular position. CT shows the lesions have a density of 20 HU and there is no enhancement with intravenous contrast medium.**

What is the most likely diagnosis?
(a) Infarction
(b) Lymphangioma
(c) Haemangioma
(d) Hamartoma
(e) Abscess

4 Emphysematous gastritis is most commonly associated with which of the following organisms?

(a) *S. pneumoniae*
(b) *C. difficile*
(c) *S. milleri*
(d) *E. coli*
(e) *S. aureus*

5 A 47 year old man undergoes a CT and subsequently an MRI. These show an area of focal fat accumulation adjacent to the falciform ligament anteriorly.

This may be attributed to flow within which of the following?

(a) Vein of Sappey
(b) Cholecystic vein
(c) Right gastric vein
(d) Anterior gastric vein
(e) Inferior epigastric vein

6 A 61 year old man has alcohol-related chronic liver disease. Which of the following conditions is he not at increased risk of developing compared with the general population?

(a) Non-specific interstitial pneumonitis
(b) Bacterial pneumonia
(c) Hydrothorax
(d) Pulmonary hypertension
(e) Acute respiratory distress syndrome

7 Enteropathy-associated T-cell lymphoma is most commonly associated with which of the following conditions?

(a) Coeliac disease
(b) Crohn's disease
(c) Lymphangectasia
(d) Whipple's disease
(e) Peutz-Jegher's syndrome

8 **An 18 year old male patient with known von Hippel Lindau disease is referred for abdominal imaging.**

Which of the following conditions would you not expect to see in association with this disease?

(a) Phaeochromocytoma
(b) Serous cystadenoma of the pancreas
(c) Neuroendocrine pancreatic tumour
(d) Pancreatic cysts
(e) Adrenocortical carcinoma

9 **With regard to radiation enteropathy, which of the following is not true?**

(a) Acute changes occur in patients who have received 1,000cGy or more
(b) Acute changes are due to damage to the blood supply
(c) Chronic changes may be seen in up to 15% of patients
(d) Multiple stenoses are a feature of chronic disease
(e) Acute radiation enteropathy refers to changes within the first 2 months

10 **A young man presents to A&E with severe central chest pain following an episode of vomiting. On questioning he reports that he has been drinking alcohol the night before. The CT shows an eccentric hyperattenuating mass within the wall of the oesophagus.**

What is the most likely diagnosis?

(a) Mallory-Weiss tear
(b) Intramural oesophageal dissection
(c) Boerhaave syndrome
(d) Transmural perforation
(e) Intramural haematoma

11 A 58 year old lady is referred for staging of a carcinoma in the middle third of the oesophagus.

Which of the following statements is true?

(a) Lymphatic drainage is likely to be via the upper abdominal lymph nodes
(b) A PET study can reliably exclude the presence of involved loco-regional nodes
(c) EUS is superior to PET-CT in the evaluation of loco-regional lymph nodes
(d) Following treatment, EUS most commonly under-stages residual disease
(e) The adrenal glands are the commonest site of metastatic disease

12 A patient with multiple medical problems is referred for CT colonography and requires intravenous hyoscine butylbromide (Buscopan) as part of the procedure.

Which of the medical conditions listed are contraindications to this?

(a) Open angle glaucoma
(b) Hypertension
(c) Ischaemic heart disease
(d) Myasthenia Gravis
(e) Parkinson's disease

13 The junction of the squamous and columnar epithelium, seen on the barium swallow, is given what term?

(a) A-ring
(b) B-ring
(c) Schatzki ring
(d) Barrett's line
(e) Z-line

14 A patient with a metastasis from a GIST tumour undergoes a contrast-enhanced CT study before and after chemotherapy. On the initial study, the lesion measures 5 cm in diameter and has a density of 100 HU. At follow up, the lesion measures 6 cm and has a density of 80 HU.

How should you classify the response to chemotherapy?

(a) Complete response
(b) Partial response
(c) Mixed response
(d) Stable disease
(e) Progressive disease

15 Regarding 2nd generation US contrast agents, which of the following statements is true?

(a) Hepatocyte-specific agents are of particular value in characterising liver lesions
(b) Microbubbles persist for 30 minutes
(c) Excretion is mainly through biliary pathways
(d) A high mechanical index setting is required for dynamic imaging
(e) Metastases are best seen in the delayed phase (2-5 min)

16 A 77 year old man presents with abdominal distension. A CT study of his abdomen and pelvis reveals nodular peritoneal thickening, omental cake and a stellate appearance within the mesentery. Some foci of calcification are evident.

What is the most likely diagnosis?

(a) Tuberculosis
(b) Lymphoma
(c) Carcinoma
(d) Pseudomyxoma
(e) Mesothelioma

17 An unenhanced CT of the liver is performed. The liver has a density of 60 HU and the spleen has a density of 50 HU.

How might you account for these findings?

(a) Normal findings
(b) Diffuse fatty infiltration
(c) Haemochromatosis
(d) Wilson's disease
(e) Budd-Chiari syndrome

18 A patient is referred for a CT of the chest, abdomen and pelvis, the clinical details read "Riedel's thyroiditis. Hyper-IgG4 disease". Are any other organs involved?'

Which of the following conditions are not associated?

(a) Cryptogenic organising pneumonia
(b) Benign pleural mesothelioma
(c) Systemic sclerosis
(d) Autoimmune pancreatitis
(e) Retroperitoneal fibrosis

19 A 50 year old man undergoes liver transplantation. A routine follow-up liver US comments that the intra-hepatic arterial Doppler has a low resistance index (0.48) and a prolonged systolic acceleration time.

What diagnosis does this suggest?

(a) Hepatic artery stenosis
(b) Portal vein occlusion
(c) Hepatic artery pseudoaneurysm
(d) Graft rejection
(e) Hepatic artery thrombosis

20 A patient with liver disease is referred for US assessment of their TIPS stent which has been in situ for 3 months. The Doppler study demonstrates a flow rate of 2.3 m/s.

What is this most likely to represent?

(a) Normal flow
(b) Arterio-venous fistula
(c) Stent stenosis
(d) Stent fracture
(e) Stent occlusion

21 Which of the following is not a recognised cause of gastric fold thickening?

(a) Adult hypertrophic pyloric stenosis
(b) Lymphoma
(c) Gastritis
(d) Menetrier's disease
(e) Zollinger-Ellison syndrome

22 A 45 year old woman with a history of diarrhoea and weight loss undergoes an endoscopy and has a duodenal biopsy. The biopsy is reported to show foamy macrophages. Granules within the cytoplasm of these macrophages stain positively with periodic acid-Schiff (PAS) stain.

What additional feature might you expect on a small bowel enema in this patient?

(a) Multiple polyps
(b) Ulceration of the mucosa
(c) Reduced mucosal folds with dilatation of the small bowel
(d) Pseudosacculation
(e) Thickening of the mucosal folds

23 A 2.3 cm adrenal lesion is noted in a 62 year old man undergoing a staging CT for colon carcinoma. A dedicated study demonstrates the lesion to have a density of –2 HU before contrast medium, 56 HU in the portal venous phase and 20 HU at 10 minutes.

What is the most likely diagnosis?

(a) Cyst
(b) Adenoma
(c) Metastasis
(d) Lipoma
(e) Adrenocortical carcinoma

24 Which of the following is true of polysplenia?

(a) It has an 80% mortality in the first year
(b) It is associated with total anomalous pulmonary venous drainage
(c) It is more common in females
(d) It is associated with right isomerism
(e) It is associated with annular pancreas

25 An 18 year old man undergoes an abdominal US and is found to have splenomegaly with multiple focal lesions.

Which of the following diagnoses is least likely to give these appearances?

(a) Sarcoidosis
(b) Lymphoma
(c) Portal hypertension
(d) Sickle cell disease
(e) Amyloidosis

26 A 40 year old man is found to have abnormal liver function whilst undergoing routine blood tests prior to abdominal surgery. Subsequent imaging demonstrates a relatively normal liver parenchyma but there is irregularity of the bile ducts with beading and short segment strictures.

What is the most likely diagnosis?

(a) Autoimmune liver disease
(b) Viral hepatitis
(c) Primary biliary cirrhosis
(d) Cholangiocarcinoma
(e) Primary sclerosing cholangitis

27 In the staging of colorectal carcinoma, inferior mesenteric lymph nodes are considered distant metastasis rather than regional drainage for which tumour site?

(a) Ascending colon
(b) Transverse colon
(c) Descending colon
(d) Sigmoid colon
(e) Rectum

28 A 46 year old man presents with abdominal pain, fever and vomiting 5 weeks after an episode of acute pancreatitis. A CT study shows a well-circumscribed collection adjacent to the pancreas with an enhancing rim.

What is the most likely diagnosis?

(a) Pseudocyst
(b) Pancreatic abscess
(c) Infective necrosis
(d) Acute pancreatitis
(e) Chronic pancreatitis

29 A 47 year old lady attends for an US of her biliary system. Three comet-tail artefacts are seen arising from the anterior wall, which is slightly thickened. The remainder of the examination was unremarkable.

What is the most likely cause?

(a) Adenomyomatosis
(b) Cholesterolosis
(c) Gallstones
(d) Chronic cholecystitis
(e) Porcelain gallbladder

30 A patient with a pyrexia of unknown origin is referred for a radio-labelled white cell scan with Tc-99m HMPAO.

At which time points should imaging of the abdomen be performed?

(a) 1 and 3 hours
(b) 1, 3 and 6 hours
(c) 1 and 6 hours
(d) 1, 3 and 24 hours
(e) 1, 6 and 24 hours

31 A patient is referred for the investigation of right upper quadrant pain. US has equivocal findings and a HIDA examination is requested. At 35 minutes, there is little uptake within the liver, but renal excretion is noted.

What is the most likely cause for these findings?

(a) Poor liver function
(b) Acute cholecystitis
(c) Poor renal function
(d) Sphincter of Oddi dysfunction
(e) Chronic cholecystitis

32 Where do gastrointestinal stromal tumours (GIST) most commonly arise?

(a) Oesophagus
(b) Stomach
(c) Small intestine
(d) Colon
(e) Appendix

33 A patient with Hodgkin's lymphoma undergoes a PET-CT which shows a 10 x 5 cm nodal mass which is PET positive. Following 2 cycles of chemotherapy, the nodal mass measures 6 x 3 cm but there is no uptake of FDG within the mass.

How should you report this study?

(a) Partial response
(b) Stable disease
(c) Mixed response
(d) Too early to assess response
(e) Complete response

34 Which of the following tumours of the vermiform appendix is encountered most commonly?

(a) Adenocarcinoma
(b) Carcinoid
(c) Lymphoma
(d) Mucinous adenocarcinoma
(e) Gastrointestinal Stromal Tumour

35 A 39 year old man presents with epigastric pain, diarrhoea, PR bleeding, exhaustion, and fatigue. He is noted to have a swelling of the jaw. On examination there are several calvarial lumps. CT head shows sebaceous cysts and bone lesions which are likely osteomas. OGD shows gastric hamartomas, colonoscopy shows multiple polyps throughout the colon.

What is the most likely diagnosis?

(a) Cowden disease
(b) Gardner's syndrome
(c) Lynch syndrome
(d) Peutz-Jegher's syndrome
(e) Turcot's syndrome

36 Which of the following is true of insulinomas?

(a) Men are affected twice as often as women
(b) Multiple lesions are seen in 25% cases
(c) They account for 25% of pancreatic endocrine tumours
(d) They are associated with MEN-I syndrome
(e) Approximately 25% cases are malignant

37 A patient is referred for an abdominal radiograph and telephones the department to ask about radiation.

What is the typical effective dose of a plain abdominal radiograph?

(a) 0.02 mSv
(b) 0.3 mSv
(c) 0.7 mSv
(d) 1 mSv
(e) 1.5 mSv

38 A patient with a 4 month history of severe upper abdominal pain undergoes an endoscopic US. This reports a combination of echogenic and echo-poor foci throughout the pancreas, an irregular contour of the pancreatic duct and thickening of the duct wall with some side duct dilatation.

What is the most likely diagnosis?

(a) Autoimmune pancreatitis
(b) Pancreatic adenocarcinoma
(c) Intraductal papillary mucinous tumour
(d) von Hippel Lindau syndrome
(e) Chronic pancreatitis

39 Hepatocellular adenomas are not associated with which of the following?

(a) Spontaneous rupture
(b) Oral contraceptive pill
(c) Hepatocellular carcinoma
(d) Androgenic steroids
(e) Cholangiocarcinoma

40 Which of the following is associated with an increased risk of developing pancreatic adenocarcinoma?

(a) Hereditary pancreatitis
(b) High alcohol consumption
(c) High coffee consumption
(d) Low fibre diet
(e) Type-1 diabetes mellitus

41 Which of the following statements regarding the internal anal sphincter is true?

(a) It is made of striated muscle
(b) Isolated injury is usually due to obstetric injury
(c) It appears hyperechoic on endo-anal ultrasound
(d) It is the termination of the circular smooth muscle of the gastrointestinal tract
(e) The deep part fuses with the puborectalis sling and levator muscles

42 A previously well 65 year old man has a myocardial infarction. Six days later he develops acute abdominal pain and distension; he feels nauseated and vomits. An abdominal film demonstrates distended proximal colon to the splenic flexure and normal colon distally. A contrast enema is performed with no abnormality seen.

What is the most likely diagnosis?

(a) Sigmoid volvulus
(b) Adhesions causing large bowel obstruction
(c) Caecal volvulus
(d) Toxic megacolon
(e) Acute colonic pseudo-obstruction

43 A 56 year old HIV-positive man presents with diarrhoea which the clinical team feel is due to a gastrointestinal infection. His CD4 count is 350.

Which of the following is most likely?

(a) Mycobacterium tuberculosis
(b) Herpes simplex virus
(c) Candida albicans
(d) Cytomegalovirus
(e) Cryptosporidium

44 How many types of caecal volvulus are described?

(a) 1
(b) 2
(c) 3
(d) 4
(e) 5

45 A 37 year old lady with longstanding constipation is referred for a defaecating proctography. The only abnormality seen on resulting images show an 8 cm anterior bulge of the anterior margin of the rectum with incomplete evacuation.

What is the diagnosis?

(a) Rectal prolapse
(b) Rectocoele
(c) Anismus
(d) Cystocoele
(e) Enterocoele

46 A patient with a biopsy proven cholangiocarcinoma undergoes imaging which demonstrates that the tumour is confined to the common bile duct.

How would you classify this?

(a) Bismuth I
(b) Bismuth II
(c) Bismuth III
(d) Bismuth IV
(e) Bismuth V

47 A 56 year old patient presents with carcinoid syndrome and is found to have liver metastases.

What is the most likely site of the primary lesion?

(a) Stomach
(b) Duodenum
(c) Small Bowel
(d) Appendix
(e) Rectum

48 A 28 year old man with cystic fibrosis and abnormal liver function is referred to you for liver imaging by his clinical team.

Which of the following are not associated with cystic fibrosis?

(a) Nodular regenerative hyperplasia
(b) Steatosis
(c) Sclerosing cholangitis
(d) Cirrhosis
(e) Cholelithiasis

49 A patient with known Crohn's disease is referred for a small bowel enema.

Which of the following features would you not expect to see?

(a) Aphthoid ulcers
(b) Kinked bowel segments
(c) Sacculation
(d) Increased number of folds in the ileum
(e) Loop separation

50 A 76 year old man with a clinical suspicion of a hernia is referred for an ultrasound. A colleague performs the study and reports: "The hernia lies lateral to the conjoint tendon and medial to the inferior epigastric artery at the inferior aspect of Hesselbach's triangle."

What type of hernia is described?

(a) Direct inguinal hernia
(b) Spigelian hernia
(c) Hypogastic hernia
(d) Femoral hernia
(e) Obturator hernia

Gastro-intestinal Practice SBA Answers

1 (b)
The clinical scenario and imaging features clearly indicate acute pancreatitis. Areas of non-enhancement >3 cm, or >30% of the pancreatic volume are considered reliable CT signs for necrosis. Imaging too early in the clinical course will reduce the sensitivity of CT for evaluating pancreatic necrosis. Sepsis tends to complicate severe pancreatitis after the first 1–2 weeks, peaking at 3 weeks, and is a common cause of mortality in these patients. A discrete abscess is less common but is suggested by the development of air within a collection. Pseudocysts are common sequelae of acute pancreatitis but take at least 4 weeks to form.

Ref: Radiology (1994); 193:297–306.

2 (c)
This describes stage IIE: localised involvement of a single extralymphatic organ or site and its regional lymph nodes with or without involvement of other lymph node regions on the same side of the diaphragm. Disseminated or multifocal extralymphatic disease would constitute stage IV disease.

Ref: TNM Atlas, 5th Ed; p. 371–382.

3 (b)
These are the typical imaging features of these asymptomatic lesions. Infarcts are usually wedge-shaped, whilst the remaining lesions usually show some enhancement.

Ref: Diagnostic Radiology, 5th Ed, p. 1763.

4 (d)
Clostridium welchii is another common cause of this unusual condition. *S. pneumoniae*, *S. aureus* (and *E. coli*) may cause non-emphysematous gastritis. *S. milleri* is a cause of liver abscesses and *C. difficile* colitis.

Ref: Diagnostic Radiology, 5th Ed, p. 638.

5 (a)
This is a common aberrant vein which drains the superior epigastric vein and/ or the internal thoracic veins and communicates with the left portal vein branches.

Ref: J Comput Assist Tomogr (2007); 31:526–33.

6 (a)
There is no increased risk of NSIP or any other interstitial lung disease as a result of cirrhosis. Patients with cirrhosis have altered immunity and undergo changes to the vascular bed both within the liver and the lungs.

Ref: Radiographics (2009); 29:825–837.

7 (a)
This is invariably seen in the underlying bowel in patients with this condition, although it may not have been diagnosed prior to the lymphoma. The other conditions do not predispose to lymphomas.

Ref: Radiol Clin North Am (2008); 46(2):287–312.

8 (e)
There are a number of abdominal manifestations in addition to these including renal cysts and renal cell carcinoma. Epididymal papillary cystadenoma may be seen on scrotal US in male patients.

Ref: Radiographics (2008); 28:65–79.

9 (b)
Acute radiation enteropathy is due to death of the mucosal cells which are dividing rapidly. Chronic enteropathy is due to the effect on the vasculature, resulting in strictures, adhesions and fistulae.

Ref: R-ITI 3_061 Small bowel: vascular conditions of the small bowel (including bleeding and ischaemia).

10 (e)
The CT features indicate an intramural haematoma. Such patients often have a history of instrumentation, vomiting or food impaction and present with sudden onset pain, dysphagia or odynophagia. Haematemesis tends to occur later in the clinical course. Mallory-Weiss tear is a longitudinal mucosal laceration at the gastro-oesophageal junction. Dissection gives a double-barrelled appearance of the lumen due to a mucosal flap. Options (c) and (d) are full-thickness injuries and demonstrate mediastinal air or fluid on CT.

Ref: Radiographics (2008); 28:1541–1553.

11 (c)
The upper and middle thirds of the oesophagus usually drain superiorly. Local staging is best performed with endoscopic US. PET-CT is the most accurate modality for distant lymph nodes or metastases but the intense uptake of the primary tumour may obscure local nodes. Following treatment, it is difficult to distinguish fibrosis from active tumour at EUS; PET is more accurate in this circumstance. The most common sites of metastases are, in order, liver, lungs bones and adrenal glands.

Ref: Radiographics (2009); 29:403–42.

12 (d)
In addition, Buscopan is contraindicated in patients with megacolon, untreated narrow angle glaucoma, tachycardia, hypertrophy of the prostate with urinary retention, and mechanical stenoses of the gastrointestinal tract.

13 (e)
The A-ring is transient and muscular. The B- or Schatzki ring is a fixed mucosal/ muscular ring which may cause dysphagia or obstruction. Barrett's stricture is a complication of gastro-oesophageal reflux disease and is premalignant.

Ref: R-ITI 3_002. The Gastro-Oeosophageal Junction, Hiatus Hernia and Reflux Disease.

14 (b)
Metastatic GIST tumours are treated with monoclonal antibody agents. These typically reduce the blood supply and metabolism of the tumours with little change in tumour size and as such, the RECIST criteria are of little value. The Choi criteria differ from RECIST in that to obtain a PR, one needs a 10% reduction in size or a 15% reduction in density. Progressive disease requires 10% tumour growth without a 15% reduction in lesion density, a new lesion or a new or growing nodule of enhancing tumour within an existing lesion. There is no mixed response category.

Ref: AJR (2004); 183:1619–1628.

15 (e)
US contrast agents are microbubbles comprising a 'shell' containing an inert gas, which is injected *i.v.* and may persist for up to 6 hours. The agents stay within the blood pool, but for an unknown reason pool in the sinusoids during the delayed (2–5 min) phase, hence metastases are well depicted. Imaging is performed using a low mechanical index (0.1–0.2) to avoid bursting the bubbles.

Ref: Contrast Enhanced US in Clinical Practice, p. 3–9.

16 (e)
These are the typical features of sarcomatous mesothelioma. Peritoneal mesothelioma represents 6–10% cases of mesothelioma, with 50% cases having had previous asbestos exposure. Radiation therapy also predisposes to this condition, which affects visceral and parietal peritoneum.

Ref: Cancer Treat Res (2008); 143:281–97.

17 (a)
The normal liver has a density of 50–70 HU. Fatty infiltration will reduce this as the atomic numbers of the elements C, H and O are low. Iron and copper deposition can raise the density, as they have high atomic numbers.

18 (c)
Hyper IgG4 is a chronic inflammatory condition that may involve a number of organs. It is characterised histologically by a lymphoplasmacytic inflammation with IgG4-positive cells and exuberant fibrosis, which leaves dense fibrosis on resolution. It may respond to corticosteroids or other immunosuppressant therapy. Sclerosing sialadenitis, retro-orbital pseudotumour, and panniculitis may also be seen.

Ref: BMC Medicine (2006); 4:23.

19 (a)
The tardus et parvus waveform described here is seen distal to a stenosis. At the stenosis, a jet phenomenon may be seen with greatly increased flow.

Ref: US of Abdominal Transplantation, p. 90–104.

20 (c)
This is a jet phenomenon at a narrow stenosis. Normal flow rates are 0.5-1.9m/s but may vary with respiration.

Ref: US of Abdominal Transplantation, p. 76–89.

21 (a)
This has similar appearances to infantile hypertrophic pyloric stenosis but may be associated with ulceration. Differentiation from malignancy in the antrum may also be difficult.

Ref: R-ITI 3_044. Non-neoplastic disorders of the stomach and duodenum.

22 (e)
These are the clinical, pathological and radiological features of Whipple's disease. This is an uncommon condition of the small bowel caused by a bacterial infection, thought to be *Tropheryma whippelli.* Antibiotic therapy needs to continue for at least a year and relapses may involve the CNS.

Ref: Digestive diseases (1995); 13:108–118.

23 (b)
An adenoma is typically a low density lesion (< 15 HU) due to fat within the lesion. It usually demonstrates a rapid wash-in and wash-out of intravenous contrast medium, thus the density at 10 minutes is less than half that seen in the portal venous phase.

Ref: Radiology (2008) 249: 756–75.

24 (c)
The remaining features are seen in asplenia, which is more commonly seen in males. Polysplenia has a mortality of 50–60% and is associated with partial abnormal pulmonary venous return, left isomerism and a semi-annular pancreas.

Ref: R-ITI 3_132. The Abnormal Spleen.

25 (d)
Sickle cell disease results in chronic sequestration with a small, occasionally calcified, spleen. The remaining diagnoses can cause splenomegaly with or without focal lesions.

Ref: R-ITI 3_132. The Abnormal Spleen.

26 (e)
Primary sclerosing cholangitis is a biliary condition of unknown aetiology that is more common in men (2:1) and often presents under the age of 45 years. It is associated with ulcerative colitis, sicca complex and retroperitoneal fibrosis and patients are at increased risk of developing cholangiocarcinoma.

Ref: R-ITI 3_103. Gall Bladder and Biliary Tract: Inflammatory Conditions of the Biliary Tract.

27 (a)
The ileocolic, right colic and middle colic lymph nodes are the regional drainage for the ascending colon (following arterial blood supply). All other nodal groups are considered distant metastases.

Ref: TNM Atlas, 5th Ed, p. 103.

28 (b)
A pancreatic abscess complicates 3% of cases of acute pancreatitis and is due to infection within a fluid collection such as a pseudocyst. Such abscesses may be found anywhere within the abdomen or pelvis and require percutaneous drainage.

Ref: Radiology (1994); 193:297–306.

29 (a)
Adenomyomatosis is caused by mucosal hyperplasia with herniations of mucosa in to the thickened muscular layer (Rokitansky-Aschinoff sinuses). Cholesterol crystals deposited in these sinuses give rise to the hyperechoic comet-tail artefacts from the anterior wall, clearly visible against the hypoechoic bile.

Ref: Ultrasound: The Requisites, p. 35-54.

30 (a)
^{99m}Tc-HMPAO begins to break down by 4 hours as it is not as stable as ^{111}In; thereafter, breakdown products may be seen within the bile and intestines.

Ref: R-ITI 7i_004. Infection 4 - Abdominal infection.

31 (a)
Liver uptake should be seen within 10 minutes. Thereafter, there is filling of the gallbladder and subsequent excretion to the bowel. Cholecystitis impairs uptake to the GB.

Ref: R-ITI 7g_005. The investigation of hepatobiliary disease-1.

32 (b)
Approximately 60% arise in the stomach, 30% in the small bowel, 7% in the ano-rectal region and the remainder in the oesophagus and colon.

Ref: R-ITI 3_059. Gastro-intestinal stromal tumours (hollow organ and mesentery).

33 (e)
If a PET positive lesion becomes PET negative, this is regarded as a CR irrespective of the size of the nodal mass. Early assessment (after 1 or 2 cycles of chemotherapy) appears to be a better predictor of long term outcome than later imaging.

Ref: Clin Rad (2008); 63:125–135.

34 (b)
Seen in up to 1.4% of histology specimens and is usually incidental. Other tumours are encountered less commonly. The presence of adenocarcinoma may necessitate a formal right hemicolectomy to resect the draining lymph nodes.

Ref: Clin Rad (2009); 64:190–99.

35 (b)
5% of colorectal carcinoma is genetic in origin; the most common inherited syndromes being familial adenomatous polyposis and hereditary non-polyposis colorectal cancer (Lynch syndrome; HNPCC). Gardner's syndrome is associated with polyposis in the colon (100%), duodenum (90%) and, rarely other bowel segments; there is an association with gastric hamartomas, osteomas in calvarium/ mandible, and soft tissue tumours (30%). Turcot syndrome is a rare condition which is also associated with CNS gliomas and medulloblastomas. Peutz-Jeghers syndrome consists of hamartomas throughout the GI system with the rare potential for malignant transformation, and perioral pigmentation. Cowden disease has hamartomas, gingival hyperplasia, oral papillomas, muco-cutaneous pigmentation and an increased risk of breast and thyroid malignancy.

Ref: Primer of Diagnostic Imaging, 4th Ed, p. 191–2.

36 (d)
Endocrine tumours account for 1-2% of all pancreatic tumours and insulinoma is the most common of these, representing 60% of cases. Approximately 5-10% are malignant; these tend to be the larger lesions (>5 cm). However, most lesions are less than 1.5 cm at presentation and only 5-10% cases have multiple lesions.

Ref: European Radiology (2000); 10(Supp 2):S203–4.

37 (c)
A chest radiograph has an effective dose of approximately 0.02mSv or 3 days background radiation. An abdominal film has a dose 35x that at 0.7mSv, equivalent to 4 months background radiation.

Ref: RCR. Making the best use of clinical radiology services, 6th Ed.

38 (e)
These are the typical findings of chronic pancreatitis at endoscopic ultrasound.

Ref: R-ITI 3_125. Pancreas: Pancreatitis Diagnosis (Chronic).

39 (e)
Hepatocellular adenomas are uncommon benign tumours which comprise hepatocytes with no portal tracts or bile ducts. They are associated with the oral contraceptive pill and androgenic steroids. On imaging, they may have a scar or a pseudocapsule and enhance avidly in the arterial phase which can make differentiation from FNH difficult. There is a tendency to bleed or rupture, whilst 1% are thought to transform in to malignant lesions (HCC).

Ref: Diagnostic Radiology, 5th Ed, p. 741–2.

40 (a)
There is a 70-fold increase in pancreatic adenocarcinoma in this condition. Dietary factors play no role, but cigarette smoking is associated. Diabetes mellitus may be a presenting feature, but is not associated with an increased risk of malignancy.

Ref: R-ITI 3_127. Pancreatic adenocarcinoma.

41 (d)
The IAS comprises smooth muscle and is not under voluntary control. It appears hypoechoic on US. Obstetric injuries involve the external anal sphincter +/- IAS. Isolated injury is due to endo-anal trauma *e.g.* haemorrhoid surgery. Answers (a) and (e) pertain to the external anal sphincter, which is under voluntary control.

Ref: R-ITI 3_071. Endoanal Ultrasound and Anal/Rectal MRI (Non-Malignant) Fistula Disease.

42 (e)
Acute colonic pseudo-obstruction (Ogilvie syndrome) is a rare condition that may be seen most commonly after trauma (including surgery), infection or with cardiac disease. The features mimic bowel obstruction and complications include perforation. Gastrograffin enema may be therapeutic; air should never be insufflated in to the colon in these cases.

Ref: Ogilvie syndrome: e-medicine Gastroenterology.

43 (a)
Extrapulmonary TB is seen as the CD4 count falls below 400. Candida and Cryptosporidium are associated with a CD4 <200; HSV and CMV are associated with a CD4 <100.

Ref: Radiographics (1995); 15:1155–1178.

44 (c)
In the axial torsion type, the caecum twists around its long axis and remains in the right lower quadrant. In the loop type, the caecum twists around its long axis and also inverts. In the caecal bascule type, the caecum folds anteromedial to the ascending colon with no torsion. In the latter two scenarios, the caecum is found in the upper abdomen.

Ref: AJR (2001); 177:95–8.

45 (b)
An anterior bulge of up to 3 or 4 cm may be normal in many cases, but beyond this, and with incomplete evacuation, the diagnosis of a rectocoele may be made. Cystocoele and enterocoele are the abnormal descent of bladder and small bowel respectively. Prolapse is the abnormal descent of the rectum. Anismus is a functional abnormality leading to poor co-ordination of the pelvic floor muscles.

Ref: R-ITI 3_072. Constipation and Obstructive Defaecation Disorders.

46 (a)
A type II stricture extends in to the 1st order ducts. A type III stricture involves 2nd order ducts in either the right (IIIA) or left (IIIB) side, whilst type IV involve 2nd order ducts bilaterally. There is no type V. This classification is used to plan surgery.

Ref: Ann Surg (2002); 215:31–38.

47 (c)
Over 40% of carcinoid tumours arise within the small intestine, with rectum (27%), appendix (24%) and stomach (8%) next most common. Duodenal carcinoids are rare. Small intestinal carcinoid tumours are often symptomatic.

Ref: Radiographics (2007); 1:237-257.

48 (a)
Cystic fibrosis produces a range of abnormalities, which may lead to fibrosis, cirrhosis and portal hypertension. A micro-gallbladder is also seen commonly.

Ref: Radiographics (2006); 26:679-90.

49 (d)
Jejunisation of the ileum is a feature of coeliac disease. In addition to the other features, transmural ulceration, fistulae, stenoses and fold thickening may be seen. Crohn's disease may affect any part of the GI tract, from mouth to anus.

Ref: R-ITI 3_054. Crohn's disease.

50 (a)
Direct inguinal hernias originate infero-medial to the inferior epigastric artery, whilst indirect originate supero-laterally. Spigelian hernias lie at the linea semilunaris, hypogastric hernias lie in the midline below the umbilicus and femoral hernias pass through the femoral canal.

Ref: R-ITI 3_009. Abdominal wall hernia.

Genito-urinary, Adrenal, Obstetrics & Gynaecology and Breast Practice SBA Questions

1 **A 62 year old female is found to have a localised 4 mm area of architectural distortion and deformity on routine screening mammography. It has multiple long, thin spicules clumped centrally with radiolucent linear structures paralleling the spicules. MRI shows a stellate lesion with equivalent signal intensity to surrounding parenchyma on T1 weighted imaging and slight enhancement after the administration of contrast medium.**

Which of the following conditions is least likely?

(a) Ductal breast carcinoma
(b) Fat necrosis
(c) Post surgical scar
(d) Radial scar
(e) Phyllodes tumour

2 **Following the administration of intravenous contrast medium for an IVU, the patient becomes rapidly unwell with hypotension, bradycardia and shortness of breath.**

Which of the following treatments should not be used?

(a) Oxygen delivered *via* a face mask
(b) Beta-2 agonist delivered *via* a nebuliser
(c) Adrenaline 1:1,000 0.3 mls intravenously
(d) Atropine 0.6 mg intravenously
(e) Normal saline intravenously

3 A 42 year old man presents with a non-tender testicular lump. On examination he is noted to have gynaecomastia. The β-HCG, α-fetoprotein and lactate dehydrogenase levels are within normal limits. US demonstrates an irregular hypoechoic nodule.

What is the most likely diagnosis?

(a) Choriocarcinoma
(b) Leydig cell tumour
(c) Lymphoma
(d) Seminoma
(e) Yolk sac tumour

4 A 56 year man presents with hypertension and headache. He undergoes renal investigations which show a small right kidney on US and prolonged nephrogenic phase on contrast enhanced CT. MRA shows a 50% stenosis in the right main renal artery 1 cm from the ostium.

What is the most likely diagnosis?

(a) Atherosclerosis
(b) Fibromuscular dysplasia
(c) Infrarenal aortic aneurysm
(d) Buerger's disease
(e) Polyarteritis nodosa

5 A 28 year old man presents with loin pain and dipstick positive haematuria. A CT KUB is arranged for further investigation.

Which of the following statements is not correct regarding this investigation?

(a) It is now the initial investigation of choice
(b) Indinavir related calculi are not well seen
(c) Urate calculi are well visualised
(d) Nephrocalcinosis may result in a false positive examination
(e) The 'comet tail' sign confirms a ureteric calculus rather than phlebolith

6 A 58 year old man presents after an occupational health check revealed a PSA of 1.1 ng/ml. He has a slightly firm left side of the prostate on digital rectal examination.

Which of the following statements is correct?

(a) Prostate biopsy is not indicated
(b) Six core biopsies should be performed during transrectal prostate biopsy
(c) Local anaesthetic is not required for transrectal prostate biopsies
(d) Antibiotic prophylaxis is mandatory for transrectal prostate biopsies
(e) A 12 MHz probe should be used for transrectal prostate biopsies

7 A 55 year old female presents with postcoital bleeding and is discovered to have cervical carcinoma. Staging investigations reveal the tumour extends beyond the uterus with parametrial invasion but does not extend to the pelvic sidewall.

What is the FIGO staging of this tumour?

(a) I
(b) II
(c) III
(d) IV
(e) V

8 A 22 year old woman is diagnosed with an extra-adrenal phaeochromocytoma and undergoes an I^{123} MIBG examination as part of his staging.

Which of the following organs does not usually take up MIBG?

(a) Adrenal glands
(b) Spleen
(c) Ovaries
(d) Salivary glands
(e) Myocardium

9 A 26 year old, otherwise fit and well female patient is referred for a pelvic US as part of her routine investigations for infertility. US shows an 8 cm right complex adnexal mass with echogenic and anechoic components. CT shows a mass of fat density floating in an interface between two water density components. MRI shows a hyperintense mass on T2W lesion with a fluid-fluid level.

What is the likeliest diagnosis?

(a) Tubo-ovarian abscess
(b) Endometrioma
(c) Ovarian carcinoma
(d) Dermoid cyst
(e) Haemorrhagic cyst

10 With regards to embolisation treatment of varicocoeles, which of the following statements is false?

(a) The right side is easier to embolise than the left
(b) Coils are the embolisation material of choice
(c) The internal spermatic vein is occluded
(d) Testicular venous rupture is a recognized complication
(e) Bilateral varicocoeles can be approached through the same puncture site

11 A 30 year old man presents with bilateral loin pain. KUB shows coarse granular calcification widely distributed in the region of the renal pyramids. US shows increased echogenicity of the renal pyramids with some posterior acoustic shadowing.

Which of the following is least likely?

(a) Alport syndrome
(b) Medullary sponge kidney
(c) Milk-alkali syndrome
(d) Hyperparathyroidism
(e) Renal tubular acidosis

12 A 24 year old female patient with a regular 28 day menstrual cycle undergoes a transvaginal US examination as part of her investigations for dyspareunia. She cannot recall when her last menstrual period began. US shows bright central line, with a markedly echogenic smooth endometrium measuring 14 mm. Mild echogenic posterior acoustic enhancement is seen with a thin hypoechoic halo of inner myometrial zone.

Which of the following statements is correct?

(a) She should be referred for biopsy/dilation and curettage
(b) She is in the proliferative phase of her menstrual cycle
(c) She is in the secretory phase of her menstrual cycle
(d) The report should not mention her unknown LMP
(e) She is in the ovulatory phase of her menstrual cycle

13 A 60 year old man presents with biliary colic. At US an incidental finding of a well-demarcated 5 cm mass of low echogenicity is noted arising from the right kidney. CT confirms a renal mass with a central low attenuation scar. MRI shows the mass to be hypointense on T1W and hyperintense on T2W with enhancement after *i.v.* gadolinium administration, although the central scar enhances less well than the remainder of the mass.

What is the likeliest diagnosis?

(a) Renal cell carcinoma
(b) Oncocytoma
(c) Transitional cell carcinoma
(d) Hamartoma
(e) Metastasis

14 A 45 year old woman undergoes a PET-CT as part of her investigations for cervical cancer.

Which of the following is the least likely to cause a false-positive result?

(a) Physiological uptake in bowel
(b) Bladder diverticulum
(c) Uterine fibroids
(d) Endometriosis
(e) Ovarian cyst

15 A 38 year woman who had undergone breast augmentation for cosmesis 5 years earlier presents complaining of loss of contour of her left breast and some associated pain. MRI shows multiple hypointense wavy lines within the implant.

What sign is described?

(a) McGregor's sign
(b) Rubber band sign
(c) Linguine sign
(d) Wire sign
(e) Ladder sign

16 A 32 year old woman with a history of multiple previous basal cell carcinomas of the skin undergoes a pelvic US. This shows a 5 cm solid-looking hypoechoic left ovarian mass. MRI shows the mass is well circumscribed, relatively homogeneous and of low signal intensity on T1 and T2.

What is the most likely diagnosis?

(a) Ovarian adenocarcinoma
(b) Cystadenocarcinoma
(c) Brenner tumour
(d) Ovarian fibroma
(e) Endometrioma

17 A 19 year old female patient presents with a history of amenorrhoea. On examination she is noted to be overweight, hirsute, the blood sugar is raised on pin-prick testing. An underlying endocrine disorder is suspected.

Which of the following features would not be in keeping with this diagnosis?

(a) Bilateral ovarian volumes of 20 mls
(b) Bilateral ovarian volumes of 5 mls
(c) 10 small peripheral 5–8 mm cystic lesions on either side
(d) Asymmetrical ovarian size
(e) Patient's age

18 With regards to MRI protocols for the assessment of endometriosis, which of the following statements is incorrect?

(a) A pelvic surface coil improves image quality
(b) T1W sequences post gadolinium administration is employed
(c) T2W spin echo sequences are routinely employed
(d) A smooth muscle relaxant improves image quality
(e) T2W gradient echo sequences are not routinely employed

19 An 80 year old woman presents with vague lower abdominal pain. AXR shows translucent linear streaky areas in the pelvis. USS shows a thickened bladder wall with echogenic foci within it. CT demonstrates areas of gas within the bladder wall.

Which of the following is not consistent with the described condition?
(a) Diabetes mellitus
(b) The patient's demographics
(c) Staphylococcal infection
(d) Tuberculosis
(e) Bladder outlet obstruction

20 A patient is diagnosed with a 4 cm right upper pole renal cell carcinoma. Staging investigations demonstrate tumour thrombus in the renal vein extending into the IVC, but no local lymphadenopathy and no evidence of distant metastases.

What is the Robson staging of this tumour?
(a) Stage II
(b) Stage IIIa
(c) Stage IIIb
(d) Stage IIIc
(e) Stage IV

21 A 24 year old with known ureteric reflux disease in childhood presents with loin pain. KUB shows an extensive calculus involving the lower pole and interpolar calyces.

What is the likeliest composition of the stone?

(a) Magnesium ammonium phosphate
(b) Xanthine
(c) Cysteine
(d) Urate
(e) Calcium oxalate

22 Regarding prostate sarcoma in adult patients, which of the following statements is correct?

(a) Rhabdomyosarcoma is the commonest subtype
(b) The PSA is usually elevated
(c) The prostate is not usually enlarged
(d) Calcification is typical
(e) Heterogeneous enhancement with cystic change is typical

23 A 23 year old man is diagnosed with a stage I germ cell tumour of the testis.

After primary treatment, what is the current method of choice for surveillance of the retroperitoneum?

(a) Serial US
(b) Serial MRI
(c) Serial CT
(d) Serial laparoscopy
(e) Serial lymphangiography

24 A 10 year old boy, recently arrived from the Indian subcontinent, presents with vague abdominal distension and discomfort. US shows bilateral multiple, non-communicating, well defined cystic lesions in the peripelvic region, renal parenchyma and in the perirenal spaces. CT shows the lesions to be homogeneous with no significant contrast enhancement. At MRI the lesions were of low signal intensity on T1W and high signal intensity on T2W, again without enhancement. Needle biopsy showed areas of connective tissue with an endothelial lining.

What is the likeliest diagnosis?

(a) Multicystic dysplastic kidney
(b) Multilocular cystic nephroma
(c) Tuberculosis
(d) Wilm's tumour
(e) Renal lymphangiectasia

25 A 30 year old patient is admitted with multiple stab wounds to the lower abdomen. His pulse is 110/ min and his blood pressure 80/40 mm Hg after fluid resuscitation. He has frank haematuria. A urethral catheter is passed freely and a normal cystogram performed in the emergency department. Initial CT in the portal venous phase with shows free fluid in the pelvis towards the right side but no major injury to the solid viscera. A ureteric injury is suspected.

Which imaging investigation would you recommend next?

(a) Single shot IVU
(b) Full IVU with delayed phase imaging
(c) Ultrasound kidneys
(d) Retrograde ureterogram
(e) Nephrostomy insertion followed by nephrostogram

26 A 60 year old man presents with frank haematuria. Cystoscopy demonstrates a transitional cell carcinoma of the bladder.

Which of the following statements is true regarding his staging investigations?

(a) CT has no role
(b) Extension of the tumour into the outer half of the muscle layer is stage T2a disease
(c) At MRI tumour is isointense to muscle on T1W and hyperintense on T2W
(d) T2W is the optimal sequence to detect extension into perivesical fat
(e) T1W is the optimal sequence to assess depth of muscle invasion

27 A number of special techniques are employed in mammography as opposed to conventional radiography.

Which of the following is not included in this category?

(a) The use of a molybdenum target
(b) The use of a tungsten target
(c) A low tube current
(d) A focal spot size of 0.3 mm
(e) The use of a grid

28 A 34 year old woman presents with left lower abdominal pain. US shows a complex adnexal lesion which cannot be fully characterised. MRI shows a 5 cm fluid filled structure with incomplete non-enhancing plicae crossing it and with areas of focal narrowing and peripheral small low signal intensity nodules on T2W. Amorphous shading of the lesion is also seen on T2W. Enhancement of the wall of the lesion after gadolinium administration is noted. Normal ovarian tissue is seen stretched around the lesion.

What is the most likely diagnosis?

(a) Endometriosis
(b) Ovarian mucinous carcinoma
(c) Fallopian tube carcinoma
(d) Pyosalpinx
(e) Lymphangioma

29 A 6 week pregnant lady presents to the early pregnancy unit with PV bleeding. As part of the US examination, crown-rump length (CRL) and mean gestational sac diameter (MGSD) measurements are recorded.

Which of the following is not correct?
(a) Lack of detectable cardiac activity in a 8 mm CRL embryo is normal
(b) MGSD of 25 mm on transabdominal US should have a detectable embryo
(c) MGSD of 20 mm on transabdominal US should have a detectable yolk sac
(d) MGSD of 20 mm on transvaginal US should have both detectable yolk sac and embryo
(e) Cardiac activity may be detected in embryos with a CRL as small as 2 mm

30 A 45 year old previously well woman presents with a breast lump. US shows a round lesion of mixed attenuation. Biopsy determines that the lesion is a metastasis and has significant areas of haemorrhage within it. The other breast is normal.

What is the most likely primary tumour?
(a) Malignant melanoma
(b) Ovarian carcinoma
(c) Lung carcinoma
(d) Kaposi sarcoma
(e) Renal oncocytoma

31 A 4 year old is found to have unilateral adrenal calcification on CT.

Which of the following is the least likely cause?
(a) Adrenal cyst
(b) Neuroblastoma
(c) Ganglioneuroma
(d) Wolman disease
(e) Adrenocortical carcinoma

32 A patient undergoes an unenhanced CT of the abdomen and suspicion of a left adrenal mass is raised.

Which of the following would not help differentiate a true adrenal lesion from a structure mimicking it?

(a) Oral contrast administration to exclude a gastric diverticulum
(b) Intravenous contrast medium to ensure homogeneity of a splenunculus with the spleen
(c) Intravenous contrast medium to ensure a pancreatic tail mass is displacing the splenic vein anteriorly
(d) CT imaging with multi-planar reconstructions to ensure that the upper pole of the left kidney is not mimicking a mass
(e) MRI to ensure the upper pole of the left kidney is not the presumed mass

33 A 30 year old man presents with recurrent loin pain. Ultrasound shows a horseshoe kidney.

Which of the following statements is incorrect?

(a) The incidence at autopsy is 1:2,000
(b) Fusion of the kidneys occurs at the lower pole in 90%
(c) It is more common in males
(d) Ascent of the kidney is arrested at the L3 level by the inferior mesenteric artery
(e) It is seen in 60% of patients with Turners syndrome

34 With regards to a ^{99m}Tc-MAG3 renogram, which of the following statements is incorrect?

(a) The pure blood flow phase lasts for 2 minutes
(b) The uptake phase should be measured 60–120 secs after tracer administration
(c) The peak of the curve represents the maximum activity in the kidney
(d) Frusemide should be administered in the presence of dilatation.
(e) A renal tumour would cause a photopaenic area within the kidney

35 A 60 year old woman undergoes a CTPA. Incidental note is made of a solitary lesion within her breast.

Which of the following is more supportive of this being a benign process?

(a) Irregular margin
(b) Irregular shape
(c) Rim enhancement
(d) Large calcifications
(e) Skin thickening

36 With regards to the normal anatomy of the breast which of the following statements is true?

(a) 30% of the lymphatic drainage is *via* the internal mammary chain
(b) Level I lymph nodes lie lateral to the medial edge of pectoralis minor
(c) Level II lymph nodes lie behind pectoralis major
(d) The breast consists of 15–20 terminal duct lobular units
(e) Increased enhancement of normal breast parenchyma during lactation is seen at MRI

37 A 37 year old female patient with suspected pelvic malignancy undergoes an MRI with diffusion weighted imaging. There is an area of slight T2 hyperintensity which shows high signal intensity on high b-value source images and decreased signal on the ADC map.

What is the most likely diagnosis?

(a) Liquefactive necrosis
(b) Fibrous tissue
(c) T2-shine through
(d) Cyst
(e) High-cellularity tumour

38 A 2 cm adrenal lesion is noted in a 52 year old woman undergoing a staging CT for lung carcinoma. A dedicated study demonstrates the lesion to have a density of 18 HU before contrast medium, 68 HU in the portal venous phase and 57 HU at 10 minutes.

What is the most likely diagnosis?

(a) Cyst
(b) Adenoma
(c) Metastasis
(d) Lipoma
(e) Adrenocortical carcinoma

39 A 53 year old female patient has recently moved to the area and you are asked to review her most recent mammogram prior to clinic review. The mammogram shows a unilateral diffuse increased density of the right breast with skin thickening, a coarse reticular pattern with prominent Cooper's ligaments and no microcalcification.

Which of the following is the least likely to cause these appearances?

(a) Radiotherapy change
(b) Lymphatic obstruction
(c) Inflammatory carcinoma
(d) Granular cell tumour
(e) Recent surgery

40 With regards to the anatomy of the retroperitoneum, which of the following statements is true?

(a) The right perirenal space communicates with the bare area of the liver
(b) The left perirenal space communicates with the scrotum
(c) The adrenal gland is in the anterior pararenal space
(d) The psoas muscle is in the posterior pararenal space
(e) The posterior pararenal space contains the ascending and descending colon

41 A 53 year old asymptomatic man is discovered to have a 1.5 cm unilateral, calcified, extrarenal solitary renal artery aneurysm.

Which of the following statements is incorrect?

(a) The lesion should be treated surgically
(b) 2/3 of renal artery aneurysms are extrarenal
(c) The likeliest cause is atherosclerosis
(d) Ehlers-Danlos syndrome is a cause
(e) It is more common in women

42 A neonate is found to have an abdominal wall defect and bilateral cryptorchidism.

Which of the following features would not support a syndromic diagnosis?

(a) Bilateral ureteromegaly
(b) Trabeculated low capacity bladder
(c) Widened prostatic urethra
(d) Urethral dilatation
(e) Asymmetric renal size

43 A 35 year old man with a history of ataxia presents unconscious after a fall. A previous unenhanced CT abdomen demonstrated multiple solid lesions within the right kidney, an absent left kidney with surgical clips nearby and multiple well-defined cystic lesions within the pancreas.

What is the most likely diagnosis?

(a) Tuberous sclerosis
(b) Amyloidosis
(c) Von Hippel Lindau syndrome
(d) Neurofibromatosis type 1
(e) Lymphoma

44 A 48 year old female patient presents to the breast clinic with a painless breast lump. Clinical examination reveals a firm 2 cm mass in the right upper outer quadrant. Mammography shows a round, well defined soft tissue opacity in the corresponding location.

Which of the following features on US suggest a malignant rather than benign cause?

(a) It is taller than it is wide
(b) It is markedly hyperechoic
(c) It has a thin echogenic capsule
(d) It has 3 lobulations
(e) It does not cast an acoustic shadow

45 A 35 year old woman presents with a history of loin pain. CT shows a large perinephric haematoma. She cannot recall any significant trauma other than whilst playing with her child.

Which of the following is the least likely cause?

(a) Multicystic dysplastic kidney
(b) Renal cell carcinoma
(c) Autosomal dominant polycystic kidney disease
(d) Polyarteritis nodosa
(e) Angiomyolipoma of the kidney

46 A 3 year old undergoes CT of the abdomen which shows an 8 cm heterogeneous enhancing mass which does not extend across the midline, but which displaces major vessels.

Which of the following conditions is not associated?

(a) Cryptorchidism
(b) Hypoplasia of the iris
(c) Hemihypertrophy
(d) Drash syndrome
(e) Proptosis

47 A 32 year old woman undergoes an IVU which demonstrates bilateral striated nephrograms.

Which of the following is least likely?
(a) Tamm-Horsfell proteinuria
(b) Hypotension
(c) Amyloidosis
(d) Acute pyelonephritis
(e) Medullary sponge kidney

48 A 50 year old man presents 4 weeks after a bout of acute epididymitis with fever, leucocytosis, a swollen foul smelling, red, tender scrotum with palpable crepitus. The degree of inflammation is observed to be rapidly spreading over a 24 hour period.

Which of the following statements is true?
(a) MRI is the best test to investigate extent of spread
(b) Ultrasound is useful in investigating the extent of spread
(c) CT is the best test to investigate the extent of spread
(d) Anaerobes are the most common responsible organism
(e) Staphylococcus is the most common responsible organism

49 A 50 year old man is found to have an incidental renal lesion. On unenhanced CT, the lesion is 2 cm, round, homogeneous, well defined, without calcification and situated in the upper pole of the right kidney. It has an attenuation of 60 Hounsfield units, which after the administration of intravenous contrast medium increases to 69 HU.

Which of the following is the likeliest diagnosis?
(a) Renal cell carcinoma
(b) Lipid poor angiomyolipoma
(c) Renal oncocytoma
(d) Simple cyst
(e) Metanephric adenoma

50 A 14 year old girl presents with lower abdominal pain. Transabdominal ultrasound shows a partially solid/partially cystic midline mass.

Which of the following radiological features would not support a diagnosis of ovarian torsion?

(a) Enhancement of the solid component on CT
(b) Free fluid in the *cul-de-sac* on US
(c) Multiple peripheral cysts on US
(d) High signal intensity on fat suppressed T1
(e) Wall thickness of 12 mm on MRI

Genito-urinary, Adrenal, Obstetrics & Gynaecology and Breast Practice SBA Answers

1 (e)
Phyllodes tumours present in the 5th-6th decades with a large firm, discrete mobile palpable mass. They demonstrate strong contrast enhancement on T1 weighted imaging. A small non-palpable stellate lesion on mammography with architectural distortion has a wide differential including primary carcinoma (up to 50%), fat necrosis, radial scar, fibrosed fibroadenoma and granular cell myoblastoma.

Ref: Radiology Review Manual, 6th Ed, p. 545.

2 (c)
Adrenaline is used in the treatment of severe contrast reactions; however the 1:1,000 concentration should only be given *via* the intramuscular route. The spectrum of contrast reactions is wide and treatments range from simple supportive measures such as leg elevation and oxygen for mild vasovagal episodes through to adrenaline and H1 antagonists with airway support for severe anaphylactic reactions.

Ref: RCR- Standards for iodinated intravascular contrast agent administration to adult patients 2005 (updated 2009).

3 (b)
Leydig cell tumours represent 1–3% of all testicular cancers, and are most common in men aged 30–60 years. They are stromal tumours, which form in the interstitial tissues that support the testes. The Leydig cells produces hormones, thus such tumours are typically hormonally active and lead to feminising or virilising syndromes; 30% secrete estradiol, resulting in gynaecomastia. β-HCG, α-FP and LDH levels are typically normal (β-HCG is 'always' raised in choriocarcinoma and in 83% of seminomas; α-FP is raised in >90% of yolk sac tumours).

Ref: Radiology Review Manual, 6th Ed, p. 975-9.

4 (a)
Overall, atherosclerosis is the commonest cause of RAS. It has a particular tendency to involve the proximal 2 cm of the main renal artery in contradistinction to fibromuscular dysplasia, the second most common cause.

Ref: Radiology Review Manual, 6th Ed, p. 956.

5 (e)
Indinavir and pure matrix calculi are the only types of stone not well visualized on CTKUB. The 'soft tissue rim' sign refers to circumferential thickening of the ureteric wall around a calculus as opposed to the 'comet tail' sign which is seen around phleboliths.

Ref: RITI 4_047 Imaging loin pain and renal colic.

6 (d)
Elevated PSA or an abnormal DRE are indications for biopsy in asymptomatic men. The sextant biopsy protocol has now been found to give too many false negatives and has been largely replaced by extended core protocols. Local anaesthesia and antibiotic cover are now standard care. A 5-7.5 MHz probe is usually used.

Ref: International Handbook of Prostate Cancer, 3rd Ed, 2007.

7 (b)
This is a FIGO II lesion, *i.e.* one where the tumour extends beyond the uterus but not to the pelvis sidewall or to the lower third of the vagina. Stage IIA lesions do not have parametrial invasion and are surgically treated lesions. Stage IIB do exhibit parametrial invasion and should be treated with chemo-radiotherapy. Stage III tumours extend to the pelvic sidewall, involve the lower third of the vagina or cause hydronephrosis. Stage IV tumours invade the bladder or rectum, or have distant metastases. Stage V does not exist.

Ref: RITI 4b_010 Staging cervical and endometrial cancer.

8 (c)
In addition to the above MIBG is taken up (to a variable extent) by liver, lung, colon, stomach and thyroid. It is uncommon to see uptake in the adrenal glands with I^{131}MIBG (<20%) but faint uptake is commonly seen with ^{123}I-MIBG. Ovaries do not take up MIBG.

Ref: Eur J Endocrinology (2002); 147(1):13–28.

9 (d)
Dermoid cysts are common congenital benign germ cell tumours that usually present in the reproductive age range. 15% are bilateral. They have a spectrum of appearances ranging from the classic fat or bone containing lesions to (less commonly) a predominantly cystic lesion with a fluid-fluid level. They can be diagnosed on plain radiographs in up to 40% of cases when the presence of fat, teeth or bone can be identified. They can be complicated by malignant degeneration (in 1-3%), torsion (4-16%) and rupture (rarely).

Ref: Radiology Review Manual, 6th Ed, p. 1034.

10 (a)
The right renal vein drains directly into the IVC thus making it harder to approach. A right internal jugular approach may help in this situation.

Ref: RITI 1c_049 Varicocoele, key facts, imaging and treatment.

11 (a)
Medullary nephrocalcinosis has a wide differential diagnosis, but options (b), (d) and (e) account for 70% of cases. Other causes include papillary necrosis and drugs such as Frusemide. Alport syndrome (hereditary chronic nephritis) typically gives rise to cortical calcification.

Ref: Radiology Review Manual, 6th Ed, p. 893.

12 (c)
An endometrial thickness of up to 16 mm may be seen in the secretory phase of the menstrual cycle. This is maximal during the mid-secretory phase. It is imperative to include the LMP, whether known or unknown as part of the report. In the proliferative phase (day 6-14), endometrial thickness is 5–7 mm and in the periovulatory phase, endometrial thickness up to 11 mm is seen.

Ref: Radiology Review Manual, 6th Ed, p. 1024.

13 (b)
In addition to the above findings, a 'spoke-wheel' appearance at angiography and a photopaenic area on ^{99m}Tc-DMSA scan may be seen.

14 (e)
^{18}FDG shows physiological uptake in brain, myocardium, liver, spleen, bone marrow, GI tract, testes, and skeletal muscle and is excreted by the kidneys. Increased uptake is also seen in healing fractures, inflammatory and granulomatous disease and infectious processes.

Ref: Radiographics (2005); 25:1031–43.

15 (c)
Implant rupture is a not uncommon complication with a prevalence of more than 50% at 12 years. US (59–70% sensitive, 57–92% specific) is less accurate than MRI (81–94% sensitive, 93–97% specific). Classically on MRI, hypointense wavy lines often parallel to the fibrous capsule are seen (linguine sign).

Ref: Radiology Review Manual, 6th Ed, p. 574.

16 (d)
Ovarian fibroma is a well defined tumour containing extensive collagen. It is associated with Gorlin's syndrome (fibromas seen in 17%) and occasionally presents as Meig's syndrome.

Ref: Essentials of radiologic imaging (1998): 763–66.

17 (d)
The diagnosis of polycystic ovary syndrome is made on the basis of clinical and biochemical findings in conjunction with the sonographic findings, which alone are non-specific. Similar sized ovaries is a key finding. The classic finding of bilaterally enlarged ovaries with multiple small peripheral follicles is seen in 50%. Hyperechoic central stroma is also usually seen. Normal ovaries are seen in 25%.

Ref: Polycystic ovary syndrome, 2nd Ed.

18 (b)
T1W imaging after the administration of intravenous gadolinium is not routinely employed for the assessment of endometriosis.

Ref: RITI 4b_013 Endometriosis.

19 (d)
Emphysematous cystitis is usually seen in women over the age of 50 with poorly controlled diabetes mellitus. Other risk factors include neurogenic bladder and recurrent UTIs. Causes other than infection include trauma, recent instrumentation and enterovesical fistula. Classically the organism is *E. coli*, but a variety of organisms including *Staphylococcus, Streptococcus, Klebsiella* and *Clostridium perfringens* have been described. TB causes an irritable hypertonic low capacity bladder and occasionally calcification of the bladder wall is seen.

Ref: Radiology Review Manual, 6th Ed, p. 926.

20 (b)
Stage I includes tumours that are confined entirely to the kidney. Stage II tumours invade the perinephric fat or adrenal gland on the same side. Stage IIIa tumours extend into the renal vein or the IVC. Stage IIIb tumours involve local LNs. Stage IIIc combines stages IIIa and IIIb. Stage IV tumours describes those with distant metastases.

Ref: Primer of Diagnostic Imaging, 4th Ed, p. 291.

21 (a)
70% of staghorn calculi are composed of magnesium ammonium phosphate (struvite stones). The remainder are cysteine or urate stones. These large calculi are often seen in patients with a history of recurrent infections.

Ref: Primer of Diagnostic Imaging, 4th Ed, p. 299.

22 (e)
Sarcoma of the prostate is a rare tumour characterized by a large heterogeneous enhancing mass. Rhabdomyosarcoma is more commonly seen in children; leiomyosarcoma more commonly in adults. The PSA is not usually affected due to the lack of epithelial involvement.

Ref: Clin Rad (2009); 64(2):171.

23 (c)
In recent times imaging surveillance of the retroperitoneum after surgery has been developed as an acceptable strategy to reduce the chance of subsequent morbidity and mortality. CT currently remains the modality most commonly used, although concerns have been raised regarding the radiation dose in this group of young patients. This has led to potential interest in MRI but as yet, this has not been widely adopted.

Ref: Clin Rad (2009); 64(4):362–7.

24 (e)
Although rare, renal lymphangiectasia has a characteristic imaging appearance resulting from the failure of the renal lymphatic tissue.

Ref: Clin Rad (2008); 63(9): 1057–62.

25 (a)
Traumatic ureteric injury is extremely rare. In this situation with an unstable patient who will imminently require emergency surgery, a one shot IVU to localize the injury should be performed. If the patient was clinically stable, either CT with delayed phase imaging or a full IVU could be performed.

Ref: Clin Rad (2008); 63(12): 1361–71.

26 (c)
MRI is the local staging investigation of choice. T2W is good for assessment of degree of muscle invasion and differentiating tumour from fibrosis, whilst T1W is good for assessing invasion into the perivesical fat. T2a disease involves the inner half of the muscle layer; T2b the outer half and T3 describes invasion of the perivesical fat.

Ref: Radiology Review Manual, 6th Ed, p. 980–1.

27 (c)
High tube currents to reduce exposure time should be used. Molybdenum targets are used most commonly as they produce a low energy spectrum providing high contrast. Although tungsten targets produce higher energy spectra they are still used in situations where there is a thicker or a denser breast.

Ref: Diagnostic Radiology, 5th Ed, p. 1173.

28 (d)
Pyosalpinx is characterized by dilatation of the fallopian tube with pus within it. It characteristically demonstrates amorphous or geographic shading on T2W.

Ref: Clin Rad (2009); 64: 815–31.

29 (a)
The discriminatory level of CRL before lack of cardiac activity becomes abnormal is 6 mm. MGSD is defined as (length + width + height)/3.

Ref: RITI 4b_005 Early pregnancy problems.

30 (a)
Haemorrhagic metastases to breast include melanoma, renal cell carcinoma, choriocarcinoma and Kaposi sarcoma. Overall, the commonest non-mammary source of non-haemorrhagic metastases is lymphoma.

Ref: Radiology Review Manual, 6th Ed, p. 575.

31 (e)
Adrenocortical carcinoma is a cause of adrenal calcification but presents in an older age group (4th –7th decade).

Ref: Radiology Review Manual, 6th Ed, p. 882.

32 (c)
The left adrenal gland lies in front of the upper pole of the left kidney and a mass within it can be confused with the upper pole itself, a gastric diverticulum, splenic lobulation, an accessory spleen or a mass in the tail of the pancreas. Such a mass in the pancreatic tail would normally displace the splenic vein posteriorly rather than anteriorly as a true adrenal mass would.

Ref: Aids to Radiological Differential Diagnosis, 4th Ed, p. 308.

33 (a)
It is the commonest fusion abnormality and is seen in 1:400 patients at autopsy. It can be complicated by obstruction, reflux or stone formation. The isthmus can contain functioning renal tissue.

Ref: RITI 4c_048 Assessment of hydronephrosis and suspected ureteric obstruction.

34 (a)
The pure blood flow phase is the first phase of the examination and lasts up to 40 secs (equivalent to an arterial phase study).

Ref: RITI 7r_003 Dynamic renography.

35 (d)
There are limited features to suggest benignity on CT examination. Rather, evaluation of these commonly seen incidental findings should be made by looking for the lack of malignant features and careful evaluation of the clinical history. Small, dystrophic calcification (which in some cases cannot be appreciated at CT resolution) rather than large, round calcifications is a predictor of malignancy.

Ref: Radiographics (2007); 27:s37–51.

36 (e)

Ref: RITI 4a_003 Breast anatomy, physiology and imaging.

37 (e)
Diffusion-weighted MRI is increasingly being used in body MRI and offers functional information over and above conventional morphological images. These features are typical of tumour.

Ref: Radiographics (2009); 29:759–778.

38 (c)
Metastases typically have a higher density (>15 HU) with less washout in the portal venous phase than an adenoma. The adrenal gland is the most common site for metastases from bronchogenic carcinoma.

Ref: Radiology (2008); 249(3):756–75.

39 (d)
These are mammographic signs of an oedematous breast and the differential diagnosis also includes venous obstruction and breast abscess. Granular cell tumour presents as an asymmetric lump with hardness, skin retraction and ulceration. It is typically a well seen spiculated mass 1–3 cm in diameter.

Ref: Radiology Review Manual, 6th Ed, p. 570.

40 (a)
The psoas lies posterior to the posterior pararenal space. The adrenal gland is in the perirenal space. The ascending and descending colon are in the anterior pararenal space.

Ref: Imaging (2000); 12:10–20.

41 (a)
A small (< 2 cm) renal artery aneurysm which is well calcified may be treated conservatively. Indications for surgery include being a woman of childbearing age (due to the increased risk of rupture in pregnancy), interval growth, emboli to kidney or diminishing renal function. Intrarenal aneurysms are most commonly congenital; true extra-renal aneurysms are caused by fibromuscular dysplasia, pregnancy and mesenchymal disease such as NF and Ehlers-Danlos, in addition to atherosclerosis.

42 (b)
The classical triad of prune-belly syndrome is abdominal wall defect/ weakness, bilateral cryptorchidism and genito-urinary abnormalities. Typically a thickened, non-trabeculated, large volume bladder is seen. Non GU abnormalities affecting the lungs (CCAM, lung hypoplasia), musculoskeletal system (scoliosis, pectus excavatum), cardiovascular (VSD, PDA, Fallots) and GI system (Hirschprung's disease, malrotation) are also seen.

Ref: Radiology Review Manual, 6th Ed, p. 950.

43 (c)
VHL disease is an autosomal dominant neurocutaneous syndrome characterised by renal cell carcinomas, often multiple and bilateral along with cystic renal and pancreatic disease, phaeochromocytomas and spinal, cerebellar and optic nerve haemangioblastomas. The cerebellar lesions can present as ataxia.

Ref: Radiology Review Manual, 6th Ed, p. 335.

44 (a)
Malignant features on US include spiculation, being taller than wide, angular margins, acoustic shadowing, being markedly hypoechoic, and having microlobulations. Benign features include being hyperechoic, having 2-3 lobulations, being ellipsoid in shape and having a thin echogenic capsule. To characterise a lesion as being sonographically benign, it must have no malignant features. If specific benign features are not found then the lesion is indeterminate.

Ref: Radiology Review Manual, 6th Ed, p. 546.

45 (a)
Occult RCC, polyarteritis nodosa, ADPKD and angiomyolipoma are well recognized causes of perinephric haematoma after innocuous trauma. MCDK do not typically bleed externally into the perinephric space.

Ref: Radiology Review Manual, 6th Ed, p. 937.

46 (e)
The features described would suggest a diagnosis of Wilm's tumour which has a number of associations including Beckwith-Wiedemann syndrome, sporadic aniridia, hemihypertrophy and other genitourinary abnormalities including Drash syndrome. Proptosis can be seen in neuroblastoma.

Ref: Radiology Review Manual, 6th Ed, p. 993.

47 (c)
Striated nephrograms are transiently seen in acute extra-renal obstruction along with hypotension and intratubular obstruction. Other causes of bilateral striated nephrograms include rhabdomyolysis and cystic renal disease. Causes of a (usually) single striated nephrogram include renal contusion and renal vein thrombosis.

Ref: Radiographics (1995); 15: 1069–85.

48 (c)
Fournier's gangrene is a rapidly spreading necrotizing fasciitis that involves the genital or peri-anal regions. It usually has an identifiable predisposing event. It is polymicrobial in origin with *E. coli* being the commonest identifiable organism. CT is the best investigation for assessing the degree of spread, and can identify complications such as abscess formation. Treatment is urgent, complete debridement.

Ref: Radiographics (2008); 28: 519–28.

49 (d)
Although most cysts are of low attenuation, by far the commonest cause of an otherwise benign appearing, non-enhancing (<10 HU increase), hyperattenuating (normal renal parenchyma approximately 40 HU on unenhanced CT) lesion is a hyperdense cyst containing proteinaceous material. Lipid poor angiomyolipomas are a rare (3–4%) subset of angiomyolipomas.

Ref: Radiographics (2007); 27: 1131–43.

50 (a)
Lack of enhancement of the solid component of the mass is seen on CT and MRI. Other features include a whorled paraovarian structure on CT, representing the ovarian pedicle.

Ref: Radiology Review Manual, 6th Ed, p. 1064.

Paediatrics Practice SBA Questions

1 **A 3 year old presents with entral epigastric pain. Blood tests reveal a raised amylase.**

Which of the following is the least likely cause?

(a) Choledochal cyst
(b) Cystic fibrosis
(c) Henoch-Schonlein purpura
(d) Non-accidental injury
(e) Rubella

2 **A 15 year old boy is under investigation for hypertension. The serum catecholamines and urinary VMAs are raised. CT abdomen confirms a left adrenal phaeochromocytoma and additionally shows multiple cysts within the liver, pancreas and both kidneys.**

Which of following additional features would you look for?

(a) Bilateral acoustic neuromas
(b) CNS haemangioblastomas
(c) Iris hamartomas
(d) Parathyroid adenomas
(e) Pulmonary lymphangioleiomyomatosis

3 **An antenatal US performed at 20 weeks demonstrated a right renal pelvis with an AP diameter of 5 mm. A 32 week scan shows the diameter to be 10 mm. The post-natal US at 4 days confirms unilateral right-sided neonatal hydronephrosis.**

What is the commonest cause of these findings?

(a) Ectopic ureterocoele
(b) Pelvi-ureteric junction obstruction
(c) Posterior urethral valve
(d) Prune-belly syndrome
(e) Vesico-ureteric junction obstruction

4 **A 1 year old boy presents with an acute history of cough, wheeze, and respiratory distress.**

Which of the following is true?

(a) Collapse of a lung or lobe is the commonest radiographic finding acutely
(b) An inhaled foreign body is equally likely to pass into either mainstem bronchus
(c) The majority of foreign bodies are radio-opaque and can be seen on CXR
(d) Mediastinal shift on expiratory radiographs/fluoroscopy is toward the lucent side
(e) Normal imaging excludes the diagnosis of inhaled foreign body

5 **The settings on the CT machine need to be optimised to reduce the dose when scanning paediatric patients. A student radiographer asks you how this can be achieved.**

Which of the following will actually increase patient dose?

(a) Reducing the gantry rotation speed
(b) Reducing the kVp
(c) Reducing the mA
(d) Reducing the scanned volume to only the abnormal region
(e) Use of automatic exposure control

6 **A 3 year old girl presents with increasing abdominal girth. US demonstrates a mass within the region of the left kidney. The patient proceeds to CT examination.**

Which of the following findings favours Wilms' tumour over neuroblastoma?

(a) Calcification within the mass
(b) Mass crosses the midline
(c) Mass encases and lifts the aorta
(d) Mass invades into the IVC
(e) Presence of bone metastases

7 **An 18 month old child presents with an unwitnessed head injury. There are elements of the history which appear inconsistent. The CT head examination demonstrates a subdural haematoma**

Which of the following findings are least specific for NAI?
(a) Associated presence of retinal haemorrhage
(b) Bilateral SDHs
(c) Interhemispheric (falx) SDH
(d) SDH of differing age
(e) SDH underlying a skull fracture

8 **A 3 year old boy presents with abdominal swelling. US and subsequent CT examination show a large 12 cm mass inferior to the liver. There is distortion of the renal parenchyma and apparent exophytic growth. There is poor enhancement and the aorta and IVC are displaced.**

Which of the following features is not a known association?
(a) Aniridia
(b) Cerebellar ataxia
(c) Horseshoe kidney
(d) Macroglossia
(e) Male pseudohermaphroditism

9 **A neonatal male patient failed to pass meconium by 48 hours and was found to have an imperforate anus of the high malformation subtype. A colostomy was formed in the neonatal period and surgical repair completed in infancy. At the age of 5 the patient presents with a UTI.**

What is the likely underlying aetiology of the UTI?
(a) Colovesical fistula
(b) Neurogenic bladder
(c) Pelvi-ureteric junction obstruction
(d) Rectourethral fistula
(e) Urethrocoele

10 A 6 week old boy with a family history of developmental dysplasia attends the department for a screening US scan of the hips.

Which of the following imaging findings constitutes an abnormal result?

(a) 60° for α-angle
(b) 60° for β-angle
(c) 60% of femoral head covered by acetabulum
(d) Femoral head lying inferio-medial to the Perkin's/ Hilgenreiner's line intersection
(e) Hypoechoic appearance of the femoral head

11 An infant presents within the first few weeks of life with stridor, respiratory distress, and wheezing. CXR shows left deviation of the trachea, the lateral view reveals increased density in the region of the hilum. A pulmonary sling is suspected and a CT chest is arranged for further evaluation.

Which of the following findings is most likely to be seen?

(a) Anterior trachea and anterior oesophageal compression
(b) Anterior trachea and posterior oesophageal compression
(c) No compression
(d) Posterior trachea and anterior oesophageal compression
(e) Posterior trachea and posterior oesophageal compression

12 An 8 month old boy presents with prolonged cough. On examination there is reduced air entry on the right side. The subsequent CXR demonstrates mediastinal shift towards the left side of the chest.

Which of the following is more likely?

(a) Congenital lobar emphysema
(b) Bronchogenic cyst
(c) Pulmonary agenesis
(d) Scimitar syndrome
(e) Swyer-James (McLeod) syndrome

13 A 2 year old boy presents with haematochezia. He is in obvious distress on examination, but the bowel sounds are normal. AXR is unremarkable, and the paediatric team suspect a Meckel's diverticulum. Your advice is sought regarding further investigation.

Which of the following would be the most sensitive radiological investigation?

(a) Barium follow-through
(b) CT
(c) MRI
(d) ^{99m}Tc-pertechnatate scintigraphy
(e) Ultrasound

14 An 18 month old boy is found to have a neuroblastoma. A subsequent CT is performed for staging purposes. This reveals the primary tumour and evidence of metastases in the skin, liver, lung and bone marrow.

What is the appropriate stage?

(a) Stage I
(b) Stage II
(c) Stage III
(d) Stage IV
(e) Stage IV-S

15 A 7 year old girl presents with lethargy, headaches and vomiting. CT shows a hyperdense lesion in the region of the posterior fossa. MR imaging confirms a midline vermian mass which abuts the roof of the 4th ventricle, displacing the brainstem anteriorly. The mass is hypointense on T2 and enhances homogeneously on T1 following *i.v.* contrast.

What is the most likely diagnosis?

(a) Brainstem glioma
(b) Ependymoma
(c) Haemangioblastoma
(d) Medulloblastoma
(e) Pilocytic astrocytoma

16 Which of the following types of craniosynostosis is correctly linked to the suture involved?

(a) Anterior plagiocephaly – unilateral lambdoidal suture
(b) Brachycephaly – metoptic suture
(c) Posterior plagiocephaly – unilateral coronal suture
(d) Scaphocephaly – sagittal suture
(e) Trigonocephaly – bilateral coronal suture

17 An 8 month old boy presents with red-currant jelly stool and abdominal distension. US confirms an intussusception and the paediatric surgeons ask you to attempt fluoroscopic reduction.

Which of the following is a contraindication to fluoroscopic reduction?

(a) Age > 12 months
(b) Evidence of small bowel obstruction
(c) Free intra-peritoneal fluid
(d) Hypovolaemic shock
(e) US demonstrates fluid in the lumen around the intussusceptum

18 A supine AXR is performed on a 4 day old neonate born at 32 weeks, who is noted to have increasing abdominal distension and appears clinically unwell.

Which of the following features is an indication for urgent surgery?

(a) Air in the portal vein
(b) Adynamic ileus
(c) Pneumatosis intestalis
(d) Pneumobilia
(e) Pneumoperitoneum

19 A 14 year old girl presents with abnormal curvature of the spine, there is no history of any back pain. On examination there is an obvious scoliosis.

Which of the following is the most likely as an underlying cause?

(a) Neurofibromatosis type I
(b) Osteoid osteoma
(c) Hemivertebrae
(d) Facet joint OA
(e) TB of psoas muscle

20 Which of the following conditions has the highest frequency of non-genitourinary anomalies?

(a) Ask-Upmark kidney
(b) Bilateral ectopia
(c) Crossed-fused ectopia
(d) Duplex kidney
(e) Horseshoe kidney

21 Antenatal US shows a RUQ cystic structure. A day 3 US shows an anechoic cyst with hyperechoic inner lining and a hypoechoic outer rim, causing superior-anterior displacement of the 1st and 2nd portion of the duodenum without bile duct dilation.

What is the most likely diagnosis?

(a) Choledochal cyst
(b) Choledochocoele
(c) Duplication cyst
(d) Mesenteric lymphangioma
(e) Pancreatic pseudocyst

22 A 15 year old boy under investigation for polyuria presents to A&E with an acute episode of dyspnoea. CXR reveals a small right-sided pneumothorax and lung cysts are noted.

What is the most likely underlying diagnosis?

(a) α1-anti-trypsin deficiency
(b) Langerhans Cell Histiocystosis
(c) Lymphangiomyomatosis
(d) Neurofibromatosis
(e) Tuberous sclerosis

23 Which of the following classifications of atria/viscera positioning relative to the midline is associated with the lowest frequency of congenital heart defects?

(a) Situs ambiguous
(b) Situs inversus/dextrocardia
(c) Situs inversus/levocardia
(d) Situs solitus/dextrocardia
(e) Situs solitus/levocardia

24 A 3 week old boy presents with high output cardiac failure. On examination he has a mass within the right upper quadrant. CT shows a large heterogeneous mass with central areas of low density, occupying the entire left lobe of the liver. The mass enhances peripherally in the arterial phase.

What is the most likely diagnosis?

(a) Haemangioendothelioma
(b) Haemangiopericytoma
(c) Hamartoma
(d) Hepatoblastoma
(e) Hepatocellular carcinoma

25 A 4 year old girl has a proven first UTI. *E. coli* is cultured and there is a good response to antibiotics. Her GP phones to ask your advice on the most appropriate way to proceed with imaging.

What should you recommend?

(a) DMSA scan at 6 months
(b) MCUG at 6 weeks
(c) No imaging
(d) US acutely
(e) US at 6 weeks

26 Which of the following types of polycystic kidney disease is associated with the greatest degree of liver fibrosis?

(a) Autosomal dominant PKD
(b) Antenatal autosomal recessive PKD
(c) Infantile autosomal recessive PKD
(d) Juvenile autosomal recessive PKD
(e) Neonatal autosomal recessive PKD

27 A 14 year old boy presents with mid/ lower back pain. He is noted to be kyphotic on examination. A lateral X-ray of the thoraco-lumbar vertebrae shows anterior wedging of the T8-10 vertebral bodies.

What is the most likely diagnosis?

(a) Ankylosing spondylitis
(b) Eosinophilic granuloma
(c) Morquio's syndrome
(d) Osteogenesis imperfecta
(e) Scheuermann's disease

28 **A 3 year old boy presents with a first seizure; he is afebrile. CT scan shows calcification within the right parietal gyri with ipsilateral skull thickening and enlargement of the choroid plexus.**

What is the likely diagnosis?
(a) Klippel-Trenaunay syndrome
(b) Neurofibromatosis type 2
(c) Sturge-Weber syndrome
(d) Tuberous sclerosis
(e) von Hippel Lindau syndrome

29 **A 2 year old boy considered at high risk for NAI. An initial skeletal survey is performed and subsequently a bone scan is requested for additional evaluation.**

Which of the following are not true regarding bone scintigraphy?
(a) It is more sensitive than plain film
(b) It is more accurate in diagnosing skull fractures
(c) It is less accurate in diagnosing metaphyseal fractures
(d) It is less specific than plain film
(e) Scintigraphy cannot reliably differentiate old and new fractures

30 **A 3 day old baby has dyspnoea. The CXR shows shift of the mediastinum to the right; the left hemithorax is filled with multiple cyst-like structures. The stomach is centrally located and there is a paucity of bowel gas within the abdomen.**

What is the most likely diagnosis?
(a) Bochdalek hernia
(b) Bronchogenic cyst
(c) Congenital cystic adenomatoid malformation
(d) Extrapulmonary sequestration
(e) Septum transverum defect

31 Which of the following features is not a feature of Juvenile Chronic Arthritis?

(a) Growth retardation
(b) Iridocyclitis
(c) Rheumatoid factor positive
(d) Spinal involvement typically precedes peripheral arthritis
(e) Oligoarthritis

32 A 3 week old, previously well baby present with cough and difficulty in breathing. On examination there is reduced air entry on the right. CXR reveals complete opacification of the right hemithorax. There is rib crowding on the right and the trachea is positioned to the right.

What is the most likely underlying cause?
(a) Congenital cystic adenomatoid malformation
(b) Congenital diaphragmatic hernia
(c) Extra-pulmonary sequestration
(d) Mucous plugging
(e) Pleural effusion

33 Regarding lung lesions in the paediatric population.

Which of the following conditions is the most likely to present as multiple pulmonary opacities?
(a) Arterio-venous malformations
(b) Congenital cystic adenomatoid malformation
(c) Extralobar pulmonary sequestrations
(d) Intralobar pulmonary sequestrations
(e) Pulmonary hamartomas

34 A 4 month old baby has a witnessed fall and head injury. The lateral skull view demonstrates no fracture, but shows multiple bones within the lambdoid suture.

Which of the following is the least likely cause?
(a) Cleidocranial dysostosis
(b) Hypoparathyroidism
(c) Normal variant
(d) Osteogenesis imperfecta
(e) Pycnodysotosis

35 A 3 year old presents with abdominal pain and vomiting. The paediatric surgeons are concerned about possible malrotation and request a plain film in the first instance.

What is the most common plain radiograph finding in malrotation?

(a) Bowel wall oedema
(b) Caecum located on left side
(c) Normal
(d) Small bowel obstruction
(e) SMA lying to right of the SMV

36 A 1 year old girl presents to A&E with a harsh cough, fever and stridor. A lateral neck X-ray shows normal supraglottic structures. The CXR shows narrowing of the sub-glottic airway.

What is the most likely diagnosis?

(a) Croup
(b) Enlarged tonsils
(c) Epiglottitis
(d) Inhaled foreign body in RLL
(e) Vocal cord palsy

37 A neonate has bile stained vomiting post feeding. The AXR shows a 'double bubble' sign?

Which of the following conditions is the least likely underlying cause?

(a) Annular pancreas
(b) Duodenal atresia
(c) Ladd's bands
(d) Pre-duodenal vein
(e) Pyloric stenosis

38 A 5 year old girl presents with a swelling on the left side of her neck. An MRI examination is subsequently arranged for investigation.

Which feature makes branchial cleft cyst more likely than cystic hygroma?

(a) Associated coarctation of the aorta
(b) Extending between ECA/ICA
(c) Extension into mediastinum
(d) High signal on T2W MR imaging
(e) Multi-loculated appearance on US

39 An antenatal US shows oligohydramnios, a protruberant abdomen, bilateral hydronephrosis and markedly dilated and tortuous ureter. The posterior urethra is dilated and there is a large distended thin-walled bladder. At birth the testicles are noted to be undescended.

What is the most likely diagnosis?

(a) Cloacal abnormality
(b) Megacystis-microcolon-hypoperistalsis (MMH) syndrome
(c) Posterior urethral valves
(d) Prostatic rhabdomyosarcoma
(e) Prune-belly syndrome

40 Which of the following causes of neonatal hydrocephalus is more likely to be communicating rather than non-communicating?

(a) Aqueduct stenosis
(b) Arnold-Chiari syndrome
(c) Dandy-Walker syndrome
(d) Encephalocoele
(e) Germinal matrix haemorrhage

41 A request is made for an MRI examination in a neonate. An antenatal US had revealed agenesis of the corpus callosum. The MRI scan shows an abnormal posterior fossa.

Which of these features make Dandy-Walker a more likely diagnosis than Chiari II malformation?

(a) Hydrocephalus
(b) Klippel-Feil anomaly
(c) Large posterior fossa
(d) Syringohydromyelia
(e) 'Towering' cerebellum

42 A pregnant mother with low α-FP, increased β-hCG and decreased unconjugated oestriol on screening is considered high risk for carrying a baby with Down's syndrome. An 18 week anomaly US is arranged.

Which of the following findings indicative of Down's syndrome is least likely to be seen?

(a) Cystic hygroma
(b) Duodenal atresia
(c) Omphalocoele
(d) Increased nuchal thickness
(e) Short femur length

43 Regarding duplication cysts of the gastro-intestinal tract in neonates.

Where is the commonest location?

(a) Duodenum
(b) Ileum
(c) Jejunum
(d) Oesophagus
(e) Stomach

44 A 9 year old child presents following an RTA. Prelimary 'FAST' scan US in A&E shows intra-abdominal free fluid. The child is resuscitated and a CT requested to help identify a bleeding site.

Which of the following is not a recognised feature of hypovolaemia with CT?

(a) Small hypodense spleen
(b) Reduced renal enhancement
(c) Small bowel dilatation
(d) Collapsed IVC
(e) Pancreatic enhancement

45 An infant is seen by the GP non-acutely, with stridor. He is systemically well and is not in distress. Tracheomalacia is suspected as a possible cause and further investigations are arranged.

Regarding tracheomalacia, which of the following statements is correct?

(a) It is associated with tracheo-oesophageal fistula
(b) It is the commonest cause of inspiratory stridor
(c) Expiratory CT is the definitive method of diagnosis
(d) Resolution occurs in late childhood
(e) The trachea typically collapses in inspiration

46 A 15 year old girl presents with gradually increasing bilateral hip pain. Pelvic X-ray reveals bilateral sclerosis of the femoral head, with lucent crescents paralleling the articular surface and subchondral cysts. The acetabulum is normal and the epiphyseal height and alignment is preserved. She had an episode of right hip pain 1 year ago and the X-ray was reported as normal.

Which of the following is the most likely diagnosis?

(a) Developmental dysplasia of the hips
(b) Diaphyseal achlasia
(c) Perthe's disease
(d) Sickle cell disease
(e) Slipped upper femoral epiphyses

47 Regarding the normal anatomy of the umbilical cord, there is:

(a) 1 umbilical artery, 1 umbilical vein
(b) 1 umbilical artery, 2 umbilical veins
(c) 2 umbilical arteries, 1 umbilical vein
(d) 2 umbilical arteries, 2 umbilical veins
(e) No 'normal number' as it is common to have different combinations of umbilical arteries/veins as an anatomical variant

48 A 4 week old baby is cyanosed and has a heart murmur. The CXR reveals pulmonary oedema with widening of the superior mediastinum to produce a 'snowman' ('cottage loaf') appearance.

What is the likely type of total anomalous pulmonary venous connection (TAPVC) present?
(a) Cardiac
(b) Infracardiac
(c) Mixed
(d) Scimitar syndrome
(e) Supracardiac

49 A 10 year old boy presents to his GP with back pain. He is found to have a scoliosis, but is also noted to be tall for his age and rather thin.

Which of the following supports the diagnosis of Marfan's syndrome over homocystinuria?
(a) Aortic aneurysm
(b) Lens dislocation
(c) Mental retardation
(d) Osteoporosis
(e) History of pulmonary emboli

50 An antenatal US shows a myelomeningocoele of the lower cord, but normal cranial appearances. A post-natal lateral skull X-ray reveals multiple ovoid lucencies with thinning of the inner table of the calvarium, clustered within in the parietal and occipital bones.

What is the most likely diagnosis?

(a) Convolutional markings
(b) Dermoid cyst
(c) Epidermoid cyst
(d) Lacunar skull
(e) Langerhans cell histiocytosis

Paediatrics Practice SBA Answers

1 (c)
Trauma (including NAI) is one of the leading causes of pancreatitis in the paediatric population. Other causes include cystic fibrosis, hyperlipidaemia syndromes, drugs, viral, hyperparathyroidism, hypercalcaemia, idiopathic, Pearson syndrome (mitochondrial disorder), Schwachman-Diamond syndrome, and anatomical anomaly (pancreas divisum).

Ref: Primer of Diagnostic Imaging, 4th Ed, p. 902.

2 (b)
VHL is associated with CNS haemangioblastomas in 50%, pancreatic/ hepatic/ renal cysts, RCC, and phaeochromocytoma (10%). Phaeochromocytomas are also associated with MEN types 2A and 2B (also medullary thyroid cancer, parathyroid adenomas), NF-1, and tuberous sclerosis. Bilateral acoustic neuromas are associated with NF-2.

Ref: Radiology Review Manual, 6th Ed, p. 943–4 & Primer of Diagnostic Imaging, 4th Ed, p. 576–80.

3 (b)
The most common causes of antenatal hydronephrosis (regardless of gender), in order of decreasing frequency are: PUJ obstruction (22%), posterior urethral valve (18%), ectopic ureterocoele (14%), Prune-belly syndrome (12%), and VUJ obstruction (8%).

Ref: Radiology Review Manual, 6th Ed, p. 931.

4 (b)
The majority of inhaled foreign bodies are food material (*e.g.* peanuts), thus are not radio-opaque. The paediatric airway diameter increases inspiration, decreases in expiration – a partial obstruction in inspiration may become complete in expiration, allowing air-trapping in expiration. The carinal angle is symmetric in infants making it equally likely that a foreign body will pass into either left or right mainstem bronchus. Radiographic evidence of air trapping is typical, however, no imaging modality can definitely exclude the diagnosis, therefore, if the history is suggestive, the child should undergo bronchoscopy.

Ref: R-ITI 5_027. Inhaled Foreign Body.

5 (a)
Increasing gantry rotation speed will reduce dose and also decreases movement artefact. Use of AEC reduces dose by automatically adjusting current in response to the attenuation of the section scanned. Reducing mA reduces dose, but noise is increased. There is an exponential relationship between kVp and dose, thus decreasing kVp greatly reduces dose, however, there are greater beam hardening artefacts and noise increases.

Ref: R-ITI 5_001. The effects of radiation on children and dose reduction.

6 (d)
Classically neuroblastoma encases vessels, whereas Wilm's tumours may invade vessels. Calcification is more common in neuroblastoma (85–95%) than Wilm's (15%), neuroblastoma commonly crosses the midline, only 10% of Wilm's tumours are bilateral. Neuroblastoma typically metastasises to bone and lymph nodes; Wilm's to the liver, lungs and lymph nodes.

Ref: Primer of Diagnostic Imaging, 4th Ed, p. 865–8.

7 (e)
SDH is the most common intracranial finding in NAI and accidental causes are rare (*e.g.* RTA) and will likely be witnessed, with other injuries apparent. Options (a) – (d) are features which strongly suggest SDH secondary to NAI. Accidental SDHs do not usually extend into the falx. A further NAI-related feature is SDH without a fracture (implying shaking injury).

Ref: Diagnostic Radiology, 5th Ed, p. 1632–5.

8 (b)
Cerebellar ataxia is associated with neuroblastoma. Wilm's is associated with WAGR (includes duplex/ horseshoe/ fused kidneys), Drash syndrome (male pseudo-hermaphroditism), and Beckwith-Wiedemann syndrome (macroglossia). It is also associated with spontaneous aniridia and hemihypertrophy.

Ref: Radiology Review Manual, 6th Ed, p. 940 & 993.

9 (b)
Anorectal malformation may be low (commonest), intermediate, or high, depending on the relation to the levator sling. High malformations are associated with fistulas and a high association with GU (50%), and VACTERL anomalies. History of surgical repair makes fistulas unlikely; post-op patients often suffer urinary incontinence; the additional association of spinal anomalies make neurogenic bladder (which predisposes to UTI) a likelihood. There is no association with PUJ obstruction or urethrocoele.

Ref: Radiology Review Manual, 6th Ed, p. 843.

10 (b)
Coronal US images are acquired with patient in the lateral decubitus position and hip flexed at 90°. The α-angle is between the acetabular roof and the iliac bone (normal = >60°). The β-angle is between the acetabular labrum and the iliac bone (normal = <55°). Also >50% of the femoral head should be covered by the acetabulum. The femoral head is unossified at this age and a hypoechoic appearance is normal. Option (d) is a plain film marker of DDH, the normal hip lies inferior and medial to the intersection of these lines.

Ref: Radiology Review Manual, 6th Ed, p. 67–8.

11 (d)
A 'pulmonary sling' refers to an aberrant left PA, which arises from the right PA and passes between the trachea and oesophagus, resulting in posterior compression of the trachea and anterior compression of the oesophagus. It may lead to tracheo-bronchiomalacia or stenosis in up to 50% patients.

Ref: Primer of Diagnostic Imaging, 4th Ed, p. 138.

12 (a)
Causes of mediastinal shift away from the abnormal side include pleural effusions, tumours, diaphragmatic hernia, tension pneumothorax, and causes of air-trapping (*e.g.* bronchial atresia, congenital lobar emphysema). Asthma may be a cause, but uncomplicated cases do not cause shift. Mediastinal shift towards the abnormal hemithorax suggests volume loss as a cause (*e.g.* lobar collapse).

Ref: R-ITI 5_016. The_dense_hemithorax.

13 (d)
Pertechnatate studies are the most sensitive test (85%), although wireless capsule endoscopy has good potential. Pertechnatate is taken up by the ectopic gastric mucosa within the Meckel's. False +ve results include AVM, haemangioma, UC, Crohn's, appendicitis; false -ve results occur if the diverticulum contains no gastric mucosa.

Ref: Clin Rad (2009); 64(2): 109–18.

14 (d)
Stage I limited to organ of origin. Stage II regional spread, but does not cross midline. Stage III tumour extends across midline, or is a unilateral tumour with contralateral LNs. Stage IV: the tumour has spread to distant lymph nodes, bone, bone marrow, liver, skin or other organs. Stage IV-S is a subset of neuroblastoma in infants < 1 year with a good prognosis.

Ref: Diagnostic Radiology, 5th Ed, p. 1647–8.

15 (d)
All are examples of posterior fossa masses in children; other causes include meningioma, and epidermoid or dermoid cysts. These features are typical for medulloblastoma (the differential diagnosis is an atypical teratoid/rhabdoid tumour). Pilocytic astrocytomas are cystic with an enhancing peripheral nodule, ependymomas arise from 4th ventricle floor and are hypodense on CT, haemangioblastomas enhance avidly.

Ref: Diagnostic Radiology, 5th Ed, p. 1677–8.

16 (d)
The most common single suture affected is the sagittal suture (scaphocephaly), others include uni-coronal (anterior plagiocephaly), bi-coronal (brachycephaly), metoptic (trigonocephaly) and unilateral lambdoidal (posterior plagiocephaly). Craniosynostosis may be part of a syndrome, with multiple sutures involved, or secondary to drugs, metabolic disease, or other causes of microcephaly.

Ref: Diagnostic Radiology, 5th Ed, p. 1674–6.

17 (d)
Hypovolaemic shock suggests ischaemic bowel, which would require surgical intervention, furthermore reduction should not be attempted in a sick infant and the patient should be appropriately resuscitated before any attempts at reduction are made. Other contraindications include pneumoperitoneum and peritonitis. The remaining options are not absolute contra-indications, but their presence reduces the chances of successful therapeutic reduction. Small bowel obstruction implies ischaemia or the presence of a tight intussusception. Free intra-peritoneal fluid or fluid in the lumen surrounding the intussusceptum suggests oedema or ischaemia of the bowel. An older age (> 12 months) suggests a pathological lead point may be the aetiology, in which case resection may be necessary.

Ref: R-ITI 5_047. Paediatric Intussusception.

18 (e)
NEC is the commonest GI emergency in premature infants. It is an infective/ ischaemic disorder of the neonatal gut in a compromised baby secondary to hypoxia. It typically presents at 2–3 days after birth and in 90% occurs before day 10. Treatment is normally conservative, surgery may be necessary due to perforation. Compared to adult patients, air in the portal system does not have such a grave prognosis. Late complications include intestinal strictures.

Ref: R-ITI 5_044. Necrotising Enterocolitis – NEC & Radiology Review Manual, 6th Ed, p. 861.

19 (c)
The patient has a 'painless' scoliosis. Congenital (*e.g.* hemi-vertebrae, wedge-shaped, or supernumerary vertebrae) and idiopathic types of scoliosis are usually painless, but can lead to secondary back pain due to the abnormal mechanics. Painful scoliosis is due to one of four primary causes: neoplastic (*e.g.* osteochondroma, GCT, osteoid osteoma), infective (*e.g.* paraspinal or psoas abscess), degenerative (facet joint OA), or traumatic.

Ref: R-ITI 5_115. Scoliosis.

20 (e)
Horseshoe kidneys are associated with other renal anomalies in 50%, and non-GU system anomalies in 30% (GI, cardiac, skeletal). In 90% of crossed ectopia there will be fusion (crossed-fused ectopia); associated anomalies are rare. Ask-Upmark kidney shows segmental hypoplasia; there is controversy over whether it is a congenital anomaly or a sequelae of severe pyelonephritis. In the cited reference, no patients with duplex kidneys were found to have non-GU related anomalies.

Ref: Primer of Diagnostic Imaging, 4th Ed, p. 856 & Radiology Review Manual, 6th Ed, p. 882 & 929 & Chang Gung Med J (2001); 24(12):779–85.

21 (c)
These cysts appear anechoic, displace the proximal duodenum supero-anteriorly. There is a double capsule: inner mucosal lining (hyperechoic) and outer rim of bowel wall (hypoechoic), this can be identified as the 'muscular rim' sign described. Choledochal cysts have 5 subtypes (type V = Caroli's disease). All bar type III involve the intra-hepatic bile ducts. Choledochocoeles arise from the duodenal portion of CBD, but other features support a duplication cyst. In mesenteric lymphangioma there is a single wall.

Ref: Radiology Review Manual, 6th Ed, p. 704 & 824–6.

22 (b)
All are causes of cystic lung disease which may present in young patients. LAM is seen in female patients. In chronic disseminated LCH (Hand-Schuller-Christian disease) there is a classic triad of exophthalmos, diabetes insipidus (due to pituitary stalk lesions) and lytic skull lesions. In 25% of these patients there are lung cysts associated, with bleb formation and spontaneous pneumothorax. The history of polyuria makes LCH the likely diagnosis.

Ref: Fundamentals of Diagnostic Radiology, 2nd Ed, p. 504–5.

23 (e)
Normal anatomy is situs solitus/levocardia. The frequency of associated CHD is: situs solitus/levocardia < 1%, situs inversus/dextrocardia 4%, situs solitus/dextrocardia 95%, situs inversus/levocardia 95%, situs ambiguous (heterotaxy syndromes) 50–100%.

Ref: Radiology Review Manual, 6th Ed, p. 593–4.

24 (a)
Infantile haemangioendothelioma typically presents in neonates (85% are diagnosed at < 6 months). 15% present with high output cardiac failure (AV shunts), consumption can lead to thrombocytopaenia/ DIC. Imaging characteristics are similar to adult haemangiomas. Haemangiopericytoma is a soft tissue sarcoma. Broadly speaking paediatric liver tumours present in 'alphabetical order' with age: haemangioendothelioma (neonates), hamartoma (15-22 months), hepatoblastoma (<3 years), and HCC (>3 years).

Ref: Radiology Review Manual, 6th Ed, p. 722–5.

25 (c)
Recent NICE guidelines recommend no imaging for simple (non-atypical) first UTIs in infants 6 months – 3 years and children over 3 years which respond to antibiotics within 48 hours. In children over 3 years with an atypical UTI, an US should be urgently arranged, in those with recurrent UTIs a 6 week US and 6 month DMSA scan should be arranged; there is no role in this age group for MCUG. An US is always performed in those < 6 months old (routinely at 6 wks), if this is abnormal, or there is an atypical organism, or recurrent UTIs, MCUG is performed. MCUG may be considered in those 6 months – 3 years if there is pelvic dilation on US, or a family history of VUR.

Ref: NICE guideline CG54 (August 2007).

26 (d)
ARPKD is associated with liver fibrosis and portal hypertension. The degree of hepatic fibrosis is inversely related to the degree of renal disease. The relative involvement is: antenatal (90%; renal disease; minimal hepatic fibrosis), neonatal (60%; mild fibrosis) infantile (20%; moderate fibrosis) and juvenile (10%; gross liver fibrosis). Juvenile type is postulated to be a primary hepatic fibrosis rather than an ARPKD.

Ref: Primer of Diagnostic Imaging, 4th Ed, p. 861–2.

27 (e)
Scheuermann's is thought to be caused by herniation of disc material through congenital end-plate defects during the adolescent growth spurt (presents 13–17 yrs). It accounts for 31% of cases of back pain in adolescent boys and is located in the thoracic (75%) or thoraco-lumbar spine (25%). At least one vertebral body needs to be involved with anterior wedging of >5° (usually 3–5 are involved), and there must be kyphosis of >35°. The posterior aspect of the vertebral body is protected by posterior articulation. The other listed conditions are potential causes of kyphosis in children.

Ref: Primer of Diagnostic Imaging, 4th Ed, p. 879 & p. 911 & Radiology Review Manual, 6th Ed, p. 223.

28 (c)
Sturge-Weber syndrome is associated with a 'port-wine stain' naevus in the distribution of the trigeminal nerve, tram-track gyral calcification (usually parietal lobe), ipsilateral choroid plexus enlargement, leptomeningeal venous angiomas, hemiparesis, seizures, mental retardation, glaucoma (30%) and choidoidal haemangiomas of the orbit.

Ref: Radiology Review Manual, 6th Ed, p. 326–7.

29 (b)
Bone scans have an increased sensitivity, but low specificity. Any fracture (accidental or non-accidental) will increase uptake on bone scan. Scintigraphy is most accurate for the evaluation of rib and long bone abnormalities. It is not accurate for the evaluation of skull fractures due to the increased activity in sutures. Bone scintigraphy is not accurate at determining the age of fractures (old fractures may have no activity); plain film is useful because different stages of healing have different radiographic features.

Ref: Primer of Diagnostic Imaging, 4th Ed, p. 873–4.

30 (a)
Congenital diaphragmatic hernias include Bochdalek (85-90%), Morgagni (5%), and rarely: septum transverum defects, hiatus hernia and diaphragmatic eventration. Bochdalek hernias are posterior, and left-sided (80%), Morgagni hernias are anterio-medial, right-sided. Differentiation from CCAM can be difficult, however, CCAM is less commonly macrocystic, the stomach will be normally sited to the left and the bowel gas pattern will be normal.

Ref: Radiology Review Manual, 6th Ed, p. 490–1.

31 (c)
JCA by definition starts <16 years old, it can be oligo- or poly- arthritis and the majority of cases are seronegative. The large joints are typically affected first, diffuse ankylosis is common and periosteal reaction is typically present. Although there is often overgrowth of the epiphyses due to increased perfusion, there is usually growth retardation due to early closure of the growth plates.

Ref: Primer of Diagnostic Imaging, 4th Ed, p. 887.

32 (d)
When there is a unilateral dense hemithorax, it needs to be decided if this is the abnormal side (usually obvious). The differential diagnosis is based on the medisatinum: if it moves towards the opaque side it suggests volume loss (collapse due to mucous plugging, asthma, CF, ET tube misplacement, pulmonary aplasia, and, rarely, pneumonectomy). Mediastinal shift away from the opaque side suggests mass effect, usually due to pleural fluid (or tumours, CCAM, etc).

Ref: R-ITI 5_016. The_dense_hemithorax.

33 (a)
AVMs are multiple in up to 35%, and are more likely to be so if associated with hereditary haemorrhagic telangiectasia. Pulmonary sequestrations and pulmonary hamartomas are considered solitary intrathoracic masses.

Ref: R-ITI 5_017. Solitary Lung Opacity & 5_018. Multiple Lung Opacities.

34 (b)
Wormian bones are intra-sutural ossicles, commonest in the lambdoid suture. They are normally found up to 6 months of age (the commonest cause). The mnemonic 'PORKCHOPS' can be used to remember other causes: Pyknodysostosis, Osteogenesis imperfecta, Rickets (healing phase), Kinky hair syndrome, Cleidocranial dysostosis, Hypothyroidism/ Hypophosphatasia, Otopalattodigital syndrome, Pachydermoperiostosis, and (syndrome of) Down.

Ref: Radiology Review Manual, 6th Ed, p. 178.

35 (c)
The commonest plain film finding in malrotation is 'normal appearances', thus a 'normal' AXR cannot exclude malrotation. Other plain film findings of malrotation include ascites, bowel wall oedema (thumb-printing, due to SMV compression), evidence of ischaemic gut (due to SMA compression), duodenal obstruction (due to Ladd's bands), SBO, right-sided small bowel, left-sided caecum/ colon.

Ref: R-ITI 5_042. Malrotation.

36 (a)
Croup is a viral infection occurring at 6 months – 3 years, mainly in winter. The 'steeple' (or inverted 'V') sign is due to oedematous narrowing of the sub-glottic airway. Epiglottitis is caused by *Haemophilus influenzae* and typically presents with stridor, fever, sore throat and drooling. It usually presents in older children (3–6 years), the key finding is thickened aryepiglottic folds on lateral neck films and it may be associated with subglottic narrowing similar to croup.

Ref: R-ITI 5_081. Stridor In Children.

37 (e)
The 'double bubble' sign describes gas within the proximal duodenum and stomach. There is often a gasless distal abdomen due to obstruction in the duodenum. Pyloric stenosis causes obstruction at the level of the pylorus. In this condition, the duodenum is usually gas-free - if gas passes into the duodenum it will also freely pass more distally.

Ref: Aids to Radiological Differential Diagnosis. 4th Ed, p. 218.

38 (b)
Branchial cleft cyst is usually in the anterior triangle. The 'beak sign', where tissue points between the ICA and ECA is described as pathognomonic. Cystic hygroma is a single or multiloculated lymphangioma and is associated with chromosomal anomalies, including Turner's syndrome (coarctation in 15%). Both are high signal on T2, cystic hygroma may be low or high signal on T1 (depending on levels of lipid/ protein/ blood products).

Ref: Radiology Review Manual, 6th Ed, p. 376–7 & p. 390.

39 (e)
Prune-belly syndrome is a triad of absent/ deficient abdominal muscules, renal dysplasia (bilateral hydroureters/ hydronephrosis), and cryptorchidism. Due to the associated absence of the prostate gland, the posterior urethra is often dilated proximally – the entire urethra may be dilated. PUVs are a key differential, but the implied abdominal wall defect, thin-walled bladder, and cryptorchidism go against this. MMH causes insufficiency of the abdominal viscera, but occurs in females. Rhabdomyosarcoma would be unusual antenatally.

Ref: Fundamentals of Diagnostic Radiology, 2nd Ed, p. 1309–10.

40 (e)
Obstructive (non-communicating) causes are more common and include spina bifida, aqueduct stenosis, Dandy-Walker syndrome, Arnold-Chiari syndrome, meningocoele, and encephalocoele. Non-obstructive causes result from reduced reabsorption within the arachnoid granulation tissue, *e.g.* infection or haemorrhage, or increased CSF production *e.g.* choroid plexus papilloma; these can also cause obstructive hydrocephalus also.

Ref: Primer of Diagnostic Imaging, 4th Ed, p. 779.

41 (c)
Dandy-Walker malformation results from congenital atresia of the foramina of Magendie and Luschka, leading to an enlarged posterior fossa, a large posterior fossa cyst, hydrocephalus and varying degrees of cerebellar hemisphere and verminian hypoplasia. Both have syringohydromyelia and hydrocephalus; Chiari II has a small posterior fossa; Chiari I is associated with Klippel-Feil.

Ref: Primer of Diagnostic Imaging, 4th Ed, p. 571–6.

42 (b)
13-50% may not have any US-detectable anomalies. Duodenal atresia is present in 50%, but is not detected before 22 weeks. Nuchal thickness is increased in 40% to ≥3 mm at 10-13 wks, ≥5 mm at 14-18 wks; CHDs are present in 40%. Other US findings include hydrops, echogenic bowel, pyelectasis, hypoplasia of the 5th digit, and 11 pairs of ribs.

Ref: Radiology Review Manual, 6th Ed, p. 70–1.

43 (b)
15% of paediatric abdominal masses are duplication cysts, they can be found anywhere along the GI tract, commonest locations are: ileum (30–33%), oesophagus (17–20%), colon (13–20%), jejunum (10–13%), stomach (7%), pylorus (4%), duodenum (4–5%), ileocaecal junction (4%), rectum (4%).

Ref: Radiology Review Manual, 6th Ed, p. 824.

44 (b)
The kidneys show enhancement, the so-called 'shock nephrogram' due to decreased excretion of contrast medium. The spleen is small and hypodense due to hypoperfusion; the small bowel is dilated with wall thickening/ enhancement due to vasoconstriction of the mesenterics, and the IVC collapsed due to decreased venous return (a very serious sign).

Ref: Radiology Review Manual, 6th Ed, p. 807.

45 (a)
Tracheomalacia can be congenital due to immaturity of the tracheal cartilage and is associated with TOF. Secondary causes include vascular rings, infective, inflammatory or post-instrumentation. It is frequently found in children who have undergone TOF repair. There is collapse of the airway on expiration with associated expiratory stridor, although rarely, if the extra-thoracic trachea is affected, there may be inspiratory collapse/ stridor. Majority have resolution of symptoms by 1 year. Chest fluoroscopy can confirm diagnosis, but bronchoscopy is more definitive; CT may not reveal its dynamic nature.

Ref: Radiology Review Manual, 6th Ed, p. 447.

46 (d)
Bilateral AVN of the femoral head is described; plain film signs may lag several months behind symptom onset. Perthe's can cause idiopathic AVN and is bilateral in 5-10% (systemic disorders are more likely to be bilateral), but typically presents at 5–10 years, and the patient was described as having a normal X-ray aged 14. Other causes to consider are trauma, collagen vascular diseases, glycogen storage diseases, drug therapy (steroids).

Ref: Radiology Review Manual, 6th Ed, p. 49–50.

47 (c)
A single UA is present in less than 1% of all births. Single UA is more common with twins and diabetic mothers, and is associated with congenital anomalies.

Ref: Radiology Review Manual, 6th Ed, p. 1063.

48 (e)
TAPVC describes return of the pulmonary veins to the RA rather than the LA; there are 3 types: supracardiac, cardiac and infracardiac. Supracardiac is the commonest; the veins drain into a common left-sided trunk which runs superiorly and drains into the left innominate vein then the SVC, widening the superior mediastinum to give the 'snowman' ('cottage loaf' or 'figure 8') appearance. Scimitar syndrome is a type of PAPVC.

Ref: R-ITI 5_033. Cardiac Shapes.

49 (a)
The conditions have a similar phenotype. In Marfan's there is MV prolapse, aortic regurgitation, coarctation, and dissecting aneurysm of the ascending aorta; lens dislocation is upwards and outwards (down/ inward in homocystinuria). Homocystinuria is an enzyme deficiency disorder, leading to homocystine build-up which causes a defect in collagen structure. Features which help distinguish it from Marfan's include the propensity for thrombo-emboli disease and osteoporosis (osteopaenia in Marfan's).

Ref: Radiology Review Manual, 6th Ed, p. 103 & 115.

50 (d)
Lacunar skull (luckenschadel) is due to defective ossification of the inner table of the skull. There are oval lucencies which are present at birth and disappear by 5 months. They are not due to increased intracranial pressure/ hydrocephalus, but are associated with Chiari II malformations, encephalocoeles, and myelomeningocoeles. Convolutional markings do not appear until 1 year; the other options are causes of lucent lesions (+/- soft tissue mass) in the neonate.

Ref: R-ITI 5_090. Skull Vault Lucencies and Bumps on the Head.

Central Nervous System and Head & Neck Practice SBA Questions

1 **A patient presents with a slowly progressive loss of vision. Enlargement of the optic nerve is seen on MR imaging.**

Which of the following features would be more in keeping with an optic nerve glioma, rather than an optic nerve sheath meningioma?

(a) Unilateral lesion
(b) Calcification
(c) Kinking of the optic nerve
(d) Hyperostosis
(e) Linear bands of enhancement following *i.v.* gadolinium

2 **A female child has problems with upward gaze. A CT head reveals a densely-enhancing pineal mass with 'exploded calcifications'. There is evidence of CSF seeding.**

Which other tumour type is this condition associated with?

(a) Retinoblastoma
(b) Teratoma
(c) Meningioma
(d) Pilocytic astrocytoma
(e) Neurofibroma

3 **A 76 year man presents with right-sided weakness. There is a low-attenuation lesion in the left basal ganglia. An MRI is arranged for further evaluation.**

Which feature would suggest a high-grade neoplasm rather than an infarct?

(a) Involvement of both cerebral cortex and juxtacortical white matter
(b) Gyriform enhancement
(c) Low signal on an apparent diffusion coefficient image
(d) Elevated choline on magnetic resonance spectroscopy
(e) Cytotoxic oedema

4 **A 45 year old female inpatient is sent to the US department for investigation of her goitre. Imaging reveals an enlarged thyroid gland with a lobulated outline. Multiple ill-defined hypoechoic areas are separated by echogenic septae. Blood results are unavailable.**

What is the most likely diagnosis?

(a) Grave's disease
(b) Hashimoto's thyroiditis
(c) Multinodular goitre
(d) De Quervain's thyroiditis
(e) Plummer's disease

5 **A young patient with learning difficulties presents with multiple skin lesions and seizures. On examination there is an erythematous facial rash in a butterfly distribution and subungual fibromas are noted in the hands. A CT head is performed.**

Which of the following is not typically associated with this condition?

(a) Sclerotic lesions in the skull
(b) Asymptomatic, calcified retinal nodules
(c) Hydrocephalus
(d) Enhancing, calcified cortical tubers
(e) Cerebral arterial ectasia

6 **A newborn child suffers respiratory distress, bradycardia and spasticity. An MRI of the brain is performed.**

Which of the following features is not associated with a Chiari II malformation?

(a) Small posterior fossa
(b) Towering cerebellum
(c) Small 4th ventricle
(d) Hyperplastic falx
(e) Stenogyria

7 A patient has radiotherapy after resection of his primary brain tumour. There is a change in his neurological symptoms.

Which imaging feature would be more supportive of tumour recurrence rather than radiation injury?

(a) Low relative cerebral blood volume on CT perfusion imaging
(b) Decreased activity on Thallium SPECT imaging
(c) Decreased amplitude of the choline peak on MR spectroscopy
(d) High signal on MR FLAIR imaging
(e) Decreased amplitude of the N-acetyl-aspartate peak (NAA) on MR spectroscopy

8 A CT reveals an intra-axial cerebral mass.

Which of the following is the most likely diagnosis?

(a) Haemangioblastoma
(b) Haemangiopericytoma
(c) Meningioma
(d) Leptomeningeal lymphoma
(e) Nasopharyngeal carcinoma

9 A young boy presents with repeated seizures. MR Imaging is normal. Surgery is being considered.

What would be the most sensitive radionuclide examination to identify the source?

(a) ^{99m}Tc-HMPAO SPECT inter-ictal imaging
(b) ^{99m}Tc-HMPAO SPECT ictal imaging
(c) ^{99m}Tc-iomazenil SPECT inter-ictal imaging
(d) ^{99m}Tc-iomazenil SPECT ictal imaging
(e) ^{99m}Tc-flumazenil SPECT post-ictal imaging

10 A patient presents with bladder dysfunction and leg weakness. MRI of the spine reveals a solitary intradural, extramedullary tumour of the thoracic spinal cord. It is posteriorly located and is of high signal intensity of T2W.

What is the most likely diagnosis?

(a) Nerve sheath tumour
(b) Leptomeningeal metastasis
(c) Chordoma
(d) Meningioma
(e) Astrocytoma

11 A patient presents with bradykinesia, rigidity and tremor. ^{123}I-ioflupane is administered and the images, acquired 4 hours post injection, reveal significant depletion of uptake in the corpus striatum.

Which of the following could not account for these appearances?

(a) Parkinson's disease whilst on levodopa treatment
(b) Lewy body dementia
(c) Progressive supranuclear palsy
(d) Shy-Drager syndrome
(e) Fronto-temporal dementia

12 An incidental cerebral arteriovenous malformation is noted on MR imaging.

Which of the following features is associated with a better prognosis?

(a) Nidus larger than 3 cm at angiography
(b) Location in eloquent brain
(c) Superficial venous drainage
(d) Osler-Weber-Rendu syndrome
(e) Surrounding areas of low T2W signal

13 A patient was discovered to have elevated serum ionic calcium on routine blood tests, and was referred for further investigations.

Which of the following appearances would be least consistent with a diagnosis of a parathyroid adenoma?

(a) A one centimetre hypoechoic mass posterior to the lower lobe of the left thyroid gland on US imaging
(b) A focus of increased uptake on ^{99m}Tc-sestamibi imaging
(c) An intensely enhancing nodule adjacent to the crico-thyroid junction on CT
(d) A high-signal lesion within the body of the thyroid gland seen on T2W MR imaging
(e) A focus of increased tracer uptake on ^{99m}Tc-Pertechnetate imaging

14 A young man with known HIV and a CD4 lymphocyte count of 300 cells/mL develops neurological symptoms. MR Imaging reveals ischaemic infarcts within the distributions of the perforator arteries of the basal ganglia and the middle cerebral artery.

What infective aetiology could account for these findings?

(a) Epstein-Barr virus
(b) Toxoplasmosis
(c) Cryptococcus
(d) Syphillis
(e) Polyomavirus

15 A 5 year old presents with symptoms of raised intracranial pressure and ataxia. A CT examination reveals hydrocephalus and a posterior fossa mass which comprises a cyst and mural nodule.

Given the most likely diagnosis, which of the following is incorrect?

(a) Surrounding vasogenic oedema is common
(b) Surgical resection is the treatment of choice
(c) Intense enhancement is typical
(d) Precocious puberty is associated
(e) Disseminated disease is rare

16 An elderly gentleman presents with a hemiplegia. CT perfusion imaging is performed. Mean transit time (MTT), cerebral blood volume (CBV) and cerebral blood flow (CBF) were calculated.

Which of the following would suggest the presence of an ischaemic penumbra?

(a) Increased MTT, increased CBV and increased CBF
(b) Increased MTT, decreased CBV and increased CBF
(c) Increased MTT, increased CBV and decreased CBF
(d) Decreased MTT, increased CBV and decreased CBF
(e) Decreased MTT, decreased CBV and decreased CBF

17 A demented, 60 year old gentleman with a gait apraxia and urinary incontinence is noted to have hydrocephalus on a CT Head. No obstructive lesion is found, and a trial of CSF withdrawal provides some clinical improvement.

Given the most likely diagnosis, which of the following would be an unexpected finding?

(a) Periventricular high signal on FLAIR imaging
(b) Radiotracer accumulation in the lateral ventricles after instillation of ^{111}In-DTPA *via* a lumbar puncture
(c) Downward bowing of the corpus callosum
(d) Normal opening pressure at lumbar puncture
(e) A prominent aqueductal flow void on MR imaging

18 An elderly, hypertensive man is found collapsed. CT imaging demonstrates a large intracerebral haematoma. The mean CT attenuation is 70 HU, and there are fluid/ fluid levels.

How old is the haematoma likely to be?

(a) 0-2 hours
(b) 3-48 hours
(c) 3-7 days
(d) 2-4 weeks
(e) 2 months

19 A child undergoes an MRI evaluation of the spine, and a thoracic, intramedullary mass is revealed. With respect to the normal cord, the lesion is hypointense on T1W, hyperintense on T2W, and enhances with the administration of *i.v.* gadolinium. The bones appear normal.

Which of the following is the most likely diagnosis?

(a) Ependymoma
(b) Astrocytoma
(c) Lipoma
(d) Metastasis
(e) Haematoma

20 A 23 year old man is involved in an RTA as a passenger and arrived in A&E with a GCS of 3/15. The initial CT head is reported as normal. Diffuse axonal injury is suspected and an MRI is arranged.

Which of the following structures are most likely to be affected?

(a) The splenium of the corpus callosum
(b) The inferior cerebellar peduncle
(c) The tegmentum
(d) The basal ganglia
(e) The hypothalamus

21 Which is the commonest type of cerebral herniation?

(a) Subfalcine
(b) Transtentorial
(c) Transalar
(d) Tonsilar
(e) Transcranial

22 A thyroid nodule is found to be malignant. The tumour is 3 cm in size and limited to the gland.

What is the local staging?

(a) T1
(b) T2
(c) T3
(d) T4
(e) T5

23 A carotid space mass is seen on MR imaging of the neck.

What feature would favour the diagnosis of a glomus body tumour rather than a schwannoma?

(a) Anterior displacement of the carotid arteries
(b) Rapid uptake of *i.v.* contrast medium
(c) An absence of flow voids on MR imaging
(d) Hypodense on CT imaging
(e) Well circumscribed lesion

24 How many of Dolan's lines can be interrupted by a 'tripod' facial fracture?

(a) 1
(b) 2
(c) 3
(d) 4
(e) 5

25 A 35 year old man presents with a focal weakness of his left arm. He had suffered from migraines in the past. A CT head reveals a lacunar stroke and white matter hypoattenuation, which particularly affects the sub-cortical regions and extends into the temporal poles. The white matter changes did not enhance after the administration of *i.v.* contrast medium.

Which of the following is the most likely underlying diagnosis?

(a) Amyloid angiopathy
(b) Moya moya
(c) Mitochondral cytopathy
(d) CADASIL
(e) Sickle cell disease

26 An elderly man is admitted for assessment of focal neurological symptoms. An incidental supratentorial cystic lesion is demonstrated.

Which of the following features would make the diagnosis of subdural hygroma, rather than arachnoid cyst, more likely?

(a) Isointense to CSF on T1W MR imaging
(b) Mass effect
(c) Isointense to CSF on T2W MR imaging
(d) Flattened sulci
(e) Bony remodelling

27 A young woman with a family history of a movement disorder presents with rigidity and bradykinesia. MR imaging reveals prominent, localised areas of central high T2W signal within both globus pallidi – although this appears to be on a background of generally decreased signal within these nuclei. Decreased T2W signal is also found in the red nuclei and substantia nigra.

What diagnosis is suggested by these appearances?

(a) Hallervoden-Spatz syndrome
(b) Huntington chorea
(c) Wilson's disease
(d) Cerebrotendinous xanthomatosis
(e) Rett syndrome

28 Incidentally, an elderly man is found to have lesions in the tails of both parotid glands. These are sharply marginated with parenchymal inhomogeneity. There are thin-walled cystic components. The solid elements display only minimal enhancement.

What is the most likely diagnosis in this asymptomatic patient?

(a) Mucoepidermoid carcinoma
(b) Pleomorphic adenoma
(c) Squamous cell carcinoma metastasis
(d) Warthin tumour
(e) Sjogren's syndrome

29 An intra-cranial cyst is seen on MR imaging.

What feature would support the diagnosis of arachnoid cyst rather than an epidermoid?

(a) Absence of enhancement
(b) Irregularity
(c) Iso-intense to CSF on DWI
(d) Cerebello-pontine angle location
(e) Calcification

30 A patient presents with thunderclap headache, vomiting and neck stiffness. A CT demonstrates blood in the subarachnoid space.

Which of the following is the next most common symptom associated with SAH?

(a) Seizures
(b) Altered consciousness
(c) Focal neurology
(d) Subhyaloid haemorrhages
(e) Vertigo

31 A CT head demonstrates cerebellar vermian hypoplasia, relatively normal cerebellar hemispheres, and a large CSF space surrounding the cerebellum. The brainstem is not disordered.

What is the diagnosis?
(a) Dandy Walker complex
(b) Dandy Walker variant
(c) Mega cisterna magna
(d) Chiari Type II
(e) Spenoidal encephalocoele

32 An MR of the spine in a neonate reveals two separate hemichords in two separate dural tubes.

Which type of split cord malformation does this represent?
(a) Type I
(b) Type II
(c) Type III
(d) Type IV
(e) Type V

33 A 55 year old has unilateral visual loss. An ocular US demonstrates an echogenic, posterior segment mass of a 'cottage loaf' appearance. Doppler imaging reveals blood flow within.

What is the most likely diagnosis?
(a) Choroidal melanoma
(b) Metastasis
(c) Retinoblastoma
(d) Vitreous haemorrhage
(e) Vitreo-retinal traction

34 An elderly man is found collapsed, and a CT head is performed. The ventricles are noted to be prominent.

Which of the following features would support the diagnosis of hydrocephalus over cerebral atrophy?

(a) Concave profile of the third ventricle on axial images
(b) Enlarged choroidal-hippocampal fissures
(c) Normal fornix-corpus callosum distance
(d) Atrophy of the corpus callosum
(e) Mammillo-pontine distance of less than 1 cm

35 A patient with facial numbness has an MRI of the brain. A lesion lying entirely within the cavernous sinus is revealed.

Given this location, which of the following cranial nerves is least likely to be involved?

(a) Oculomotor nerve
(b) Trochlear nerve
(c) Abducens nerve
(d) The first division of the trigeminal nerve
(e) The third division of the trigeminal nerve

36 An immunocompromised patient develops progressive neurological deficits. Confluent, bilateral white matter lesions are seen in the parieto-occipital region on MR imaging. Progressive multifocal leukoencephalopathy is suspected.

Which of the following conditions is not known to be associated with PML?

(a) Whipple disease
(b) Migraine
(c) AIDS
(d) Cancer
(e) Sarcoid

37 A middle aged man is found collapsed, with a GCS of 5/15. A CT head (performed without *i.v.* contrast medium administration) reveals increased attenuation material within the basal cisterns, superior cerebellar cistern and cortical sulci.

Which of the following conditions is not associated with the likely underlying diagnosis?

(a) Intra-cerebral arterio-venous malformation
(b) Eclampsia
(c) Hypertension
(d) MELAS
(e) Tumour

38 A patient presents with headache. A CT head is performed. After the administration of intravenous contrast medium, a dural pattern of enhancement is noted.

Which of the following is most likely to produce this pattern?

(a) Infarction
(b) Intracranial hypotension
(c) Subarachnoid haemorrhage
(d) Sturge-Weber syndrome
(e) A normal variant

39 Plain skull radiographs are performed. A possible abnormality is identified, and a CT head is requested.

Which of the following measurements is abnormal?

(a) The tip of the odontoid process is 7 mm above McGregor's Line
(b) The basal angle is 130 degrees
(c) There are 3 Wormian bones
(d) The largest Wormian bone is 3 x 3 mm
(e) The basal angle is 125 degrees

40 A man is brought into A&E unconscious after near-drowning. His GCS was 5/15. A CT head was performed.

Which of the following imaging features would be unusual for this condition?

(a) Diffuse cerebral oedema
(b) Loss of grey-white distinction
(c) Surface blood vessels which appear dark relative to brain
(d) Relative sparing of the cerebellum
(e) Generalised decrease of the attenuation of the cerebral parenchyma

41 A patient presents with suspected neurofibromatosis type 1.

Of the following lists of features, which would not be sufficient to make the diagnosis?

(a) 6 *cafe-au-lait* macules and two neurofibromas
(b) A Lisch nodule and an optic nerve glioma
(c) Thinning of long bone cortex and axillary freckling
(d) A first-degree relative with NF-1 and inguinal freckling
(e) A plexiform neurofibroma and a sphenoid dysplasia

42 An adolescent presents to A&E after trauma and facial radiographs are taken. No fracture is seen, but incidental note is made of a cystic lesion, related to the crown of an un-erupted tooth. It is unilocular.

What is this most likely to represent?

(a) Radicular cyst
(b) Dentigerous cyst
(c) Primordial cyst
(d) Aneurysmal bone cyst
(e) Osteoclastoma

43 An elderly patient presents with confusion. A CT head reveals a lesion involving the corpus callosum and invading both frontal lobes. There is enhancement of the lesion periphery after the administration of intravenous contrast medium.

What is the most likely diagnosis?

(a) Abscess
(b) Radiation necrosis
(c) Meningioma
(d) Infarction
(e) Glioblastoma multiforme

44 A young man presents with a fever, stiff neck and headache. CSF studies reveal a raised protein concentration, a predominance of polymorphonuclear leukocytes and a low glucose concentration.

Which of the following would be the most atypical imaging appearance for the most likely diagnosis?

(a) Normal unenhanced CT
(b) Normal unenhanced MR
(c) Hypointense plaques on T2W MR imaging
(d) Obliteration of the basal cisterns on contrast-enhanced CT
(e) Increased attenuation of the subarachnoid space on unenhanced CT

45 A young patient suffers seemingly trivial trauma to the neck and subsequently presents with acute onset focal weakness. Arterial dissection is suspected.

Regarding arterial dissection of the head and neck, which of the following is incorrect?

(a) Dissection of the internal carotid artery is more common than vertebral artery dissection
(b) Vertebral dissection is commonest at the C4-5 level
(c) Stroke occurs earlier with intracranial, rather than extracranial dissection
(d) Periarterial rim of high signal can be seen on T1 W
(e) Neck pain and headache are present in the majority

46 A middle aged lady presents with bilateral proptosis. There is eyelid retraction and lid lag on downgaze. CT demonstrates bilateral enlargement of the extraoccular muscles with sparing of the tendons.

Given the most likely disease process, which of the following would one expect to be affected last?

(a) Superior rectus
(b) Inferior rectus
(c) Medial rectus
(d) Lateral rectus
(e) Oblique muscles

47 A pregnant lady patient presents with headache and a focal neurological deficit. A non-enhanced CT shows increased attenuation in the superior sagittal sinus. Following the administration of intravenous contrast medium, the dura surrounding the sinus enhances but the sinus itself does not. MR imaging is performed.

Given the most likely diagnosis, which appearances would be unusual for this condition?

(a) Low T2W signal intensity at 2 days
(b) Iso/high T1W signal intensity in 20 days
(c) High T1W signal intensity in 10 days
(d) Low T2W signal intensity in 20 days
(e) High T2W signal intensity in 10 days

48 An MRI examination of the brain reveals multiple metastases which affect the superior orbital fissure, the optic canal and foramen ovale.

Which of the following structures is least likely to be affected?

(a) 3rd cranial nerve
(b) Accessory meningeal artery
(c) 6th cranial nerve
(d) 2nd division of the 1st cranial nerve
(e) 4th cranial nerve

49 A patient presents with unilateral hearing loss. CT demonstrates a non-dependent expansile mass within the middle ear with bony erosion of the sigmoid sinus plate, scutum and ossicles. MR imaging reveals that the mass has high signal on both T1 weighted fat saturation and T2 weighted acquisitions.

What is the diagnosis?

(a) Glomus tumour
(b) Cholesteatoma (congenital)
(c) Cholesteatoma (acquired)
(d) Cholesterol granuloma
(e) Schwannoma

50 A CT head demonstrates a dilated lateral and third ventricle with a normal sized fourth ventricle.

Which of the following would most likely account for this appearance?

(a) Colloid cyst
(b) Pinealoma
(c) Tonsillar herniation
(d) Choroid plexus papilloma
(e) Basilar impression

Central Nervous System and Head Practice SBA Answers

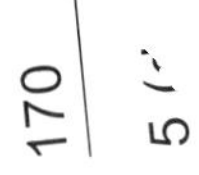

1 (c)
Optic nerve glioma is the most common cause of diffuse optic nerve enlargement. NF-1 is present in 25%. Kinking and buckling of the optic nerve is common. Calcification, hyperostosis, and the 'tram-track' sign (linear bands of enhancement) are features more typical of meningioma.

Ref: Aids to Radiological Differential Diagnosis, 4th Ed, p. 383.

2 (a)
Pinealoblastomas are associated with bilateral retinoblastomas (the combination producing the so-called 'trilateral retinoblastoma').

Ref: Primer of Diagnostic Imaging, 4th Ed, p. 546.

3 (d)
MR spectroscopy interrogates the chemical environment of intra-cerebral lesions: elevated choline is associated with high cellular turnover as found in neoplasms. Tumours are often centred upon white matter with relative sparing of the overlying cortex. Gyriform enhancement is unusual in neoplasms unless there is meningeal disease. In the acute stage, an infarct will demonstrate restricted diffusion: high signal on the DWI image and low signal on the ADC image. Cytotoxic oedema is typical of infarcts, whilst vasogenic oedema is typical of neoplasms.

Ref: Aids to Radiological Differential Diagnosis, 4th Ed, p. 402 & Neuroradiology: the requisites, 2nd Ed, p. 22.

4 (b)
Hashimoto's thyroiditis is the most common cause of goitrous hypothyroidism. Diagnosis is usually biased on serology rather than imaging. The appearances depend upon the stage of the disease: small avascular hypoechoic foci in the acute phase, followed by the chronic appearances described in the question and then by a small, end-stage, heterogeneous gland. None of the other conditions are associated with fibrous, echogenic septae.

Ref: RITI 6a_058 Ultrasound of the Thyroid and Parathyroid Glands.

)
The CNS features of tuberous sclerosis include: subependymal nodules which increase in number and calcification with time; parenchymal tubers which are *non-enhancing* and *rarely calcifed*; hydrocephalus; giant cell astrocytomas; retinal phakomas; arterial ectasia.

Ref: Aids to Radiological Differential Diagnosis, 4th Ed, p. 620.

6 (d)
A complex of anomalies secondary to a small posterior fossa. The falx is hypoplastic/ fenestrated, with concomitant gyral interdigitation. A summary of the major features: the 4th ventricle and brainstem are caudally displaced, there is tonsillar herniation, a myelomenigiocoele, syringohydromelia, dygenesis of the corpus callosum, obstructive hydrocephalus, absence of the septum pellucidum, and stenogyria.

Ref: Radiology Review Manual, 6th Ed, p. 275-276.

7 (e)

	Radiation injury	**Tumour recurrence**
MR spectroscopy	Decreased choline peak	Decreased NAA peak Increased choline peak
CT perfusion: relative cerebral blood volume (rCBV)	rCBV low	rCBV high
Thallium SPECT	Deceased activity	Increased activity

Ref: RITI 6b_122 Radiation injury.

8 ([illegible])
Haemangiopericytoma is the only intra-axial mass listed.

Ref: RITI 6b_120 Intracranial metastases: Imaging and differential diagnosis.

9 (b)
99mTc-HMPAO SPECT ictal imaging is the most sensitive examination.

Ref: RITI 7n_005 HMPAO 2.

10 (d)
Of the listed options, only nerve sheath tumours, meningiomas and leptomeningeal metastasis are typically intradural and extramedullary (chordomas are extradural and astrocytomas are intramedullary). Although nerve sheath tumours are more common, meningiomas are more likely if the tumour is solitary, posterior and does not contain areas of low signal intensity on T2W.

Ref: RITI 6b_126 Spinal extramedullary tumours.

11 (e)
Parkinson's disease, Lewy-body dementia and 'Parkinson's plus' syndromes (*e.g.* progressive supranuclear palsy, corticobasal degeneration and multiple system atrophy) all cause a significant reduction of uptake of ^{123}I-ioflupane in the corpus striatum.

Ref: RITI 7n_001 Theory and practice of imaging in Parkinson's Disease.

12 (c)
The Spetzler-Martin scheme is used to grade AVMs. Points are allocated according to size of the nidus (< 3 cm, 1 point; 3 – 6 cm, 2 points; > 6 cm 3 points), location (non-eloquent brain, 0 points; eloquent brain, 1 point), and venous drainage (superficial drainage only, 0 points; deep, 1 point). The more points, the worse the prognosis. Surrounding areas of low T2W signal are likely to be due to old haemorrhage.

Ref: Clinical Neuroradiology: A Case-Based Approach, 1st Ed, p. 133–4.

13 (e)
^{99m}Tc-Pertechnetate localises to the thyroid but not the parathyroid gland. This feature is exploited in combined studies where the ^{99m}Tc-Pertechnetate scintigram is subtracted from a similarly acquired study using thallium-201 (which localises to both thyroid and parathyroid tissue).

Ref: Clin Rad (2004); 59:967–976.

14 (d)
Neurosyphillis causes a large and medium sized vessel arteritis, which can result in infarcts in the brain stem, basal ganglia and MCA territory. Syphillitic gummas are a further imaging manifestation.

Ref: Clin Rad (2006); 61:393–401.

15 (a)
A pilocytic astrocytoma is the most likely diagnosis. This is the most common paediatric glioma, and the characteristic appearance is of a cyst with an intensely enhancing mural nodule. Surrounding oedema is rare. 40% of patients with both NF-1 and an optic pathway glioma also suffer from precious puberty.
Ref: Radiographics (2004); 24:1693–1708.

16 (b)
The ischaemic penumbra is indicated by increased mean transit time (MTT) with either moderately decreased cerebral blood flow (CBF) and normal / increased cerebral blood volume (CBV) or markedly reduced CBF and moderately reduced CBV. Infarcted tissue has an increased MTT with severe reductions in both CBF and CBV.
Ref: Radiographics (2006); 26:S75-95.

17 (c)
This patient is suffering from normal pressure hydrocephalus, a potentially treatable cause of dementia in the elderly. Appearances are of communicating hydrocephalus, with ventricles dilated out of proportion to sulcal effacement, upward bowing of the corpus callosum, a pronounced aquaductal flow void on MRI, periventricular hyperintensity, and reflux of indium ^{111}In-DTPA into the lateral ventricles.
Ref: Neuroradiology: the requisites, 2nd Ed, p. 376.

18 (b)

Time	CT appearances
0–2 hours (hyperacute)	Mean attenuation 40-60 HU
3–48 hours (acute)	Mean attenuation 60-80 HU ± fluid / fluid levels
3–7 days (subacute)	High density 'core' with low density periphery (vasogenic oedema)
2–4 weeks (chronic)	Density decreases from periphery to centre ± peripheral enhancement

Ref: Aids to Radiological Differential Diagnosis, 4th Ed, p. 404.

19 (b)
Astrocytomas and ependymomas can have similar MR appearances, but astrocytomas are much more common in the paediatric population. Intramedullary metastases are relatively rare.

Ref: Aids to Radiological Differential Diagnosis, 4th Ed, p. 91.

20 (a)
Diffuse axonal injury is most likely to affect the lobar grey/ white matter junction, the corpus callosum, the dorso-lateral brainstem and the internal capsule. There is relative sparing of the cortex.

Ref: RITI 6b_060 Diffuse Brain Injury.

21. (a)
Subfalcine is the commonest type of herniation.

Ref: RITI 6b_060 Diffuse Brain Injury.

22 (b)
The staging is: T1: tumour 2 cm or less, confined to the thyroid. T2: tumour > 2 cm but < 4 cm, confined to the thyroid. T3: tumour > 4 cm, limited to the thyroid; or any tumour with limited extension. T4: a) extension into the subcutaneous tissues, larynx, trachea, oesophagus or recurrent laryngeal nerve; b) extension into the prevertebral fascia or encases the carotid artery/ mediastinal vessels. There is no T5.

Ref: Neuroradiology: the requisites, 2nd Ed, p. 741.

23 (b)
The glomus body tumours classically splay the internal and external carotid arteries apart. They are highly vascular, and therefore typically enhance rapidly and demonstrate flow voids on MRI. They are usually isodense on CT imaging.

Ref: Neuroradiology: the requisites, 2nd Ed, p. 725.

24 (c)
Dolan only defined three lines (orbital, zygomatic and maxillary) – all can be disrupted by a tripod fracture.

Ref: RITI 6a_024 Trauma of the face, orbit and mandible.

25 (d)
This patient suffers from 'Cerebral autosomal dominant arteriopathy with subcortical infarcts and leukoencephalopathy' (CADASIL). Symptoms include migraine in the 3rd decade, recurrent stroke, and early-onset dementia. The extension of white matter hypoattenuation into the temporal poles is virtually pathognomonic of CADASIL.

Ref: RITI 6b_081 - Unusual causes of stroke.

26 (e)
Scalloping of the adjacent bone, possibly through transmitted pulsations, is often seen in arachnoid cysts. This is never seen in subdural hygromas, but can be seen with epidermoid cysts or porencephaly.

Ref: Neuroradiology: the requisites, 2nd Ed, p. 417.

27 (a)
The basal ganglia has the 'eye of the tiger' appearance. In combination with the hereditary movement disorder, this suggests Hallervodern-Spatz disease. Other causes of this sign include: CO poisoning, corticobasal ganglionic degeneration, Leigh syndrome, neurofibromatosis, progressive supranuclear palsy, Shy-Drager syndrome, toxins.

Ref: Neuroradiology: the requisites, 2nd Ed, p. 393.

28 (d)
Although pleomorphic adenoma are the most common lesion, well circumscribed multiple/ bilateral parotid masses in an asymptomatic patient should be considered Warthin's tumours.

Ref: Diagnostic Imaging: Head and Neck, 1st Ed, p. III-7-20.

29 (c)
The content of an arachnoid cyst has the same characteristics as CSF on all MR imaging sequences.

Ref: Primer of Diagnostic Imaging, 4th Ed, p. 624.

30 (c)
There are focal neurological signs in approximately one third of cases of subarachnoid haemorrhage. Seizures occur in 6–16% of cases, altered consciousness in 2%, subhyaloid haemorrhages in 10%; vertigo is a recognised feature but rare.

Ref: RITI 6b_093 SAH: Acute investigation, treatment and prevention.

31 (b)
The above is a description of Dandy Walker variant. By contrast, in Dandy Walker complex the cerebellar hemispheres and vermis are both absent or hypoplastic and the brainstem is compressed by a cyst. In mega cisterna magna, the cerebellum is normal and there is a simple dilatation of the CSF space posterior to the cerebellum.

Ref: RITI 6b_151 Craniospinal congenital malformations.

32 (a)
This is a type I malformation, also known as diastematomyelia. A type II malformation comprises two hemicords within a single dural tube, also known as diplomyelia. There are no type III, IV or V malformations.

Ref: RITI 6b_151 Craniospinal congenital malformations.

33 (a)
The 'cottage loaf' appearance derives from the tumour breaking through the basal lamina of the choroid, and is said to be specific for choroidal melanoma.

Ref: RITI 6a_028 Orbits (2) Ocular ultrasound.

34 (e)
Indicators of hydrocephalus include: dilatation of the recesses of the third ventricle, convexity of the third ventricle, expansion of the temporal horns, effacement of sulci, narrowing of the mamillopontine distance, and enlargement of the ventricles out of proportion to the sulcal dilatation. Specific MR findings include: transependymal CSF exudation (seen as high signal on FLAIR imaging), and accentuation of the aqueductal flow void in normal pressure hydrocephalus.

Ref: Neuroradiology: the requisites, 2nd Ed, p. 371.

35 (e)
The cavernous sinus contains the III, IV, V_1, V_2 and VI cranial nerves.

Ref: Clinically Oriented Anatomy, 5th Ed, p. 914.

36 (b)
Other associated conditions include: autoimmune diseases, immunosuppressive therapies, Lympho- and myeloproliferative disorders, nontropical sprue, transplantation, and tuberculosis.

Ref: Neuroradiology: the requisites, 2nd Ed, p. 350.

37 (d)
Subarachnoid haemorrhage is described. It is associated with a ruptured aneurysm in 70% of cases, and an AVM in 10%. Other causes include: hypertension, tumour haemorrhage, embolic infarction, blood dyscrasia, eclampsia, and intracranial infection. SAH is cryptogenic in approximately 5%.

Ref: Radiology Review Manual, 6th Ed, p. 327.

38 (b)
A 'dural', rather than 'leptomeningeal', pattern of enhancement can be seen in: infection, tumour, intracranial hypotension, post-operative states, idiopathic pachymeningitis, venous thrombosis, sarcoidosis, extramedullary haematopoesis, and rheumatoid arthritis.

Ref: Aids to Radiological Differential Diagnosis, 4th Ed, p. 431.

39 (a)
The tip of the odontoid process should lie less than 5 mm above McGregor's Line. The basal angle (the angulation between the floor of the anterior cranial fossa and the clivus) should be less than 140 degrees. Wormian bones should be less than 10 in number and less than 6 x 4 mm in size. Cranial sutures should be < 10 mm at birth, < 3 mm at 2 years old, and < 2 mm at 3 years old.

Ref: Aids to Radiological Differential Diagnosis, 4th Ed, p. 421.

40 (c)
In profound hypoxia, the surface blood vessels can appear bright relative to the brain parenchyma, an appearance which may be confused for subarachnoid blood. The cerebellum is often relatively spared, which leads to the 'bright cerebellum' sign.

Ref: Clin Rad (2007); 62:404-15.

41 (c)
At least two of the following seven criteria must be fulfilled for a diagnosis: ≥ 6 *cafe-au-lait* spots, ≥ 2 neurofibromas of any type (or one plexiform neurofibroma), freckling of the axillary or inguinal region, optic glioma, ≥ 2 Lisch nodules, a distinctive osseous lesion such as sphenoid dysplasia or thinning of long bone cortex, a first-degree relative with NF-1.

Ref: Clin Rad (2005); 60:960–7.

42 (b)
This is most likely to be a dentigerous cyst, which occurs when there is cystic degeneration of tooth enamel before eruption. They are usually unilocular and (unlike the more common radicular cyst) are intimately related to the crown.

Ref: A Textbook of Radiology and Imaging, 5th Ed, p. 1542.

43 (e)
A ring-enhancing lesion that crosses the midline may represent, amongst other conditions, a glioblastoma multiforme ('a butterfly glioma'), astrocytoma or lymphoma. Abscesses rarely cross the midline. An infarct is less likely as the above distribution does not correspond to a single arterial territory.

Ref: Radiology Review Manual, 6th Ed, p. 247.

44 (c)
Hyperintense, rather than hypointense plaques are a recognised T2-weighted MR imaging finding in bacterial meningitis. Most cases of bacterial meningitis will have normal non-enhanced MR imaging.

Ref: Radiology Review Manual, 6th Ed, p. 308.

45 (b)
Vertebral dissection is most common at the C1-2 level. Stroke may be delayed for several hours in extracranial dissections. The periarterial rim of high signal on T1W represents intramural haematoma.

Ref: Emergencies in Clinical Radiology, 1st Ed, p. 220.

46 (e)
The patient is suffering from thyroid-associated orbitopathy. The muscles are affected in the following order: inferior, medial, superior, lateral, oblique muscles (mnemonic "I'M SLO").

Ref: Diagnostic Imaging: Head and Neck, 1st Ed, p. II-1-70.

47 (d)
This patient has suffered a venous sinus thrombosis. The pattern of signal intensities is as follows: Acute (< 5 days): T1W isointense, T2W low; Subacute: T1W high, T2W high; Chronic: T1W isointense/ high, T2W, isointense/ high.

Ref: Emergencies in Clinical Radiology, 1st Ed, p. 213.

48 (d)
The 2nd division of the 1st cranial nerve (the maxillary nerve) passes through the foramen rotundum.

Ref: Clinically oriented anatomy, 5th Ed, p. 846.

49 (c)
A cholesterol granuloma is an inflammatory mass of granulation tissue due to recurrent haemorrhage into the middle ear. Characteristically, there is high signal on both T1-fat saturation imaging and on T2-weighted imaging.

Ref: RITI 6a_017b Petrous temporal bone: infection, cholesteatoma and glomus tumour.

50 (b)
The pattern of dilatation is consistent with obstruction at the level of the aqueduct – of the options listed, a pinealoma is most likely to cause obstruction at this level.

Ref: Clinical Imaging: An Atlas of Differential Diagnosis, 4th Ed, p. 1040.

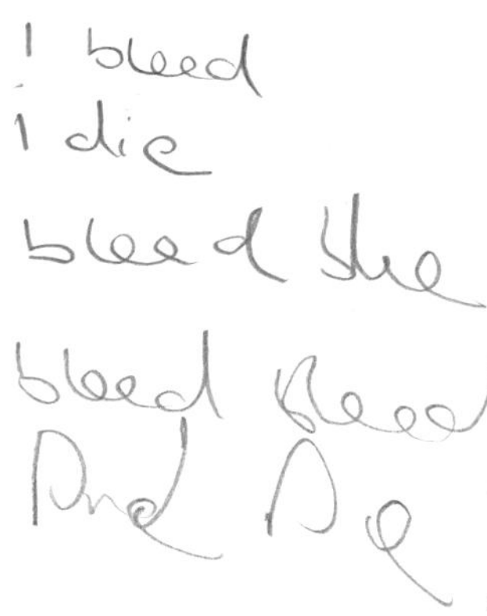

Section 2:
Mock Papers

Cardiothoracic and Vascular Mock Paper Questions

1 **A 36 year old man has returned from a long adventure holiday in South-Eastern USA. He had an episode of fever, dry cough and polyarthralgia. He still has dyspnoea and on examination is noted to have erythema nodosum on his shins. CXR shows diffuse bilateral tiny calcific nodules, some with central calcification, and hilar and mediastinal 'popcorn' calcified lymphadenopathy.**

What is the most likely diagnosis?
(a) Acute sarcoidosis
(b) Histoplasmosis
(c) Langerhans Cell Histiocytosis
(d) TB
(e) Varicella pneumonia

2 **A 35 year old Japanese man with a long history of mouth ulceration and a recent diagnosis of posterior uveitis presents to the emergency department with breathlessness. A CTPA is performed which demonstrates bilateral pulmonary emboli.**

What is the most likely diagnosis?
(a) Sarcoidosis
(b) Systemic Lupus Erythematosus
(c) Behcet's disease
(d) Polyarteritis nodosa
(e) Amyloidosis

3 A 27 year old woman is under investigation for renovascular hypertension. Selective angiograms of the renal arteries show bilateral stenoses of the mid main renal artery with further focal stenoses more distally and multiple aneurysmal dilations of the arteries.

What is the most likely sub-type of fibromuscular dysplasia in this patient?

(a) Adventitial fibroplasias
(b) Intima fibroplasia
(c) Medial dissection
(d) Medial fibroplasia
(e) Medial hyperplasia

4 Regarding lung transplantation, which of the following conditions would not be suitable for a single lung transplant, and would necessitate a double-lung transplantation?

(a) Bronchiectasis
(b) Emphysema
(c) Idiopathic pulmonary fibrosis
(d) Primary pulmonary hypertension
(e) Sarcoid

5 You are asked to report the CXR of a 58 year old man. The request form simply states 'shortness of breath', there are no previous films available for comparison. There is bibasal atelectasis and pleural calcification is seen within the right hemithorax.

What is the least likely of the following diagnoses?

(a) Berylliosis
(b) Prior haemothorax
(c) Radiation therapy
(d) Talcosis
(e) Tuberculosis

6 **Which of the following is not an accepted indication to choose CO_2 angiography?**

(a) EVAR stent procedure
(b) Fluoroscopic angiography where DSA unavailable
(c) IVC filter placement
(d) Previous anaphlaxis post-IVU
(e) Serum creatinine of 190 μmol/L

7 **A 64 year old woman presents with dyspnoea. CXR shows reticulonodular opacities and coarsened bronchovascular marking only within the right lower zone. HRCT shows focal RLL thickening of peribronchovascular interstitium, interlobular septa and fissures with preservation of normal parenchymal architecture.**

What is the most likely underlying cancer?
(a) Bronchogenic
(b) Cervical
(c) Gastric
(d) Ovarian
(e) Thyroid

8 **After squamous cell carcinoma, which is the next most common tumour of the trachea?**

(a) Adenoid cystic carcinoma
(b) Muco-epidermoid tumour
(c) Carcinoid
(d) Squamous cell papilloma
(e) Lymphoma

9 A 45 year old man is referred from chest clinic with a cough and intermittent breathlessness. A CT of his thorax demonstrates ill-defined centrilobular nodules and a mosaic attenuation pattern, exacerbated on expiratory phase imaging.

What is the most likely diagnosis?

(a) Respiratory bronchilitis-interstitial lung disease
(b) Chronic pulmonary thrombo-embolism
(c) Sarcoidosis
(d) Extrinsic allergic alveolitis
(e) Lymphocytic interstitial pneumonitis

10 A diagnostic lower limb angiogram is to be performed. Which of the following guidewires is appropriate in order to site the pigtail catheter in the aorta following a standard retrograde common femoral artery puncture?

(a) Amplatz
(b) J-wire
(c) Mandrel
(d) Straight wire
(e) Terumo

11 A 67 year old lady presents with chest pain and shortness of breath ten days after hip replacement surgery. She is known to have COPD. A CT-pulmonary angiogram is requested.

Which of the following factors is more likely to increase the risk of a severe idiosyncratic reaction to iodinated contrast medium?

(a) Asthma
(b) Creatinine > 133 μmol/L
(c) Metformin
(d) NSAIDs
(e) Type-2 diabetes mellitus

12 A 32 year old man presents to his GP with increasing shortness of breath. He has never smoked. The initial bloods show a normal full blood count, but abnormal liver function. A CXR is requested and shows emphysematous change within both lower zones only. A subsequent CT is requested.

What sub-type of emphysema is likely to be seen?

(a) Centriacinar emphysema
(b) Centrilobular emphysema
(c) Panacinar emphysema
(d) Paracicatricial emphysema
(e) Paraseptal emphysema

13 Which of the following drugs used in treating patients with haematological malignancy is not associated with pulmonary haemorrhage?

(a) Bleomycin
(b) Cytarabine
(c) Amphotericin B
(d) Rituximab
(e) Cyclophosphamide

14 A 63 year old smoker presents with pain in the right arm. On examination there is wasting of the small muscles in the right hand, ptosis and miosis of the right eye. CXR shows right apical pleural thickening and an associated mass.

What is the most likely tumour type?

(a) Large cell
(b) Mesothelioma
(c) Oat cell
(d) Reed-Sternberg cell
(e) Squamous cell

15 A man with a long smoking history is found to have a subpleural 2.5 cm lesion in the left lower lobe. His FEV-1 is 1.5 L and clotting is normal. He is consented for a CT-guided biopsy of the lesion.

What is the commonest occurring complication from this procedure?

(a) Air embolism
(b) Haemoptysis
(c) Infection
(d) Pneumothorax
(e) Tumour seeding

16 Which of the following CT signs is the most specific for a diagnosis of pulmonary hypertension?

(a) Aorta:pulmonary artery ratio > 1.0
(b) Main pulmonary artery diameter ≥ 2.9 cm
(c) Mosaic perfusion pattern
(d) Reflux of contrast into IVC
(e) Segmental artery:bronchus ratio > 1.0 in ≥ 3 lobes

17 A 25 year old woman has a CXR for insurance purposes. There is a 2 cm well-circumscribed lesion in the periphery of the RLL. The subsequent CT demonstrates fat and calcification within the lesion; no other lesions are identified.

What two further conditions, if present, would make the diagnosis part of Carney's triad?

(a) Atrial myxoma and extra-adrenal paraganglioma
(b) Atrial myxoma and pituitary adenoma
(c) Breast fibroadenoma and pituitary adenoma
(d) Gastric leiomyosarcoma and breast fibroadenoma
(e) Gastric leiomyosarcoma and extra-adrenal paraganglioma

18 A 2 day old neonate presents with difficulty in breathing. On examination there are widespread crepitations. The CXR shows florid pulmonary oedema.

Which of the following congenital heart anomalies would be the most likely cause of these appearances?

(a) Atrial septal defect
(b) Hypoplastic Left Heart Syndrome
(c) Pulmonary atresia
(d) Tetralogy of Fallot
(e) Ventricular septal defect

19 An adolescent male patient presents with dyspnoea, cough, and complains of feeling increasingly tired. The subsequent CXR shows a mass located within the anterior mediastinum.

Which of the following is the most likely diagnosis?

(a) Bochdalek hernia
(b) Bronchopulmonary foregut malformation
(c) Extramedullary haemopoeisis
(d) Germ cell tumour
(e) Neuroblastoma

20 With regard to cardiac MRI, which of the following is not true?

(a) In balanced-steady state free precession images stationary blood is bright
(b) Gradient echo sequences are not flow-sensitive
(c) In balanced-steady state free precession images flowing blood is bright
(d) Triple inversion recovery sequences are sensitive for myocardial oedema
(e) T1-weighted spin-echo sequences show blood as black

21 A 58 year old patient has a chest CT 6 months after resection of a primary lung tumour. There are noted to be new ipsilateral superior mediastinal and supraclavicular lymph nodes measuring 6–8 mm. An ^{18}FDG-PET/CT is requested for further evaluation.

Which of the following is not a routine part of the pre-scan preparation?

(a) Inject FDG tracer 15 minutes prior to imaging
(b) Check blood glucose level prior to tracer injection
(c) No food for 6 hours prior to imaging
(d) No talking for 30 minutes prior to imaging
(e) No jogging for 24–48 hours prior to imaging

22 Regarding coronary artery fistulas, which of the following statements is true?

(a) They are seen in 1% of cases undergoing coronary angiography
(b) They account for 5% of congenital cardiac abnormalities
(c) They are seen more commonly in men
(d) They are most commonly congenital
(e) They most commonly drain in to the right atrium

23 A 53 year old man presents with right calf swelling. He had a previous right leg DVT treated 5 years previously at another hospital and describes the current symptoms as being similar. US shows echoic material extending 5 cm within the mid right SFV.

What feature most strongly supports a diagnosis of acute DVT over chronic changes from his previous DVT?

(a) Enlarged vein diameter
(b) Hyperechoic material in the vein
(c) Non-compressible vein
(d) Presence of collateral veins
(e) Vein wall thickening

24 A patient undergoing induction chemotherapy for the treatment of acute myeloid leukaemia undergoes a chest CT. This shows several foci of consolidation with a halo of ground glass opacification.

What is the most likely diagnosis?

(a) Leukaemic infiltrate
(b) Mycobacterium avium infection
(c) Klebsiella spp. infection
(d) Pulmonary thromboembolic disease
(e) Angioinvasive aspergillosis

25 With regard to coronary artery calcium scoring, which of the following is not true?

(a) The absence of calcification makes atherosclerotic disease very unlikely
(b) Calcification is highly specific for atherosclerotic disease
(c) Calcium is expressed as the Hounsfield score
(d) Calcification may progress at up to 25% per year
(e) Lipid lowering drugs may stop progression of calcification

26 A 64 year old man undergoes nephrectomy for a right renal tumour. A year later he presents with haemoptysis. CT of the chest shows 3 lesions in the right hemithorax measuring 20 × 10 mm, 20 × 12 mm and 10 × 10 mm. Biopsy confirms these are metastases. After a course of chemotherapy, the lesions measure 18 × 8 mm, 17 × 10 mm and 10 × 8 mm.

By RECIST criteria the status of the disease is?

(a) Stable disease
(b) Partial response
(c) Good response
(d) Excellent response
(e) No response

27 **A 68 year old man presents with a lower GI haemorrhage. He is fluid resuscitated and an angiogram is performed to localise the site of bleeding. Initial selective angiogram of the IMA shows a distal bleeding point within the pelvis.**

Which of the following arteries is the more likely source of the bleed?

(a) Median sacral
(b) Middle rectal
(c) Sigmoid
(d) Inferior epigastric
(e) Internal pudendal

28 **A routine CXR in a 30 year old man demonstrates bilateral inferior rib notching.**

Which of the following is least likely to cause this?

(a) Normal variation
(b) Coarctation of the aorta
(c) Hyperparathyroidism
(d) Neurofibromatosis type 2
(e) Thalassaemia

29 **A 62 year old otherwise well woman presents with chronic and progressive dysponea. CXR reveals fine reticular opacification in the upper zones bilaterally with volume loss.**

Which of the following is the likeliest diagnosis?

(a) Tuberous sclerosis
(b) Extrinsic allegic alveolitis
(c) Sarcoidosis
(d) Usual interstitial pneumonitis
(e) Ankylosing spondylitis

30 A 24 year old lady, 27 weeks pregnant, presents with chest pain and you are contacted for imaging advice.

Which of the following is not a risk factor/ indicator of pulmonary embolism?

(a) Raised D-dimer
(b) Gestational diabetes
(c) Thrombophilia
(d) Obesity
(e) Multiparity

31 A 55 year old man undergoes a CT to assess pleural thickening previously noted on a chest radiograph.

Which of the following features is not an indicator of malignancy?

(a) Involves mediastinal pleural surface
(b) Depth greater than 1 cm
(c) Volume loss
(d) Nodularity
(e) Pleural effusion

32 Plain radiographic signs seen more commonly in patients with acute pulmonary embolism include all but which of the following?

(a) Cardiomegaly
(b) Decreased vascularity
(c) Pulmonary oedema
(d) Pleural opacity
(e) Atelectasis

33 An 18 year old woman with proven hydatid disease of the liver presents with chest pain and fever. She has a CXR which shows an 8 cm cystic lesion in the right lung.

Which of the following features would be least expected in lung echinococcosis?

(a) Calcification of the cyst wall
(b) Water lily sign
(c) An air/fluid level within cyst
(d) Ground glass change around the cyst
(e) The size of the lesion

34 A 50 year old woman with a history of scleroderma and a 30 pack per year smoking history presents with a cough. CXR shows a 1.2 cm peripheral nodule in the right lower lobe. CT confirms the nodule is solitary and is of mixed attenuation with a ground glass appearance. There is no mediastinal lymphadenopathy. Repeat interval CT at 6 weeks, after treatment with antibiotics, shows the lesion has remained stable in size but there is some evidence of cavitation. ^{18}FDG-PET is performed and found to be negative.

The likeliest diagnosis is?

(a) Bronchoalveolar carcinoma
(b) Squamous cell carcinoma
(c) Atypical infection
(d) Carcinoid
(e) Adenocarcinoma

35 Which of the following is considered an absolute indication for an IVC filter?

(a) DVT/PE and limited cardiopulmonary reserve
(b) Iliocaval DVT
(c) High risk of DVT/PE in peri-operative setting
(d) High risk of DVT/PE following trauma
(e) PE/DVT and complication of anticoagulation

36 A 58 year old man undergoes an uncomplicated pneumonectomy for lung cancer.

Which of the following signs on CXR is considered abnormal?

(a) Opacification of 1/3 of the pneumonectomy hemithorax within 24 hours
(b) Depression of the hemidiaphragm on the pneumonectomy side
(c) Apical herniation of the unaffected lung to the pneumonectomy side
(d) Shift of the mediastinum to the pneumonectomy side
(e) Opacification of 2/3 of the hemithorax on the pneumonectomy side within 7 days

37 A 3 year old boy who has recently arrived in the UK presents to A&E. His mother explains that he has suffered repeated respiratory infections from the neonatal period. CXR shows bilateral lower zone bronchiectasis and dextrocardia.

What is the likeliest diagnosis?

(a) Cystic fibrosis
(b) Kartagener's syndrome
(c) Yellow nail syndrome
(d) Pulmonary sequestration
(e) Tuberculosis

38 Regarding catheters used for interventional angiography.

Which of the following catheters is inappropriate for imaging the respective artery?

(a) Bernstein – superior mesenteric artery
(b) Cobra – renal artery
(c) Pigtail – abdominal aorta
(d) Sidewinder (Simmons) – coeliac axis
(e) Straight catheter – iliac artery

39 A 74 year old man presents with progressive dyspnoea. CXR shows bilateral, lower zone, peripheral subpleural reticulation.

Which of the following is least likely?

(a) Amiodarone toxicity
(b) Usual interstitial pneumonitis
(c) Asbestosis
(d) Rheumatoid arthritis
(e) Chronic extrinsic allergic alveolitis

40 A 50 year old man is found to have a 3.5 cm round, well-defined, right lower lobe nodule on CXR. CT examination shows the lesion is solitary and contains areas of fat.

The likeliest diagnosis is?

(a) Carcinoid
(b) Bronchoalveolar carcinoma
(c) Pulmonary teratoma
(d) Pulmonary hamartoma
(e) Pulmonary lipoma

41 Which of the following is not a risk factor for developing radiation pneumonitis?

(a) Withdrawal of steroids
(b) Increasing interval between radiotherapy fractions
(c) Concomitant chemotherapy
(d) Pulmonary fibrosis
(e) Smoking

42 A 67 year old male non-smoker presents with cough, dyspnoea and weight loss. The CXR shows a large right-sided pleural effusion which occupies three quarters of the hemithorax. There is no mediastinal shift. The film is otherwise normal.

What is the most likely diagnosis?

(a) Congestive cardiac failure
(b) Bronchogenic carcinoma
(c) Meig's syndrome
(d) Mesothelioma
(e) Pancreatitis

43 A tall, thin 18 year old man with no medical history presents with acute pleuritic chest pain and shortness of breath. On examination there is reduced air entry on the right side, with hyper-resonant percussion.

Which of the following signs would you not expect?
(a) Continuous diaphragm sign
(b) Deep sulcus sign
(c) Increased sharpness of the cardiomediastinal border
(d) Double diaphragm sign
(e) Ipsilateral hypochondrial transradiancy

44 Which of the following conditions is not associated with Raynaud's phenomenon?

(a) Atherosclerosis
(b) Rheumatoid arthritis
(c) Sarcoid
(d) Takayasu disease
(e) Trauma

45 A 28 year old man has a Barium swallow to investigate dysphagia. The RAO views show a 'reverse 3' indentation in the mid oesophagus.

Which of the following features would make the diagnosis of true coarctation more likely than pseudocoarctation?
(a) Ejection systolic murmur
(b) His lack of symptoms
(c) Inferior rib notching
(d) No gradient on pressure studies
(e) Widening of the superior mediastinum

46 A 36 year old man presents with cough, shortness of breath, fever and night sweats. The eosinophil count is 1.3×10^9/l. The CXR shows bilateral interstitial infiltrates. Subsequent CT chest shows diffuse ground-glass opacities and interlobular septal thickening.

Which of the following is the least likely underlying diagnosis?

(a) Allergic broncho-pulmonary aspergillosis
(b) Churg-Strauss syndrome
(c) Lofgren's syndrome
(d) Schistosomiasis
(e) Wegener's granulomatosis

47 Which of the following is the earliest radiological feature of asbestos-related lung disease?

(a) Pleural thickening
(b) Asbestosis
(c) Pleural effusion
(d) Folded lung
(e) Pleural calcification

48 A 20 year man has recently completed chemotherapy for NHL. A follow-up PET-CT scan is arranged. There is increased uptake within the region of the thymus. Subsequent MRI shows intermediate signal within the thymus on T1 and T2-weighting and signal drop out on in/out of phase imaging.

What is the most likely diagnosis?

(a) Lymphomatous infiltration
(b) Thymic carcinoma
(c) Thymic hyperplasia
(d) Thymic lipoma
(e) Thymoma

49 A CT examination in a 56 year old patient shows bronchial dilatation due to retained secretions and appearing as V- or Y-shaped tubular or branching structures.

What term should be used to describe this appearance?

(a) Bronchiectasis
(b) Bronchiolectasis
(c) Tree-in-bud
(d) Traction bronchiectasis
(e) Bronchocoele

50 Which of the following is not a feature of amyloidosis?

(a) Tracheobronchial strictures
(b) Recurrent pneumothoraces
(c) Calcified parenchymal nodules
(d) Septal thickening
(e) Lymphadenopathy

51 A 35 year old lady undergoes a screening CXR. This shows unilateral transradiancy with reduced vessel markings on the affected side. A subsequent CT of the thorax reveals the changes are bilateral but asymmetrical, with areas of bronchiectasis.

What is the most likely diagnosis?

(a) Bronchial atresia
(b) Congenital lobar emphysema
(c) Panacinar emphysema
(d) Swyer-James (McLeod) syndrome
(e) Primary ciliary dyskinesia

52 A 29 year old women presents with pain in her left forearm. She has previous been investigated for hypertension, arthralgias, and weight loss. The arm BPs are unequal. Aortic angiogram reveals long-segment smooth stenoses at the origin of the left subclavian artery, within the abdominal aorta and in the right renal artery.

What is the most likely diagnosis?

(a) Buerger's disease
(b) Giant cell arteritis
(c) Polyarteritis nodosum
(d) Syphilitic aortitis
(e) Takayasu disease

53 Which of the following causes of pneumoconiosis is considered a fibrogenic dust?

(a) Silver
(b) Coal dust
(c) Tin
(d) Silica
(e) Iron oxide

54 During a CT-guided lung biopsy the patient becomes acutely dyspnoeic with a 'gasp' reflex and retrosternal chest pain; the ECG monitor shows dysrythymias. An air embolism is suspected.

Which position should the patient be placed in immediately for treatment?

(a) Erect
(b) Left lateral decubitus
(c) Prone
(d) Right lateral decubitus
(e) Supine

55 What is the most common cause of eosinophilic lung disease in developed countries?

(a) Allergic bronchopulmonary aspergillosis
(b) Drug-induced disease
(c) Churg-Strauss syndrome
(d) Hypereosinophilic syndrome
(e) Rheumatoid disease

56 A 37 year old lady with Sjögren's syndrome presents with a 2 year history of progressive breathlessness, low-grade fever and malaise. A CT of the thorax demonstrates diffuse ground glass opacification and a number of discrete thin-walled cysts within the lungs. The CT is otherwise normal.

What is the most likely diagnosis?
(a) Pneumocystis infection
(b) Non-specific interstitial pneumonitis
(c) Cryptogenic organising pneumonia
(d) Desquamative interstitial pneumonitis
(e) Lymphocytic interstitial pneumonitis

57 What is the most common thoracic complication of HIV worldwide?

(a) Bacterial pneumonia
(b) Kaposi's sarcoma
(c) Pneumocystis infection
(d) Lymphoma
(e) Tuberculosis

58 A 36 year old man has recurrent episodes of haemoptysis. Investigations reveal a solitary pulmonary AVM in the right lower lobe. An elective embolisation procedure is planned.

What is the most appropriate embolisation agent to use?
(a) Autologous blood clot
(b) Coils
(c) Ethyl alcohol
(d) Gelfoam
(e) Polyvinyl alcohol

59 A 35 year old female is under investigation for known sarcoidosis. Her most recent CXR and HRCT show widespread mid and upper zone reticular opacification with multiple small nodules and no mediastinal or hilar lymphadenopathy.

What is the stage of her disease?

(a) 0
(b) I
(c) II
(d) III
(e) IV

60 A 57 year old man with biopsy proven lung cancer attends for a PET-CT study. This demonstrates a 4 cm tumour in the left lower lobe, not abutting the pleural surface. There are enlarged, PET positive nodes in the left hilar, sub-carinal and cervical nodes.

How would you stage this tumour?

(a) T3 N3 M0
(b) T2 N2 M0
(c) T2 N3 M0
(d) T2 N2 M1
(e) T2 N3 M1

61 Which of the following statements regarding MUGA studies is not true?

(a) Acquisition requires a minimum of 16 frames per cardiac cycle
(b) It is a more accurate measure of ejection fraction than echocardiography
(c) Images are acquired in the LAO position
(d) Images are gated to the r-wave of the cardiac cycle
(e) Attenuation correction is applied to reduce errors

62 A 72 year old woman with a history of recent surgery presents with shortness of breath and pleuritic chest pain. On examination there is a slight swelling of the right leg compared to the left. The D-dimer level is raised.

Which imaging investigation should be performed next?

(a) Chest X-ray
(b) CTPA
(c) Pulmonary angiogram
(d) Ultrasound bilateral lower leg veins
(e) V/Q scan

63 A 48 year old man undergoing a CT of the abdomen has an anaphylactoid reaction to *i.v.* contrast medium, with bronchospasm and hypotension. You need to administer adrenalin.

What dose and via which route should this be done?

(a) 0.15 mg 1:1,000 (0.15 mls)intravenously
(b) 0.15 mg 1:10,000 (0.15 mls) intramuscularly
(c) 0.15 mg of 1:10,000 (0.15 mls) subcutaneously
(d) 0.5 mg of 1:1,000 (0.5 mls) intramuscularly
(e) 0.5 mg of 1:10,000 (0.5 mls) intravenously

64 Which of the following statements is most accurate regarding IVC filters?

(a) Bilateral iliac vein thrombosis is a contraindication
(b) Cannot be placed above the renal veins
(c) Filter migration is common
(d) Post-procedural anti-coagulation is required for 6 weeks
(e) Retrieval is performed *via* the SVC

65 A 37 year old man presents with non-specific symptoms of malaise. A whole body CT demonstrates a mass of soft tissue density within the right atrium. No other abnormality is seen.

What is the most likely diagnosis?

(a) Myxoma
(b) Rhabdomyosarcoma
(c) Thrombus
(d) Metastasis
(e) Lymphoma

66 Regarding a trans-jugular intrahepatic porto-systemic shunt procedure.

Which of the following is incorrect?

(a) A 10 mm x 6 cm stent is appropriate
(b) A cobra catheter is used to select the hepatic vein
(c) CO_2 angiography is an accepted technique to outline the portal vein
(d) Portal vein patency should be demonstrated before the procedure
(e) The preferred route is *via* the left hepatic vein

67 After a prolonged stay on ITU for pancreatitis, a 53 year old patient develops bilateral pleural effusions along with sepsis of unknown origin.

Which of the following US features suggests a transudate rather than an exudate?

(a) Homogeneously hyperechoic material
(b) Anechoic material
(c) Complex septated material
(d) Complex non-septated material
(e) Parenchymal hyperechogenicity

68 A 54 year old man presents with a cough and breathlessness 1 year after bone marrow transplantation. A CT study demonstrates bronchial wall thickening and dilatation, with gas trapping on expiratory phase images.

What is the most likely diagnosis?

(a) Organising pneumonia
(b) Non-specific interstitial pneumonitis
(c) Extrinsic allergic alveolitis
(d) Obliterative bronchiolitis
(e) Engraftment syndrome

69 Which of the following is not a cause of a mismatch on V/Q imaging?

(a) Acute pulmonary embolism
(b) Pulmonary hypertension
(c) Bronchial carcinoma
(d) Pneumothorax
(e) Idiopathic pulmonary fibrosis

70 At a multidisciplinary team meeting, the pathologist shows a surgical specimen with destroyed and fibrotic tissue. It contains numerous cystic airspaces with thick fibrous walls and complete loss of acinar architecture.

How might you best describe this at CT?

(a) Interlobular septal thickening
(b) Idiopathic pulmonary fibrosis
(c) Honeycombing
(d) Panacinar emphysema
(e) Non-specific interstitial pneumonitis

71 Which of the following is not a feature of high kV chest radiographs?

(a) Greater detail of the airways
(b) Sharper outline of pulmonary structures
(c) Increased focus-to-film distance with an air gap
(d) Reduced obscuration of lung by skeletal structures
(e) Better delineation of calcified pleural plaques

72 A 23 year old patient presents with acute dyspnoea and pleuritic chest pain. The CXR shows a right-sided pneumothorax and multiple bilateral cystic changes. Following successful treatment, a CT chest is requested.

Which feature favours a diagnosis of lymphangioleiomyomatosis over Langerhans cell histiocytosis?

(a) Chylous pleural effusion
(b) Pulmonary nodules
(c) Smoking history
(d) Thin-walled cysts > 1 cm
(e) Upper lobe predominance

73 In the assessment of a thoracic CT, which of the following features is least supportive of a diagnosis of non-specific interstitial pneumonitis?

(a) Traction bronchiectasis
(b) Volume loss
(c) Ground glass opacification
(d) Thin-walled cysts
(e) Reticular abnormality

74 A follow-up CT is performed in a patient 12 months after an endovascular aneurysm repair (EVAR) stenting for an enlarged AAA. There is enlargement of the aneurysm sac, with retrograde blood flow entering the sac *via* lumbar arteries, but with a complete seal around the graft attachment zones.

What sub-type of endoleak does this represent?

(a) Type I
(b) Type II
(c) Type III
(d) Type IV
(e) Type V

75 A 63 year old man previously treated for lung cancer presents with a gradual onset of dyspnoea, headache and facial swelling with prominent veins over the preceding weeks. A CT is requested.

Which of the following collateral veins are least likely to be enlarged?

(a) Azygous vein
(b) Hemiazygous veins
(c) Internal thoracic veins
(d) Lateral thoracic veins
(e) Pericardial veins

Cardiothoracic and Vascular Mock Paper Answers

1 (b)
Histoplasmosis is endemic in certain areas of the USA, particularly Ohio, Mississippi, and the St Lawrence river valley. Acute infection produces flu-like symptoms (polyarthralgia, fever). Acute CXR findings may be non-specific, but include diffuse subsegmental opacities, +/- lymphadenopathy. Sub-acute infection results in small calcific nodules and there may be hilar or mediastinal LNs which can display popcorn calcification. The 'target lesion' with central calcification is said to be pathognomonic.

Ref: Fundamentals of Diagnostic Radiology, 2nd Ed, p. 468-9 & Radiology Review Manual, 6th Ed, p. 234.

2 (c)
Behcet's disease is an autoimmune condition that is characterised by oro-genital ulceration and uveitis. There are numerous systemic complications which include vasculitis, arterial and venous thrombosis, pulmonary artery aneurysms and pulmonary haemorrhage.

Ref: e-medicine: Behcet's disease.

3 (d)
FMD involves the renal artery in 60% of cases and extracranial carotid artery in 30%, there are 6 sub-types. FMD accounts for 35% of cases of RAS and 25% of all cases of renovascular hypertension (most common cause in those < 30 years; 3x more common in females. Medial fibroplasia is the commonest type of FMD accounting for 60-85% of cases and gives the classic 'string of beads' appearance (alternating areas of stenoses and aneurysms) which is typically bilateral and affects mid and distal renal artery and branches.

Ref: Radiology Review Manual, 6th Ed, p. 957.

4 (a)
Suppurative lung disease, such as cystic fibrosis and bronchiectasis, necessitates double lung transplant to prevent the spread of infection from native lung to the graft. The other conditions can be treated with single lung transplantation, although patients with PPH or emphysema may also be offered double lung transplantation.

Ref: R-ITI 1b_059. Thoracic Imaging in Heart and Lung Transplantation.

5 (a)
Pleural calcification can be due to infection (TB, healed empyema), trauma (healed haemothorax), radiation therapy, pneumoconioses (asbestosis), talcosis, hyperparathyroidism. Berylliosis rarely involves the pleura.

Ref: Radiology Review Manual, 6th Ed, p. 440.

6 (b)
The main advantages of CO_2-angiography is its use in patients where iodinated agents are contraindicated, *e.g.* renal failure or previous contrast reaction, or for long procedures in order to limit contrast burden (*e.g.* EVAR placement). CO_2 is not diluted by blood thus can opacify central veins more readily from a peripheral approach, which is advantageous when placing IVC filters. The overall quality of CO_2 images is reduced as there is decreased density compared to Iodine, thus DSA is essential. Additionally, multiple injections are usually required, thus radiation exposure may be increased.

Ref: Clin Rad (2005); 60(3): 123–5.

7 (a)
The findings described are consistent with lymphangitis carcinomatosis. Although the appearance of LC on HRCT scans is nonspecific, the features in a symptomatic patient with history of malignancy is highly suggestive. A number of primary tumours are associated with this finding within the lung, including cervix, colon, stomach, breast, pancreatic, thyroid and larynx. Focal, unilateral disease is particularly associated with underlying bronchogenic carcinoma (breast cancer can also produce this pattern).

Ref: Khan AN (2008) e-medicne article: Lymphangitic carcinomatosis Imaging.

8 (a)
More than 90% of tracheal neoplasms are malignant, with adenoid cystic carcinomas second most common. Squamous cell papillomas, related to human papilloma virus infection, are the most common benign lesions.

Ref: R-ITI. 1b_037. Tracheal and bronchial stenoses.

9 (d)
The clinical features are non-specific, but many patients with EAA (also known as hypersensitivity pneumonitis) have exacerbation of symptoms on exposure to the antigen, *e.g.* returning to the workplace. EAA has acute, sub acute and chronic phases which may progress to widespread pulmonary fibrosis. The mosaic attenuation with gas trapping described here is a characteristic finding.

Ref: R-ITI 1b_018. Hypersensitivity pneumonitis.

10 (b)
Guidewires have a central stiff steel core with a 'floppy' end; most are coated with Teflon to reduce friction. Wires are sized according to their outer diameter, measured in 1/1000 of an inch (typical measurements are 0.018 – 0.035). 'J' wires are often described in terms of the radius of the curve they form (*e.g.* 3 mm) and are routinely used for access. The other wires vary in their properties and are useful in different situations.

Ref: Interventional Radiology: A Survival Guide, 2nd Ed, p. 63–5.

11 (a)
Factors that increase the risk of an idiosyncratic contrast reaction include: Atopy, asthma, B-blockers (all increase x3), cardiac disease (x5), age >50 years (x2) and previous allergic reaction to iodine or shellfish (x10). The other listed answers will increase the chance of contrast-related nephrotoxicity rather than allergic reaction.

Ref: Interventional Radiology: A Survival Guide, 2nd Ed, p. 12–4.

12 (c)
α1-anti-trypsin deficiency is a genetically inherited disorder. In individuals with the PiZZ phenotype there is insufficient α1AT to protect the lungs from neutrophil elastase. Even non-smokers develop emphysema in the lower zones which involves the pulmonary acinus diffusely (another cause is *i.v.* methylphenidate abuse). Liver fibrosis/cirrhosis can also occur in this condition. Centriacinar emphysema (centrilobular and focal subtypes) occurs in smokers. Paracicatricial emphysema is often seen in scar tissue (*e.g.* in pulmonary fibrosis).

Ref: R-ITI module: 1b_038 – Emphysema.

13 (a)
Bleomycin may result in one of two conditions: an organising pneumonia with multiple foci of consolidation or tree-in-bud opacification, or diffuse alveolar damage which gives appearances akin to ARDS.

Ref: Clin Rad (2009); In press. doi:10.1016/j.crad.(2009).04.006

14 (e)
The lesion described is that of a Pancoast tumour. This is a superior sulcus tumour that is most commonly due to a primary lung tumour, but can result from breast cancer, myeloma, mesothelioma, lymphoma, or metastases. Overall 3% of bronchogenic cancers present this way, the commonest being squamous cell; adenocarcinoma is the second commonest. Symptoms result from local involvement of the brachial plexus (arm pain, hand muscle wasting) and the sympathetic chain (Horner's syndrome: ipsilateral enophthalmos, ptosis, miosis and anhidrosis).

Ref: Radiology Review Manual, 6th Ed, p. 476.

15 (d)
Published complication rates vary widely, and technique and practice differs according to the centre. The below study showed that small pneumothoraces are common but rarely require treatment (overall rate 16.4%); the number requiring chest drain was only 2.4%. Haemoptysis occurred in 4.8%, but major haemoptysis requiring blood transfusion was only 0.15%. Further rare complications include death (0.15%), air embolism (0.02%) and tumour seeding (0.02%).

Ref: BJR (2002); 75:731–735.

16 (b)
There is a good correlation between a main PA ≥2.9 cm and right heart catheter studies in demonstrating PHT. Some argue that the PA diameter is affected by body habitus, thus the ratio of aorta to main PA is more specific (note this is a *PA : aorta* ratio > 1). Segmental artery : bronchus ratio >1 in 3 of 4 lobes (RUL, RLL, LUL and LLL) has been used by some authors, however, this ratio may exceed 1 in normal individuals and, rarely, a ratio of ≥1.25 can be within normal limits. Mosaic perfusion is indicated of small vessel disease which can lead to PHT but is not specific, and reflux of contrast into the IVC is indicative of tricuspid regurgitation which may be secondary to PHT, but is not specific. A combination of 2 or more features greatly increases specificity.

Ref: Clin Rad (2009); 64: 751–60.

17 (e)
Pulmonary hamartomas, gastric leiomyosarcomas (GISTs) and functioning extra-adrenal paragangliomas make up this rare triad. Almost all patients are female (80%) aged 10-30 years. Pituitary adenomas, cardiac myxomas, along with myxoid fibroadenomas of the breast and testicular tumours are associated with the autosomal dominant Carney complex.

Ref: Radiology Review Manual, 6th Ed, p. 850.

18 (b)
The overall incidence of CHD is 1%, the most common are structural defects bicuspid aortic valve and MVP. The most common types of CHD presenting in the first month of life are: hypoplastic left heart syndrome (35%), TGA (25%), coarctation (20%), multiple defects (15%), pulmonary atresia/stenosis (10%), severe Tetralogy of Fallot's (10%). HLHS describes underdevelopment of LA, LV, MV, AV and aorta, survival requires a large ASD and PDA to allow admixing of the left and right circulations. CXR shows marked pulmonary oedema and right heart enlargement. HLHS and the '5 Ts' present at 0-2 days, but HLHS is more common and more likely to produce marked CCF. Coarctation and AS present at 7-14 days; VSD and PDA presents in infancy and ASD in adulthood.

Ref: Primer of Diagnostic Imaging, 4th Ed, p. 140-1 & 154.

19 (d)
The other options are either exclusively or typically found within the posterior mediastinum. The anterior mediastinum is the third most common site of primary germ cell tumour, after gonadal and sacrococcygeal location.

Ref: Radiology Review Manual, 6th Ed, p. 534–5.

20 (b)
Cardiac MRI demands rapid and complex sequences which are evolving continually. Gradient echo sequences are flow sensitive and may be used to show jets or regurgitation.

Ref: R-ITI 1a_002. Cardiac MRI anatomy and MRA.

21 (a)
Imaging should not be performed until at least 30 minutes, and more typically 60 minutes after tracer administration to allow clearance from the background blood pool. Patient preparation is key in order to minimise artefacts from physiological uptake. Muscle uptake is reduced by keeping serum insulin levels low, thus patients are fasted for 6 hours prior to the study. It is important to check blood glucose prior to the study as elevated blood glucose competes with FDG for transport, increasing background activity; above a certain level (often quoted as 13 mmol/ml) the procedure may have to be postponed. For imaging in the head/neck region it is advisable to avoid talking for 30-60 minutes prior in order to minimise muscle uptake in this region, similarly strenuous exercise should be avoided 24-48 hours prior to reduce whole-body muscle uptake. Additional avoidance of caffeine is recommended in cardiac/chest imaging as it will increase heart rate, hence increasing heart size and myocardial uptake.

Ref: Clin Rad (2007); 62(2): 97–108.

22 (d)
CAF have a prevalence of 0.0002% in the population, are seen in <0.25% patients undergoing angiography and account for approximately 0.3% of congenital cardiac abnormalities. Approximately 50% arise from the RCA, 42% from the LCA, 5% from both; drainage is almost always into a low pressure venous structure, most commonly right ventricle (41%) and right atrium (26%) and the vast majority are single. There is no predilection for race or sex.

Ref: Radiographics (2009); 29:781–9.

23 (a)
It may be difficult to distinguish acute from chronic DVT, and previous imaging if available can be helpful. Signs more in keeping with chronic DVT include wall thickening, collateral vessels, and echogenic material of the same or increased echoreflectivity as compared to surrounding tissue; vein diameter is often reduced. Acute thrombus is of lucent-to-intermediate echogenicity as compared to surrounding tissues, is seen to expand the vein, is often 'free-floating' within the lumen in the first week, and may be compressible in the early stages.

Ref: Radiol Clin North Am (2007); 45(3):525–47.

24 (e)
This group of patients are severely immuno-suppressed and are particularly prone to fungal chest infections, which need to be recognised early and treated aggressively.

Ref: Eur J Radiol (2006); 59:371–83.

25 (c)
Coronary artery calcification is expressed as the Agatston score. The greater the degree of calcification, the greater the risk of a cardiac event.

Ref: R-ITI 1a_006. Normal cardiac CT.

26 (a)
Baseline is defined as the sum of the long diameters of the target lesions where up 2 target lesions per organ and 5 overall can be used. Partial response involves a decrease of 30% or more in the sum of the long diameters. Complete response implies the disappearance of all lesions. Disease progression involves an increase in the sum of the long diameters of 20%. Good response, no response and excellent response are not part of the RECIST criteria.

Ref: EJC (2009); 45:228–47.

27 (c)
Branches of the IMA include left colic, sigmoidal branches, superior rectal, and marginal arteries. Medial sacral comes directly off the aorta; middle rectal and internal pudendal arteries are branches of the IIA; the inferior epigastric arteries are branches of the EIA.

Ref: Radiology Review Manual, 6th Ed, p. 791.

28 (d)
The causes can be divided into arterial, venous (including SVC obstruction), neurogenic (including polio, paraplegia, Neurofibromatosis type 1) and osseous. Neurofibromatosis type 2 is not a recognised cause.

Ref: Radiology Review Manual, 6th Ed, p. 19.

29 (c)
Tuberous sclerosis and UIP typically affect the lower zones. Lung volumes are preserved in EAA. Ankylosing spondylitis is a possibility but is much less common than sarcoid.

Ref: Radiology Review Manual, 6th Ed, p. 417.

30 (a)
In addition, increasing age, prolonged bed rest, familial disposition, previous venous thromboembolism, varicose veins and smoking are all risk factors. D-dimer is often elevated in pregnancy and the test is not indicated in this situation.

Ref: Clin Rad (2006); 61:1–12.

31 (e)
Pleural effusions are seen in both benign and malignant pleural disease. In addition to the other signs, encasement of the lung by pleural disease is a feature of malignancy.

Ref: R-ITI 1b_072-Malignant mesothelioma.

32 (c)
Pulmonary oedema is seen in patients with PE rarely (4% vs 13% in patients without PE). Other signs include pleural effusion.

Ref: Radiology Review Manual, 6th Ed, p. 524.

33 (d)
Lung involvement occurs in 15-25% of hydatid cases with a lower lobe preponderance. The cystic lesion is solitary in up to 75% of cases. It has a sharply defined ovoid/ spherical appearance and can measure up to 20 cm. It is characterised by varying degrees of collapse of the endocystic membrane leading to the so called 'water lily', 'serpent' and 'cumbo' signs. Rib and vertebral erosion is rarely seen.

Ref: Radiology Review Manual, 6th Ed, p. 500.

34 (a)
BAC is a slow growing peripheral tumour associated with chronic lung disease and ground glass appearance on HRCT. It can cavitate and is PET negative in 55%.

Ref: Radiology Review Manual, 6th Ed, p. 474.

35 (e)
The Society of Interventional Radiology consensus statement indications for IVC filter insertion classify the indications as being prophylactic, answers (c) and (d), absolute, or relative. Other absolute indications include a contraindication to anticoagulation, inability to achieve/maintain therapeutic anti-coagulation or recurrent DVT/PE despite anti-coagulation. Relative indications include answers (a) and (b), also free-floating proximal DVT, massive PE/ileocaval DVT treated with thrombolysis/thrombectomy, high risk of complications from anti-coagulation, or likely poor compliance with anti-coagulation.

Ref: Clin Rad (2009); 64(5): 502–10.

36 (b)
Ipsilateral mediastinal shift and elevation of the hemidiaphragm are normally seen after pneumonectomy. Depressions of the hemidiaphragm or contralateral mediastinal shift are abnormal and may indicate haemorrhage, empyema or a bronchopleural fistula.

Ref: Radiology Review Manual, 6th Ed, p. 520.

37 (b)
Kartagener's syndrome is due to abnormal ciliary motility. There is a high familial incidence and in addition to the above, is associated with chronic sinusitis, conductive deafness and other congenital abnormalities such as pyloric stenosis.

Ref: Radiology Review Manual, 6th Ed, p. 504.

38 (a)
Catheters are sized using the French system: the circumference in mm (diameter is roughly this measurement divided by 3, *i.e.* 6 Fr has approximately 2 mm diameter). Sheaths are sized in French measurement of their internal diameter (*i.e.* a 4Fr sheath can hold a 4 Fr catheter). Bernstein catheters are upwards pointed, thus they are ideal for accessing branches of the aortic arch. Access to the downwardly orientated mesenteric vessels would be technically very challenging with a Bernstein catheter - the downward facing sidewinder, or even the side-facing cobra catheters can be used.

Ref: Interventional Radiology: A Survival Guide, 2nd Ed, p. 52–6.

39 (e)
The acute and subacute forms of EAA can cause lower zone reticular change but the chronic form typically has an upper lobe distribution. Other drugs that can cause lower zone reticulation include bleomycin, methotrexate and nitrofurantoin. Asbestosis refers specifically to interstitial fibrosis in the context of asbestos exposure rather than the benign pleural asbestos related diseases. UIP is the commonest histological type of pattern found in idiopathic pulmonary fibrosis.

Ref: RITI module 1b -23 Chest x-ray: reticular patterns (differential).

40 (d)
Fat in a round well defined pulmonary lesion measuring up to 4 cm is virtually diagnostic of pulmonary hamartoma. Calcification, classically in a “popcorn” distribution, is seen in 15–20%.

Ref: Radiology Review Manual, 6th Ed, p. 497.

41 (b)
Giving higher doses (>2Gy), more frequent fractions, or a total dose in excess of 10 Gy to the lung are also treatment-specific risk factors. Patient-specific risk factors are increasing age and decreasing performance status.

Ref: R-ITI. 1b_048 - Acute and chronic radiation changes.

42 (d)
Mesothelioma more typically produces a unilateral pleural effusion (only 10% of effusions will be bilateral) which is exudative and may be haemorrhagic. There is classically no mediastinal shift (‘frozen’ hemithorax) due to fixation by the pleural rind of neoplastic tissue. 5-10% of workers exposed to asbestos will develop mesothelioma (30x increased risk), with a latency period of 35 years; an occupational exposure history is not always present. Crocidolite is the most carcinogenic of the asbestos fibres (> amosite, > chrysotile).

Ref: Radiology Review Manual, 6th Ed, p. 513–4.

43 (a)
In the erect film, a pneumothorax can be easily diagnosed when the visceral pleural can be seen separated from the chest wall by a transradiant zone devoid of vessels. In supine films, more subtle signs may be present, including ‘deep sulcus sign’, due to pleural air tracking anterior to the hemidiaphragm into the costophrenic angle, ‘double-diaphragm’ sign describes air outlining the anterior costophrenic angle combined with aerated lung outlining the diaphragmatic dome. There may also be a relative hyper-lucency in the ipsilateral hemithorax/ hypochondrial region or increased sharpness of the cardiomediastinal border due to anteromedial collection of air. The continuous diaphragm sign is due to pneumomediastinum or pneumopericardium.

Ref: Ellis S, Riti module 1b_067 - Signs of Pneumothorax and Pleural, Effusions & Diagnostic Radiology, 5th Ed, p. 228-9.

44 (c)
Raynaud's disease is the primary form of vasospasm induced digital ischaemia following cold or emotional stimuli. The colour changes typically seen are pallor, cyanosis, then eventually redness with re-perfusion. Raynaud's phenomenon is secondary vasospasm with obstruction, causes include atherosclerosis (most frequent; either *in situ* or due to emboli), arterial trauma, Buerger's, Takayasu's, drugs (ergot), and collagen vascular diseases (RhA, scleroderma, SLE). Radiological investigations include angiograms performed at ambient temperatures, followed by 'stress angiogram' performed after immersing the hand in ice water for 20 seconds. Sarcoidosis is not associated.

Ref: Radiology Review Manual, 6th Ed, p. 653.

45 (c)
Pseudocoarctation is an acute kink/ anterior buckling just distal to the left SCA origin. Patients are asymptomatic and there is no pressure gradient (hence collateral vessels with subsequent rib-notching are not seen). There is an ESM on auscultation and the superior mediastinum appears widened due to elongated, redundant ascending aorta and elongated aortic arch. Both true and pseudocoarctation produce the 'figure 3' sign on angiogram ('reverse 3' on RAO projections at Barium swallow) due to notching at the ligamentum arteriosum.

Ref: Radiology Review Manual, 6th Ed, p. 651.

46 (c)
Eosinophilia is defined as a peripheral eosinophil count > 0.44×10^9/l. Causes of eosinophilia and pneumonia include acute eosinophilic pneumonia (Loeffler's syndrome), drugs (nitrofurantoin, sulfonamides), parasitic (ascariasis, schistosomiasis), fungal (ABPA), and those associated with angiitis/granulomatosis (WG, Churg-Strauss, RhA, scleroderma, Sjogren's). Lofgren's syndrome is acute sarcoidosis, and has a triad of erythema nodosum, bilateral hilar adenopathy and arthritis and is associated with a good prognosis.

Ref: Radiology Review Manual, 6th Ed, p. 493-4.

47 (c)
A pleural effusion develops in up to 3% of workers, often occurring between 10 and 20 years after the initial exposure; effusions can be unilateral or bilateral. The effusion is usually small, with the fluid serous or mildly blood stained. The effusion persists up to 6 months, and recurs in up to of 30% cases. Some workers are left with blunting of the costo-phrenic angle, diffuse pleural thickening or round atelectasis. Mesothelioma appears to be unrelated to benign pleural effusions.

Ref: R-ITI. 1b_014 - Benign Asbestos Related Disease.

48 (c)
Rebound hyperplasia is seen in recovery from illness, after chemotherapy or radiotherapy. PET may be positive in all the given options. MRI chemical shift ratio can be used to distinguish thymic hyperplasia and thymoma, as the latter contains no fat. Thymic lipoma would also show this but would have high (not intermediate) signal on T1W and T2W. Thymoma typically appears asymmetrical with a lobulated contour.

Ref: Radiology (2007); 243:869-876.

49 (e)
This mucoid impaction is usually due to proximal obstruction by congenital (*e.g.* bronchial atresia) or acquired (*e.g.* carcinoma) abnormalities. Bronchiectasis and Bronchiolectasis are abnormal, irreversibly dilated bronchi or bronchioles. Traction bronchiectasis is dilatation due to adjacent fibrosis. Tree-in-bud pattern is seen in a spectrum of endo- and peribronchiolar disorders; airway dilatation is not a feature.

Ref: Radiology (2008); 246:697-722.

50 (b)
Amyloidosis is an uncommon condition in which there is deposition of amyloid protein in the tissues. Its manifestations are manifold and may be localised or diffuse.

Ref: Imaging of diseases of the chest, 3rd Ed. p. 609-615.

51 (d)
These are the typical features of Swyer-James (McLeod's) syndrome, a form of obliterative bronchiolitis that follows an insult (most commonly viral) to the developing lung. The CT findings are often more extensive than the plain film, with bilateral changes common.

Ref: Imaging of diseases of the chest, 3rd Ed, p. 917–9.

52 (e)
Takayasu ('pulseless') disease is a granulomatous inflammation of unknown aetiology affecting mainly elastic arteries, *i.e.* aorta and its major branches and the pulmonary arteries causing stenoses and occasionally aneurysms. It is more common in female patients (x 8) and presents at a young age (90% < 30 years). In up to 50% the early phase is marked by systemic symptoms such as fever, weight loss, night sweats, arthralgia; mean time from disease development to diagnosis is 8 years.

Ref: Radiology Review Manual, 6th Ed, p. 655–6.

53 (d)
Silica and Beryllium are considered fibrogenic dusts, *i.e.* they elicit a fibrogenic response in the lung parenchyma. The remaining dusts are inert within the lung parenchyma and cause very few clinical symptoms even though the radiographs may appear quite dramatic.

Ref: R-ITI. 1b_015. Pneumoconiosis.

54 (b)
VAE is a rare complication of lung biopsy. VAE can only occur if there is direct communication between air and the circulation and a pressure gradient favouring passage into the circulation. 'Gasp' reflex is described as a gasp induced when a bolus of air enters the pulmonary circulation causing acute hypoxia. Treatment is to place the patient in the left lateral decubitus (Durant manoeuvre) and Trendelenburg (head down) positions, which helps prevent air travelling through the right heart into the pulmonary arteries, which can lead to right ventricular outflow obstruction (air lock). 100% O_2 is also given to try and reduce the size by decreasing the nitrogen content of the air bubble.

Ref: Natal BL (2009) e-medicine article: Venous air embolism.

55 (a)
This accounted for 78% of cases in one large series. The importance of this condition is that repeated episodes lead to progressive lung damage that may be controlled by corticosteroids.

Ref: Imaging of diseases of the chest, 3rd Ed, p. 590–6.

56 (e)
Histopathologically characterised by a lymphocytic infiltrate in the lung parenchyma, LIP has an insidious onset and is often diagnosed many months after onset of non-specific symptoms. LIP is also seen in HIV patients, presumably as a consequence of impaired immune function.

Ref: R-ITI 1b_016. Idiopathic interstitial pneumonias.

57 (e)
Tuberculosis co-infection is the commonest complication worldwide. In the UK, bacterial infection is commonest, with unusual organisms seen more commonly than in the general population.

Ref: R-ITI 1_057. HIV AIDS in the thorax.

58 (b)
Pulmonary AVMs may be multiple if associated with Osler-Weber-Rendu syndrome, and they are more common in the lower lobes (70%). Symptoms are rare, but they are an indication for treatment, and include epistaxis, dyspnoea, and cyanosis. There is a theoretical risk of embolisation material particles passing into the systemic circulation, thus large materials such as coils or detachable balloons are used when embolisation is attempted (*NB:* in the USA only coils are licensed by the FDA, balloons are yet to gain approval).

Ref: Primer of Diagnostic Imaging, 4th Ed, p. 668 & p. 712–3.

59 (d)
There is a normal CXR in stage 0. Stage I shows hilar and mediastinal lymphadenopathy only. Stage II shows lymphadenopathy and parenchymal disease. Stage III shows parenchymal disease only. Stage IV is characterized by pulmonary fibrosis.

60 (d)
T2 lesions are those greater than 3 cm not invading the parietal pleura and more than 2 cm away from the carina. N1 nodes are hilar, N2 nodes include ipsilateral mediastinum and sub-carinal, N3 nodes are supraclavicular and contralateral mediastinum. Nodes outside these regions are considered to be M1.

Ref: TNM Atlas, 5th Ed, p. 158–168.

61 (e)
Attenuation correction is not used in MUGA imaging. MUGA images sum all the data from points on a cardiac cycle and these may be viewed as a cine loop.

Ref: R-ITI. 7c_003. Basics of cardiac radionuclide imaging.

62 (a)
The patient is at high risk for a PE. The CXR is less likely to be diagnostic, but may provide a differential diagnosis in some cases (*e.g.* spontaneous pneumothorax) and forms an important part of the diagnostic flow chart. A normal CXR means a V/Q scan would be the next appropriate investigation, abnormal CXR requires CTPA. The right leg swelling may be post-operative rather than due to a DVT, but regardless, it is important to diagnose a PE over a DVT as most clinicians recommend a longer treatment period for the former. Pulmonary angiography is invasive and is now rarely used in the context of PE diagnosis.

Ref: Radiology Review Manual, 6th Ed, p. 523–6.

63 (d)
Intramuscular adrenaline is the treatment of choice for patients having an anaphylactic reaction. Adrenaline *i.v.* must only be given in certain situations and by those skilled and experienced in its use. The recommended intramuscular dose is 0.5 mg of 1:1,000 (0.5 mls) for those > 12 years, 0.3 mg for those 6–12 years and 0.15 mg for those < 6 years.

Ref: www.resus.org.uk

64 (e)
Retrieval is performed *via* the SVC (left or ideally right IJV approach) to snare the retrieval hook at the top of the filter. IVC filters should be sited below the renal veins to reduce the chance of renal vein thrombosis, however, they can be sited supra-renally if the DVT extends above the renal veins. Filter migration is very rare (0.2% of patients in the below study). Post-procedural anticoagulation is not necessary as the filter is expecting to be effective immediately. Bilateral iliac vein thrombosis is a contraindication to a femoral approach for filter placement, but they can still be placed in the IVC *via* a superior approach (IJV and SVC).

Ref: Clin Rad (2009); 64(5): 502-10.

65 (a)
Myxomas are by far the commonest cardiac tumours, typically arising on a pedicle from the interatrial septum. They may prolapse in to the ventricle and obstruct the mitral or tricuspid valves.

Ref: R-ITI 1a_024. Cardiac tumours.

66 (e)
Access is ideally *via* the right IJV to the right (or middle) hepatic vein, with the shunt running from the RHV to the right portal vein; this may not be possible in conditions such Budd-Chiari syndrome where the RHV may be thrombosed. Stents are typically of 8–12 mm diameter, length 6 cm. Portal vein patency should be confirmed pre-procedure by US, CT or angiography. Portal vein position and patency can be demonstrated during the procedure, CO_2 may be used for this, as its lower viscosity allows for easier diffusion (and reduces iodinated contrast burden).

Ref: Interventional Radiology: A Survival Guide, 2nd Ed, p. 222-6 & Clin Rad (2009); 64(7): 664-74.

67 (b)
Hyperechoic effusions can be difficult to discriminate from normal lung but can be differentiated by observing movement with respiration.

Ref: RITI module 1b – 71 Ultrasound scan to diagnose empyema.

68 (d)
These are the typical features of OB, which is a late complication (>100 days) after BMT. Organising pneumonia typically has patchy peribronchovascular consolidation and may be secondary to drugs or infection. Engraftment syndrome is an early complication which manifests as diffuse lung injury.

Ref: R-ITI. 1b_058 - Pulmonary complications following bone marrow transplantation.

69 (d)
A pneumothorax will be neither ventilated nor perfused and thus would give a matched defect.

Ref: Imaging of diseases of the chest, 3rd Ed, p. 409–420.

70 (c)
This is the pathological correlate of honeycombing, a descriptive term only, which is seen in end-stage fibrosis from a number of causes. It is an important criterion for IPF, but is not exclusive to it, and it is not a dominant feature of NSIP.

Ref: Radiology (2008); 246:697–722.

71 (e)
High kV radiographs penetrate the skeleton and mediastinum better, enabling improved lung images; a shorter exposure time gives sharper images. Low kV images allow better appreciation of calcified nodules or pleural plaques.

Ref: Imaging of diseases of the chest, 3rd Ed, p. 1–2.

72 (a)
LAM occurs in young women and is a *forme fruste* of tuberous sclerosis. There is a proliferation of smooth muscle cells along the lymphatics (which may also result in chylothorax). The cysts are < 5-10 mm, thin-walled and surrounded by normal lung. Abdominal and pelvic LAM is associated and renal angiomyolipomas may be present. LCH occurs in young heavy-smoking men, there is an evolution from pulmonary nodules through to thin-walled small, then large cysts, often with a bizarre shape.

Ref: Primer of Diagnostic Imaging, 4th Ed, p. 37–8.

73 (d)
Thin-walled cysts are not a feature of NSIP but should raise the possibility of LIP. The remaining features are typical. Consolidation, honeycombing and nodules are variably reported in the literature as being present or absent.

Ref: Radiographics (2009); 29:73–87.

74 (b)
There are 4 types of endoleak. Type II is also termed 'retrograde' or 'non-graft related' endoleak. Type I is due to inadequate or ineffective seal at the graft ends. Type III is due to a defect in the graft fabric (mechanical graft failure). Type IV is a minor blush of contrast due to contrast diffusion across the pores of the graft fabric; it is usually an inherent part of the graft design.

Ref: Primer of Diagnostic Imaging, 4th Ed, p. 693–4.

75 (e)
The extent and location of collateral opacification in SVCO at CT depends on the location/ degree of obstruction and the site/ timing of contrast injection. Major collateral pathways include the azygous, hemiazygous, internal thoracic, lateral thoracic veins, and the thoraco-acromioclavicular venous complex. Minor collateral pathways include the anterior jugular, the pericardial and umbilical veins; the parascapular, pericardial superficial, thoraco-abdominal and epigastric veins may also be opacified.

Ref: R-ITI 1b_094 - Superior Vena Cava Obstruction – CT Imaging Findings of Pathology and Anatomy.

Musculoskeletal and Trauma Mock Paper Questions

1 **You review a plain radiograph of the left femur of a 16 year old patient and note a lesion with a wide zone of transition and a marked 'sunburst' periosteal reaction.**

Which of the following is the most likely diagnosis?
(a) Aneurysmal bone cyst
(b) Ewing's sarcoma
(c) Osteosarcoma
(d) Fibrosarcoma
(e) Osteoid osteoma

2 **A gentleman presents to A&E after trauma. Plain radiographs of the cervical spine are taken. There is an abrupt transition in the alignment of the cervical spine at C5-6, with anterolisthesis of C5 on C6 by 3/4 of a vertebral body's width.**

Which of the following is incorrect?
(a) There is a high incidence of cord injury
(b) This is a stable dislocation
(c) The posterior ligament complex is disrupted
(d) The anterior longitudinal ligament is disrupted
(e) The facets may be in a 'batwing' or 'bow-tie' configuration

3 **A patient presents with joint pain and plain radiographs are taken.**

Which of the following features would favour the diagnosis of osteoarthritis over rheumatoid arthritis?
(a) Marginal erosions
(b) 'High-riding' shoulder
(c) Periarticular osteoporosis
(d) Superolateral migration of the femoral head
(e) Involvement of the proximal joints of the hand

4 **A 40 year old man with chronic renal failure is involved in an RTA and presents with abdominal pain. Unenhanced CT shows a small volume of free intra-abdominal fluid of mixed attenuation.**

Which of the following is the likeliest source of haemorrhage?

(a) Right lobe of the liver
(b) Left lobe of the liver
(c) Spleen
(d) Body of pancreas
(e) Small bowel mesentery

5 **An MRI examination of the lumbar spine demonstrates 5 mm of intravertebral disc tissue protruding beyond the margin of the vertebral body over 60% of the vertebral body circumference.**

What is the most appropriate diagnosis?

(a) Annular disc bulge
(b) Broad based disc herniation
(c) Focal disc herniation
(d) Intravertebral herniation
(e) Disc sequestration

6 **You review a series of plain radiographs of a male patient taken over the course of 25 years. There is irregular, solid, bilateral, symmetrical periosteal proliferation of the distal long bones. These appearances developed in his adolescence, and have been stable since. You are told that this is relatively pain-free.**

What is the most likely diagnosis?

(a) Pachydermoperiostitis
(b) Diffuse idiopathic skeletal hyperostosis
(c) Fluorosis
(d) Secondary hypertrophic osteoarthropathy
(e) Vascular insufficiency

7 **A 20 year old man presents after a fall with anatomical snuff box tenderness.**

Which of the following statements is incorrect?
(a) 40% of scaphoid fractures are visible on initial radiographs
(b) Interval radiographs at 7–10 days detect the majority of initial occult fractures
(c) The MRI sequences of choice are coronal T1 and STIR
(d) 80% of fractures occur through the waist of the scaphoid
(e) Distal radius fractures can present in this manner

8 **A 23 year old woman complains of anterior chest wall pain. CXR shows a large expansile mass arising from the left 3rd rib. CT confirms the mass is solitary and demonstrates whorled areas of 'rings and arcs' calcification with no soft tissue component.**

Which of the following is the most likely diagnosis?
(a) Osteosarcoma
(b) Osteoblastoma
(c) Chondrosarcoma
(d) Askin tumour
(e) Plasmacytoma

9 **The radiographs of an elderly patient demonstrate the expansion of a long bone, with cortical bone thickening and coarse trabeculation. Pagets's disease is suspected. Further investigations were performed in the nuclear medicine department.**

Which of the following is not typical?
(a) Marginal uptake of ^{99m}Tc-MDP in lytic lesions
(b) Deformity of bones
(c) Normal uptake of ^{99m}Tc-MDP in some sclerotic lesions
(d) Increase uptake of ^{99m}Tc-MDP in the active phase
(e) Increased uptake of ^{99m}Tc-sulphur colloid by bone marrow

10 A gentleman presents with knee swelling, pain and stiffness. Plain radiographs and subsequent MR imaging were performed, and a diagnosis of pigmented villonodular synovitis is suspected.

Which of the following is not typical of this disease?

(a) Preservation of bone density
(b) Synovial low signal intensity on gradient echo MR imaging
(c) Well-defined erosions on both sides of the joint
(d) Joint space narrowing early in the disease
(e) Joint effusion

11 A patient presents with a painless, slow growing mass of the finger. On clinical and radiographic grounds, this is likely to be a giant cell tumour of the tendon sheath.

Regarding this condition, which of the following are incorrect?

(a) The lesion is typically non-calcified
(b) The lesion is typically hypointense to muscle on T1W
(c) Most lesions are associated with bony erosion
(d) The lesion is not usually centred on a joint
(e) The lesion is often painless

12 A CT is performed following major trauma. A cervical burst fracture is suspected.

Regarding this condition, which of the following statements is incorrect?

(a) Interpedicular widening is common
(b) Injury to the spinal cord is common
(c) There are commonly fragments within the spinal canal
(d) There is loss of posterior vertebral body height
(e) This is considered an unstable fracture

13 An elderly patient has increasing back pain and weight loss. There is local tenderness over the upper lumbar vertebrae. Plain radiographs and MR imaging is performed. A history of tuberculosis is noted.

Which of the following features would be more supportive of a pyogenic, rather than tuberculous spondylodiscitis?

(a) Marked vertebral collapse
(b) Early bridging of affected vertebrae
(c) A large paravertebral abscess
(d) A pulmonary lesion
(e) Slow progression

14 A 32 year old woman undergoes a CXR after developing a cough. The CXR is unremarkable except for bilateral superior rib notching affecting multiple ribs.

Which of the following is least likely?

(a) Hypoparathyroidism
(b) Rheumatoid arthritis
(c) Scleroderma
(d) Systemic lupus erythematosus
(e) Marfan's syndrome

15 A patient with a hereditary haemoglobinopathy has multiple skeletal abnormalities evident from his plain radiographs.

Which feature is typically more marked in sickle-cell anaemia than thalassaemia major?

(a) 'Hair-on-end' appearance of the skull
(b) Obliteration of the paranasal sinuses
(c) 'Erlenmeyer flask' deformity of the long bones
(d) Square-shaped compression infarcts of the vertebral end plates
(e) Widening of the skull diploe

16 A middle aged man presents with low back pain and faecal incontinence. MR imaging of the lumbar spine is performed and a diagnosis of chordoma is subsequently made.

Regarding the chordomas, which of the following is incorrect?

(a) They typically have poor uptake of ^{99m}Tc-MDP
(b) They usually cause extensive local bone destruction
(c) They most frequently arise in the sacrum or coccyx
(d) They may have a narrow zone of transition
(e) Metastasis is common

17 A young man avulses his anterior inferior iliac spine whilst kicking a football.

The origin of which muscle will be affected?

(a) Adductor magnus
(b) Iliopsoas
(c) Rectus femoris
(d) Sartorius
(e) Tensor fasciae latae

18 A man falls from a balcony and is brought into A&E. There is clinical shortening of the left leg and plain radiographs demonstrate fractures through the left sacroiliac joint and the left pubic rami.

What is the most appropriate description of this fracture?

(a) Bucket-handle
(b) Duverney
(c) Open-book
(d) Malgaigne
(e) Wide-swept pelvis

19 A plain radiograph of a 20 year old's knee shows a well defined lesion in the distal femoral epiphysis. It is lytic, with a narrow zone of transition and a well defined sclerotic rim. The lesion does not reach the articular surface, and is not expansile.

Which of the following conditions is the most likely?

(a) Aneurysmal bone cyst
(b) Chondroblastoma
(c) Giant cell tumour
(d) Simple bone cyst
(e) Metastasis

20 A young man sustains blunt trauma to the chest. There is a suspicion of thoracic aortic injury.

With this in mind, which of the following measurements is considered abnormal?

(a) The mediastinum is 6 cm wide at the level of the origin of the left subclavian artery
(b) The left paraspinal stripe is 3 mm wide
(c) The right paratracheal stripe is 2 mm wide
(d) There is depression of the left mainstem bronchus of 60° below the horizontal
(e) The right hemidiaphragm is higher than the left

21 On MR imaging, an elderly gentleman is noted to have an acute compression fracture of a lumbar vertebra.

Which of the following features would be more suggestive of a malignant, rather than benign cause for the fracture?

(a) The vertebral body returns low signal on T1W in the acute phase
(b) Enhancement after *i.v.* gadolinium
(c) The vertebral body returns intermediate signal on T1W two months after the fracture
(d) Involvement of the anterior elements
(e) The overall mass of the vertebral body is increased

22 A 35 year old man involved in an RTA falls from a motorcycle and injures his forearm. Plain radiographs show a comminuted displaced radial head fracture with dislocation of the radioulnar joint.

What is the eponymous term for this injury?

(a) Monteggia fracture
(b) Reverse Monteggia fracture
(c) Essex-Lopresti fracture
(d) Galeazzi fracture
(e) Maisonneuve fracture

23 A 15 year old girl presents with a history of several months leg pain, worse at night which is relieved by salicylates. Plain films show a 1.3 cm lesion in the proximal tibial shaft which has a round central lucency with surrounding sclerosis.

What is the likeliest diagnosis?

(a) Osteosarcoma
(b) Brodie abscess
(c) Aneurysmal bone cyst
(d) Osteoid osteoma
(e) Stress fracture

24 CT imaging is performed on a patient with known malignancy who is unwell. There appears to be fluid within the abdominal cavity. This has an attenuation of 40 HU. The images were acquired in the portal venous phase after the administration of *i.v.* contrast medium.

What type of fluid/ tissue is this most likely to represent?

(a) Fat
(b) Serum
(c) Fresh unclotted blood
(d) Clotted blood
(e) Active arterial extravasation

25 A CT is performed after blunt abdominal trauma. Images were acquired in the portal venous phase after the administration of *i.v.* contrast medium. Clinically, the patient is thought to be hypovolaemic.

Which of the following is not a CT imaging feature of hypovolaemia?
(a) Normal enhancement of the adrenal gland
(b) Normal enhancement of the spleen
(c) Flattening of the IVC
(d) Dilatation and mural enhancement of the bowel
(e) Normal enhancement of the pancreas

26 A 32 year old previously well woman presents with a 4 week history of unilateral hip pain. There is no history of trauma or evidence of sepsis. Plain film shows marked unilateral osteoporosis of the femoral head and neck with loss of the subchondral cortex of the femoral head and neck.

Which of the following statements is incorrect with regard to the most likely diagnosis?
(a) This condition is more common on the left side
(b) Joint space narrowing is a common feature
(c) Increased uptake on bone scintigraphy is typical
(d) It is more common in men
(e) A small joint effusion on MRI is often seen

27 You are reporting plain films from the outpatient clinic. A request states "...chronological age 6 years, please assess bone age". The film shows the fingers are nearly equal in length and are divergent at the first interphalangeal joint, leading to a separation of the 2nd and 3rd digits.

What is the underlying diagnosis?
(a) Achondroplasia
(b) Down's syndrome
(c) Holt-Oram syndrome
(d) Hurler's syndrome
(e) Morquio's syndrome

28 A patient has lateral ankle pain and a feeling of hindfoot instability. MR imaging reveals a torn lateral collateral ligament and obliteration of the normal fat between the talus and calcaneus; no ligaments are visualised in this space.

What is the most likely diagnosis?

(a) Fibrous tarsal coalition
(b) Sinus tarsi syndrome
(c) Longitudinal split tears of peroneus brevis
(d) Lateral gutter syndrome
(e) Osteomyelitis

29 A lesion is noted within the marrow of a vertebral body. MR imaging reveals high signal intensity on both T1 and T2W imaging.

Which of the following processes would be consistent with these appearances?

(a) Lytic bone metastases
(b) Sclerotic bone metastases
(c) Modic type I changes
(d) Lymphoma
(e) Haemangioma

30 A pelvic radiograph reveals sacroilitis. This is most prominent on the lower and middle thirds of the joints, particularly on the iliac side. The changes are bilateral and symmetrical.

These appearances are most commonly seen in which of the following conditions?

(a) Reiter's syndrome
(b) Rheumatoid arthritis
(c) Gouty arthritis
(d) Osteoarthritis
(e) Ankylosing spondylitis

31 A patient has widespread metastatic disease. The skeletal metastases are sclerotic.

Which of the following primary cancers most commonly produce sclerotic metastases?

(a) Renal cell carcinoma
(b) Carcinoid
(c) Wilm's tumour
(d) Ovarian carcinoma
(e) Melanoma

32 A 32 year old workman presents with wrist pain. Plain radiographs show sclerosis and deformity of the lunate.

Which of the following statements is incorrect?

(a) This condition is more common on the right
(b) There is an association with positive ulnar variance
(c) Despite the presence of pain, the radiographs can initially be normal
(d) Scapholunate separation is a complication
(e) It is more commonly bilateral

33 A 14 year old boy has a CXR which shows clear lungs, no cardiomegaly, an indistinct right heart border, decreased heart density and leftward displacement of the heart.

Which of the following conditions is not associated with these findings?

(a) Prematurity
(b) Down's syndrome
(c) Noonan's syndrome
(d) Marfan's syndrome
(e) Homocystinuria

34 Which of the following is a contraindication to percutaneous vertebroplasty?

(a) Myeloma metastasis
(b) Vertebral body haemangioma
(c) Previous vertebroplasty in an adjacent vertebra
(d) Fractures involving the posterior elements
(e) Sclerotic metastases

35 A 28 year old man undergoes a CXR for occupational purposes. The lung parenchyma is clear, but the ribs are noted to be diffusely sclerotic.

Which of the following does not cause bone sclerosis?

(a) Fibrous dysplasia
(b) Acromegaly
(c) Mastocytosis
(d) Tuberous sclerosis
(e) Fluorosis

36 A 35 year old man involved in an RTA presents to A&E with lower neck pain. The mechanism of injury is thought be one of flexion. Cervical and thoracic spine films are obtained.

Which of the following flexion fractures would you describe as being unstable?

(a) Anterior subluxation
(b) Clay-Shoveler's fracture
(c) Flexion teardrop fracture
(d) Unilateral facet joint dislocation
(e) Wedge compression fracture

37 A 32 year old woman presents after minor trauma with a lump over the midshaft of her left tibia. Plain films show an 8 cm multilocular, slightly expansile, predominantly lytic lesion with a sclerotic margin, and a narrow zone of transition. The lesion is orientated longitudinally along the anterior tibial diaphysis.

What is the most likely diagnosis?

(a) Adamantinoma
(b) Eosinophilic granuloma
(c) Fibrous dysplasia
(d) Non-ossifying fibroma
(e) Chondromyxoid fibroma

38 A teenager presents with recurrent patella dislocations. Radiographs reveal hypoplastic patellae and bilateral posterior iliac horns.

Which of the following is an unlikely association?

(a) Renal dysfunction
(b) Short 5th metacarpal
(c) Hypoplastic radial head
(d) Scoliosis
(e) Hypoplastic recessed anterior iliac spines

39 A 56 year old man presents with weight loss, skin changes and sensory symptoms. He is found to have a polyneuropathy, and areas of hyperpigmentation and thickening of the skin. A CT is requested which gives the clinical details and also states "…?paraneoplastic phenomenon, ?scleroderma, ?POEMS syndrome".

Which two features at CT support the diagnosis of POEMS syndrome?

(a) Eosinophilic granuloma and hepatosplenomegaly
(b) Eosinophilic granuloma and multiple exostoses
(c) Hepatosplenomegaly and plasmacytoma
(d) Multiple exostoses and synovitis
(e) Plasmacytoma and synovitis

40 A 36 year old active male patient presents with medial foot pain. AP foot x-ray shows a triangular bone fragment projected adjacent to the medial aspect of the navicular bone, which is itself irregular in outline with a sclerotic rim. Subsequent MR imaging shows bone marrow oedema within the medial navicular and the adjacent bone seen on x-ray; additionally there is high signal within the posterior tibial tendon on T2W imaging.

What is the likely underlying diagnosis?

(a) Cornuate navicular bone
(b) Avulsion fracture of the medial navicular tuberosity
(c) Stress fracture of the navicular
(d) Os tibiale externum
(e) Type 2 accessory navicular bone

41 A 35 year old woman presents with gradually progressive knee pain over several years with locking of the joint. Plain radiographs show multiple round, well defined calcified loose bodies in the joint with no osteoporosis, and widening of the joint space.

Which of the following is the likeliest diagnosis?

(a) Synovial osteochondromatosis
(b) Pigmented villonodular synovitis
(c) Lipoma arborescens
(d) Synovial sarcoma
(e) Osteochondritis dissecans

42 A 33 year old sportsman presents with knee pain following a twisting injury. He has previously had a stainless steel screw in his knee as a result of reconstructive surgery of the anterior cruciate ligament, and the orthopaedic team request an MR examination of the knee for further assessment. You consider techniques that can be employed to reduce artefact from the metal.

Which of the following will actually increase the artefact?

(a) Utilising fast spin echo sequences rather than conventional spin echo sequences
(b) Utilising STIR sequences rather than spectral fat saturation sequences
(c) Use of a high resolution matrix
(d) A decrease in the echo train length
(e) Imaging with a 3.0 Tesla magnet rather than a 1.5 Tesla magnet

43 A 70 year old woman presents with a longstanding right sided painless swelling on her back. US shows a lesion with an array of linear strands against an echogenic background. MRI shows the lesion lies between the posterior chest wall and the inferomedial border of the scapula. It is well defined, has signal characteristics similar to surrounding skeletal muscle and has linear areas of high signal. It enhances heterogeneously after the administration of *i.v.* gadolinium.

What is the likeliest diagnosis?
(a) Liposarcoma
(b) Extra-abdominal desmoid
(c) Metastasis
(d) Elastofibroma
(e) Lipoma

44 A child presents with knee pain, without a history of trauma. Plain radiographs of the knee demonstrate expansion of the distal end of the femur.

Which of the following do not cause this appearance?
(a) Hyperphosphatasia
(b) Fibrous dysplasia
(c) Gaucher's disease
(d) Pyle disease
(e) Osteopetrosis

45 A 25 year old man presents with chronic back pain. X-rays show bilateral irregularity of the sacro-iliac joints and paravertebral ossification on the AP view. Radiographs of the feet demonstrate destruction of the interphalangeal joint of the great toe with an exuberant periosteal reaction and bony proliferation at the distal phalangeal base.

Which of the following is the likeliest diagnosis?
(a) Ankylosing spondylitis
(b) Rheumatoid arthritis
(c) Psoriatic arthritis
(d) Reiter's syndrome
(e) Inflammatory bowel disease

46 A 65 year old man has a pelvic X-ray following a fall. No fracture is identified. However, incidental note is made of thickening of the trabeculae in the ilium along with acetabular protrusion and thickening of the iliopectineal line.

Which of the following features are not seen in this condition?

(a) Picture frame vertebra
(b) Ivory vertebra
(c) Diploic widening of skull
(d) 'Cotton wool' appearance of the skull
(e) 'Hair-on-end' appearance of skull

47 A patient presents following a head injury. CT confirms an intracranial bleed.

Which of the following more accurately describes a subdural, rather than epidural haematoma?

(a) It is biconvex in shape
(b) It commonly associated with skull fractures
(c) It may cross the midline
(d) It separates the venous sinuses from the inner table of the skull
(e) It is usually arterial in origin

48 An infant has an incidental finding of bone within bone appearance within the thoracic vertebrae.

Which of the following is not a recognised cause of this appearance?

(a) Gaucher's disease
(b) Normal variant
(c) Caffey's disease
(d) Osteopetrosis
(e) Melorheostosis

49 A 35 year old man presents with leg weakness. Plain films and MRI demonstrate a lesion involving the posterior elements of the L4 vertebra only.

Given the location, which of the following lesions is least likely?

(a) Eosinophilic granuloma
(b) Aneurysmal bone cyst
(c) Osteoblastoma
(d) Renal cell carcinoma metastases
(e) Osteoid osteoma

50 An epileptic patient complains of left shoulder pain after a seizure. A posterior dislocation is suspected.

Which part of the humeral head is at risk of a compression fracture?

(a) Anteromedial
(b) Anterolateral
(c) Posteromedial
(d) Posterolateral
(e) Surgical neck

51 A patient presents with wrist pain subsequent to a fall. Carpal instability is suspected and a lateral radiograph is taken of the wrist in neutral alignment. The scapholunate angle is 70° and the capitolunate angle is 10°.

What is the most appropriate description?

(a) Normal
(b) Scapholunate dissociation
(c) Volar intercalated segment instability
(d) Dorsal intercalated segment instability
(e) Scapholunate advanced collapse

52 A 31 year old previously well woman presents with pain just above the knee. Plain radiographs show a fracture through a well circumscribed, expansile, solitary lytic bone lesion with a narrow zone of transition. The lesion involves the articular surface but does not extend into the joint space.

What is the likeliest diagnosis?

(a) Chondroblastoma
(b) Fibrous dysplasia
(c) Giant cell tumour
(d) Eosinophilic granuloma
(e) Aneurysmal bone cyst

53 A 15 year old boy presents with a history of right knee clicking, locking and intermittent swelling. There is no clear history of trauma. MRI shows a focus of abnormal signal in the subarticular marrow, a defect in the overlying cartilage, a loose intra-articular body and a small effusion.

What is the likeliest site of the cartilaginous defect?

(a) Medial aspect of the lateral condyle
(b) Lateral aspect of the lateral condyle
(c) Medial aspect of the medial condyle
(d) Lateral aspect of the medial condyle
(e) Posterior surface of the patella

54 A wrist radiograph in a child demonstrates a carpal angle of 110°.

Which of the following is not a recognised cause?

(a) Hurler's syndrome
(b) Down's syndrome
(c) Madelung deformity
(d) Turner's syndrome
(e) Morquio's syndrome

55 A 3 year old child of short stature is found to have numerous bony exostoses on plain radiography.

Which of the following statements is not true?

(a) Hereditary transmission is autosomal dominant
(b) Malignant transformation to osteosarcoma occurs in 1%
(c) The distal femur and proximal tibia are most commonly involved bones
(d) It is more common in males
(e) There is an association with polydactyly

56 A 50 year old man presents with gradual onset pain in multiple joints. Radiographs and MRI examinations show bilateral olecranon bursal effusions along with well defined, homogeneous, enhancing soft tissue masses which are isointense to muscle on T1W and hypointense on T2W which involve the wrist, ankle and knee joints.

What is the likeliest diagnosis?

(a) Rheumatoid arthritis
(b) Gout
(c) Pseudogout
(d) Psoriasis
(e) Amyloidosis

57 A 34 year old woman is found to have bilateral hilar lymphadenopathy on CXR along with elevated serum ACE levels.

Which of the following radiological features would not be in keeping with the likely diagnosis?

(a) Acro-osteolysis of the distal phalanges
(b) Erosions involving the joints of the hand
(c) A lacelike trabecular pattern in the metaphysis of the metacarpals
(d) More advanced changes in the middle and distal phalanges than the proximal phalanges and the metacarpal bones
(e) Sclerosis of multiple vertebral bodies

58 **A 30 year old patient presents with multiple bilateral renal angiomyolipomas, one of which has bled. She is also found to have a giant cell astrocytoma in her brain and bilateral interstitial lower lobe fibrosis on CXR.**

Which of the following bone lesions is most commonly associated with this condition?

(a) Bone cysts
(b) Osteochondroma
(c) Giant cell tumour
(d) Fibrous dysplasia
(e) Adamantinoma

59 **A 27 year old man presents with ongoing pain in the region of the sternum. There is no history of trauma. On examination there is tenderness, pain and swelling over the sternoclavicular joints; he is systemically well but is noted to have yellowish intradermal blisters on his hands. There is sclerosis and ankylosis of the right SCJ, with hyperostosis and hypertrophy of the left SCJ noted.**

What is the likely diagnosis?

(a) Ankylosing spondylitis
(b) Caffey's disease
(c) Osteomyelitis
(d) Paget's disease
(e) SAPHO syndrome

60 **A 30 year old man is hit by a car sustaining a 'bumper' type injury. Radiographs show a bicondylar tibial plateau fracture with an 'inverted Y' appearance.**

In the Schatzker classification, which type of fracture is this?

(a) I
(b) II
(c) III
(d) IV
(e) V

61 A 10 year old girl presents with precocious puberty and café au lait spots. McCune-Albright syndrome is suspected.

Which of the following features would you not expect to see?
(a) A ground glass lesion in the medullary cavity of the femur
(b) Champagne glass appearance of the pelvis
(c) Endosteal scalloping of the femur with intervening normal cortex
(d) Cortical expansion of the ribs
(e) Increased uptake of a rib lesion on bone scintigraphy

62 A 45 year old woman has hand radiographs for multiple joint pains. The radiographs show fusion of the distal interphalangeal joints.

Which of the following is the least likely diagnosis?
(a) Erosive osteoarthritis
(b) Reiter's syndrome
(c) Rheumatoid arthritis
(d) Psoriatic arthropathy
(e) Ankylosing spondylitis

63 An 8 year old child presents with exquisitely tender hands. Blood films demonstrate a haemolytic anaemia.

Which of the following are not plain film manifestations of this condition?
(a) H-shaped vertebrae
(b) Rib notching
(c) Hair on end appearance of the skull
(d) Cortical thickening
(e) Osteoporosis

64 A man with lower back pain has a plain lumbar radiograph. The L5 vertebral body has slipped forward on S1 by 60% of the body diameter.

What grade spondylolisthesis does this represent?

(a) I
(b) II
(c) III
(d) IV
(e) V

65 An active 48 year old woman presents with pain and paresthesia between the 3rd and 4th metatarsals, which radiates to the toes. On examination, direct pressure between the metatarsal heads replicates the pain. On axial compression of the forefoot a 'click' is heard. MR shows a well demarcated 'teardrop-shaped' mass arising between the 3rd and the 4th metatarsal heads. The lesion is isointense to muscle on T1W and hypointense to fat on T2W, and enhances on T1W following *i.v.* gadolinium.

What is the likely diagnosis?

(a) Freiberg's disease
(b) Morton's neuroma
(c) Rheumatoid nodule
(d) Schwannoma
(e) Tendon sheath ganglion

66 A 20 year old man presents with a swelling in his thigh. He recalls innocuous trauma at this site a few weeks earlier. Plain films suggest a soft tissue mass with peripheral calcification at the level of the mid femur with a radiolucent zone separating the lesion from cortex. MRI shows a heterogeneous, well defined soft tissue mass, isointense to muscle on T1W and hyperintense on T2W, with curvilinear peripheral areas of low signal intensity.

Which of the following is the likeliest diagnosis?

(a) Myositis ossificans
(b) Parosteal sarcoma
(c) Tumoural calcinosis
(d) Rhabdomyosarcoma
(e) Chondrosarcoma

67 A 60 year old man who had a THR a year previously presents with discomfort and a clicking sensation in that hip.

Which of the following features are considered normal?

(a) 3 mm radiolucent zone at the cement bone interface
(b) Endosteal sclerosis at the tip of the femoral component
(c) 5 mm subsidence of the femoral component
(d) Progressive metal bead shedding
(e) Cement fracture

68 A 47 year old man presents with severe pain of the left shin; there is no history of trauma. On examination there is thickening and fibrosis of the overlying skin. X-rays show cortical thickening of the tibia with patchy areas of exuberant longitudinal subperiosteal bone formation and streaky endosteal new bone formation in the diaphysis and distal epiphysis. A skeletal survey reveals similar changes in the left femur, but no other abnormalities.

What is the likely diagnosis?

(a) Engelmann's disease
(b) Melorheostosis
(c) Osteopetrosis
(d) Osteopoikilosis
(e) Pyknodysostosis

69 A young man was involved in an RTA 48 hours ago and is currently an inpatient in the trauma centre. He becomes dyspnoeic. Fat embolism is suspected.

Which features would be very unusual in this condition?

(a) A normal chest radiograph at 48 hours
(b) Bilateral diffuse alveolar infiltrates at 48 hours
(c) Petechiae
(d) Neurological symptoms
(e) Cardiomegaly

70 A 35 year old intravenous drug abuser presents complaining of pain in his great toe. On questioning, he has been using foot veins to inject drugs.

Which of the following statements is incorrect regarding his risk of osteomyelitis?

(a) *Staphylococcus aureus* is the likeliest organism
(b) Initial plain radiographs may be normal
(c) Localised soft tissue swelling occurs within 2 weeks
(d) A sequestrum is not seen until at least a month after the insult
(e) Radiographs are not sensitive detectors of osteomyelitis

71 A 62 year old man presents with a history of a lump in his thigh which he feels has enlarged over several months. On plain films a soft tissue mass with punctuate calcification and adjacent cortical erosion is seen. At MRI the mass is confirmed to be in the soft tissues, is heterogeneous in signal intensity but is generally isointense to muscle on T1W and hyperintense on T2W.

What is the likeliest diagnosis?

(a) Parosteal sarcoma
(b) Liposarcoma
(c) Lipoma
(d) Malignant fibrous histiocytoma
(e) Rhabdomyosarcoma

72 A 56 year old woman is found to have uniform osteopaenia, cortical thinning, acetabular protrusion, indistinct trabeculae and pseudofractures involving the femoral necks on a pelvic radiograph.

Which of the following is least likely to cause these appearances?

(a) Paraneoplastic syndrome
(b) Biliary disease
(c) Phenobarbitone
(d) Dietary phosphorous deficiency
(e) Renal tubular acidosis

73 A 30 year old undergoes a shoulder x-ray following a fall. No fracture is identified. However, note is made of acromio-clavicular joint erosion.

Which of the following is least likely?

(a) Lymphoma
(b) Hyperparathyroidism
(c) Rheumatoid arthritis
(d) Scleroderma
(e) Fibrous dysplasia

74 A CT is performed for polytrauma. A Jefferson fracture is suspected.

Which of the following appearances is consistent with this diagnosis?

(a) Bilateral anterior arch fractures
(b) Bilateral posterior arch fractures
(c) Unilateral anterior and posterior arch fractures
(d) Bilateral fractures of the superior articular facets
(e) Bilateral transverse process fractures

75 A 13 year old boy presents with a long history of a dull ache in his hip. Plain radiographs show a 4cm eccentric lytic lesion of the proximal femoral epiphysis extending to involve the proximal metaphysis. It has a lobulated, well-defined sclerotic margin and areas of calcification within it. There is significant surrounding periosteal reaction.

Which of the following is the likeliest diagnosis?

(a) Enchondroma
(b) Chondromyxoid fibroma
(c) Chondrosarcoma
(d) Chondroblastoma
(e) Giant cell tumour

Musculoskeletal and Trauma Mock Paper Answers

1 (c)
Of the above list, osteosarcoma is the most likely. The periosteal reaction (and wide zone of transition) indicates an aggressive lesion. Ewing's sarcoma is more common in the 1–10 year old age group, and fibrosarcoma in the 30–60 year old age group.

Ref: Musculoskeletal Imaging: the Requisites, 3rd Ed, p. 413.

2 (b)
Given the extent of anterolisthesis (>50% of a vertebral body), this is most likely to represent bilateral, rather than unilateral facet dislocation, and therefore an unstable injury.

Ref: Musculoskeletal Imaging: the Requisites, 3rd Ed, p. 174.

3 (d)
In rheumatoid arthritis, the femoral head tends to migrate axially, whilst in osteoarthritis, it tends to migrate superolaterally.

Ref: Fundamentals of Skeletal Radiology, 3rd Ed, p. 117.

4 (c)
The spleen is the most commonly injured organ in blunt abdominal trauma. Second most common is the liver (20%), then the GI tract (5%), pancreas (3%), and gallbladder (2%). The right lobe of the liver is more commonly injured than the left.

Ref: Radiology Review Manual, 6th Ed, p. 809.

5 (a)
In an annular disc bulge, disc tissue extends beyond the adjacent vertebral bodies by at least 3mm for more than 50% of the disc circumference. This is associated with degenerative disease and is not regarded as a true herniation.

Ref: RITI 6b_149 Degenerative Lumbar Spine Disease.

6 (a)
Pachydermoperiostosis, also known as primary hypertrophic osteoarthropathy, is an autosomal dominant condition resulting in a bilateral, symmetrical periosteal reaction of the distal long bones. This typically develops in young men and spontaneously arrests in adulthood. Compared to secondary hypertrophic osteoarthropathy, the periosteal reaction is more solid and relatively painless.

Ref: Musculoskeletal Imaging: the Requisites, 3rd Ed, p. 358.

7 (a)
85% of scaphoid fractures are detectable initially using scaphoid views. Repeat views are commonly obtained but detection of occult fractures are unreliable. Nuclear imaging is sensitive but non-specific. MRI is the best test for detection of occult fracture. However, lack of availability means that other tests are still used.

Ref: RITI 2_045 Snuffbox tenderness after fall.

8 (c)
Rings and arcs of calcification indicate a chondroid matrix. Chondrosarcoma is the likeliest primary rib tumour in this age group. Other primary malignant tumours include plasmacytoma and lymphoma.

Ref: Radiology Review Manual, 6th Ed, p. 18.

9 (e)
Uptake of ^{99m}Tc-sulphur colloid is reduced due to the replacement of bone marrow by fibrovascular tissue.

Ref: Radiology Review Manual, 6th Ed, p. 144.

10 (d)
Pigmented villonodular synovitis is a proliferation of synovium that occurs in joints, bursae and tendon sheaths. The joint space is well preserved until late in the disease.

Ref: Aids to Radiological Differential Diagnosis, 4th Ed, p. 59.

11 (c)
Giant cell tumours of the tendon sheath are histologically identical to pigmented villonodular synovitis. They usually occur in the hand, where they are the second most common benign tumour (the most common are ganglia). Only 10% of lesions are associated with bony erosion.

Ref: Musculoskeletal Imaging: the Requisites, 3rd Ed, p. 506.

12 (e)
This is considered to be a stable fracture. All patients require CT to identify fracture fragments (most commonly from the posterior, superior margin) within the spinal canal.

Ref: Radiology Review Manual, 6th Ed, p. 211.

13 (b)
It is difficult to differentiate tuberculous from pyogenic spondylodiscitis, however a number of features may point towards TB: slower progression, marked vertebral collapse, a large paravertebral abscess (which may be calcified) and a reduced osteoblastic response. In addition, pyogenic infection tends to result in earlier bridging of the affected vertebrae.

Ref: Aids to Radiological Differential Diagnosis, 4th Ed, p. 76.

14 (a)
Hyperparathyroidism is a cause of both superior and inferior rib notching, but not hypoparathyroidism.

Ref: Radiology Review Manual, 6th Ed, p. 19.

15 (d)
Marrow hyperplasia and extramedullary haematopoiesis are less severe in sickle-cell anaemia than thalassaemia major, and may not be evident on radiographs. The 'hair-on-end' appearance, obliteration of the paranasal sinuses, 'Erlenmeyer flask' deformity and widening of the skull diploe are all more common in thalassaemia major. Square shaped compression infarcts of the vertebral end plates are virtually diagnostic of sickle-cell anaemia.

Ref: Aids to Radiological Differential Diagnosis, 4th Ed, p. 612.

16 (e)
Chordomas arise from notochord remains and are therefore limited to the clivus, spine, sacrum and coccyx. Metastasis is uncommon, but when it does occur, lung secondaries are typical. Tumour size (the average size of a sacrococcygeal chordoma is 10 cm), lytic nature and location are important clues to the diagnosis.

Ref: Musculoskeletal Imaging: the Requisites, 3rd Ed, p. 526.

17 (c)
The anterior inferior iliac spine is the origin of rectus femoris.

Ref: Radiology Review Manual, 6th Ed, p. 36.

18 (d)
A Malgaigne fracture typically involves two fractures, both on the same side of the pelvic ring: one anterior to the acetabulum (*e.g.* both pubic rami) and one posterior to the acetabulum (*e.g.* through the ilium, or the SI joint).

Ref: Primer of Diagnostic Imaging, 4th Ed, p. 406.

19 (b)
Chondroblastomas almost invariably occur in the epiphyses, and 90% occur in those under 30 years old. Lesions to consider in this location and age group include: infection, chondroblastomas, GCTs and, less commonly, ABCs and eosinophilic granulomas. With regards to the other conditions mentioned: GCTs abut the articular surface; ABCs are almost always expansile; simple bone cysts are not epiphyseal; metastases are unlikely in a 20 year old.

Ref: Fundamentals of Skeletal Radiology, 3rd Ed, p. 24.

20 (d)
Signs of aortic injury include: depression of the left mainstem bronchus > 40° below the horizontal; mediastinal widening >8 cm at the level of the origin of the left subclavian artery; an indistinct aortic contour at the arch; obscuration of the aortopulmonary window; a widened left paraspinal stripe > 5 mm; a widened right paratracheal stripe > 4-5 mm; an apical pleural cap.

Ref: Radiology Review Manual, 6th Ed, p. 659.

21 (e)
In the acute phase, low T1W signal is returned from the vertebral body in both malignant and benign causes. In benign disease, the low signal will return to normal over 4-6 weeks; in malignant disease the low T1W signal is retained. Enhancement with *i.v.* gadolinium is non-specific. In benign disease, the overall mass of the vertebral body is diminished, in contra-distinction to malignancy, where it is increased.

Ref: Neuroradiology: the requisites, 2nd Ed, p. 826.

22 (c)
A Galeazzi fracture is radial shaft fracture with subluxation/ dislocation of the distal radioulnar joint. A Monteggia fracture is a fracture of the ulnar shaft with dislocation of the radial head. The reverse version refers to the angulation/ displacement of the ulnar fracture and radial head dislocation. A Maisonneuve fracture refers to a fracture of the upper third of the fibula with a tear of the distal tibiofibular syndesmosis.

Ref: Radiology Review Manual, 6th Ed, p. 87.

23 (d)
The classical finding is that of a central, usually lucent nidus of less than 1.5 cm in size with varying degrees of surrounding sclerosis. There is often a typical clinical picture which enables differentiation from a Brodie abscess.

Ref: Radiology Review Manual, 6th Ed, p. 137.

24 (c)

CT Attenuation	Type of fluid
0–20	Serum/ascites
30–45	Fresh unclotted blood
60–100	Clotted blood
>180	Active arterial extravasation

Ref: Radiology Review Manual, 6th Ed, p. 807.

25 (b)
The spleen tends to be small and hypodense in hypovolaemia. As well as the features above, there may be a 'shock nephrogram', and the aorta and mesenteric arteries may be small.

Ref: Radiology Review Manual, 6th Ed, p. 807.

26 (b)
Transient osteoporosis of the hip is a self limiting disease of unknown aetiology typically affecting one joint at a time. Bone marrow oedema is seen on MRI. Joint space narrowing is not a feature. It is associated with pregnancy although still more common overall in middle aged men.

Ref: Radiology Review Manual 6th Ed, p. 170.

27 (a)
The findings described are those of a 'trident' hand which is seen in achondroplasia.

Ref: Radiology Review Manual, 6th Ed, p. 42.

28 (b)
The sinus tarsi is the space between the talus and calcaneum that contains several ligaments conferring some hindfoot stability. In sinus tarsi syndrome there is obliteration of the normal fat and disruption of at least one of the ligaments.

Ref: Fundamentals of Skeletal Radiology, 3rd Ed, p. 216.

29 (e)
Haemangiomas tend to return high signal on both T1 and T2 weighted sequences. All the other options listed would return low signal on T1 sequences.

Ref: Aids to Radiological Differential Diagnosis, 4th Ed, p. 64.

30 (e)
Ankylosing spondylitis typically produces a bilateral, symmetrical sacroiliitis, whilst the other conditions typically result in bilateral but asymmetrical disease. Other conditions producing bilateral, symmetrical sacroiliitis include: inflammatory bowel disease, psoriatic arthropathy, osteitis condensans ilii, hyperparathyroidism and paraplegia.

Ref: Aids to Radiological Differential Diagnosis, 4th Ed, p. 101.

31 (b)
Sclerotic metastases are typically the result of: prostate carcinoma, carcinoid, transitional cell carcinoma, breast (mixed), medulloblastoma, colon (occasionally), and lymphoma.

Ref: Aids to Radiological Differential Diagnosis, 4th Ed, p. 18.

32 (b)
AVN of the lunate (Kienbock's disease) is associated with negative ulnar variance in 75%. Manual labour is a predisposing factor. Other complications include ulnar deviation of the triquetrum and degenerative joint disease in the radiocarpal and midcarpal compartments.

Ref: Radiology Review Manual 6th Ed, p. 51.

33 (c)
These findings are those of pectus excavatum which is most usually an isolated abnormality, but in addition to the above is also associated with foetal alcohol syndrome. Other radiological signs include a horizontal course of the posterior portion of the ribs along with an accentuated downward course of the anterior ribs.

Ref: Radiology Review Manual, 6th Ed, p. 17.

34 (d)
Other absolute contraindications include bleeding diathesis, acute fractures not responding to bisphosphonate treatment within 2 weeks and those where the level of collapse cannot be clearly defined.

Ref: RITI 2_020 – Painful osteoporosis vertebroplasty.

35 (b)
Acromegaly, along with Cushing's disease and scurvy are acquired causes of lucent ribs. Other causes of dense ribs include osteopetrosis, subperiosteal rib resection, chronic infection and trauma.

Ref: Radiology Review Manual, 6th Ed, p. 19.

36 (c)
Neutral films infer stability based on fracture type; stability is a function of ligamentous injury and thus cannot be implied with 100% accuracy, if doubt remains MRI or flexion/ extension views should be obtained. The other type of unstable flexion injury is a bilateral facet joint dislocation. Unstable extension injuries include Hangman's fracture and hyperextension-dislocation fracture; stable extension injuries include posterior arch of C1 fracture, laminar fracture, Pillar fracture, and extension teardrop fracture. Jefferson's fracture is an unstable compression fracture, burst fracture a stable one. 'Complex' unstable fractures include odontoid fracture and atlanto-axial disassociation.

Ref: Primer of Diagnostic Imaging, 4th Ed, p. 380.

37 (a)
These are locally aggressive lesions which tend to recur and after several recurrences can metastasize to lungs. The main differential diagnosis for this 'soap-bubble' like appearance is fibrous dysplasia, but this usually presents in a slightly younger age group.

Ref: Radiographics (2008); 28:1215–20.

38 (e)
Nail-patella syndrome (also known as Fong's disease) is described. This is a rare autosomal dominant disorder characterised by symmetrical meso- and ecto-dermal anomalies. Bilateral posterior iliac horns (seen in 80%) are diagnostic. Renal dysfunction is the commonest serious complication. A flared iliac crest with protuberant anterior iliac spines are seen.

Ref: Radiology Review Manual, 6th Ed, p. 127.

39 (c)
POEMS syndrome (Polyneuropathy, Organomegaly, Endocrinopathy/ Edema, Monoclonal gammopathy, and Skin changes) is a rare multi-systemic disease. There may be an overlap with Castleman's disease. All patients have a polyneuropathy; most authors state that a minimal of 3 of the listed features need to be present for diagnosis. There is usually a plasma cell dyscrasia: most have osteosclerotic myeloma, plasmocytomas and/ or a monoclonal gammopathy of unknown significance. Skin changes include hyper-pigmentation, hypertrichosis, plethora, and haemangiomata.

Ref: POEMS syndrome: e-Medicine article.

40 (e)
3 types of accessory navicular bones have been described; they have a collective incidence of 4–21%. Type 1 (os tibiale externum) is a small, round sesamoid bone within the posterior tibial tendon. Type 2 is a triangular ossification centre adjacent to the navicular tuberosity and connected by a synchondrosis (which is often irregular). Type 3 (cornuate navicular bone) describes an enlarged medial horn of the navicular. Types 2 and 3 are associated with PTT tears, but can independently cause pain also. Type 2 accounts for 70% of accessory navicular bones and are the dominant type in symptomatic patients. In types 2 or 3, the PTT inserts onto the accessory ossicle, leading to a more proximal insertion, reducing the leverage of the malleolus on the PTT and increasing the stress on the tendon.

Ref: JBR–BTR (2004); 87 (5): 250–1.

41 (a)
Cross sectional imaging shows a soft tissue mass of near water attenuation on CT containing calcifications, and a lobulated intra-articular mass which is isointense to muscle on T1W and hyperintense on T2W with foci of low signal intensity.

Ref; Radiographics (2007); 27:1465–88.

42 (e)
A small field of view, high gradient strength and thin sections reduce artefact as does the use of a lower strength magnet.

Ref: Radiographics (2007); 27:791–803.

43 (d)
Elastofibroma is benign tumour forming as a reaction to mechanical friction most commonly seen in the subscapular area. Recent evidence suggests a genetic component. It is bilateral in 25%. Its site, presentation and imaging characteristics are usually typical, however, excision is still performed if there is any doubt with regards to malignant transformation.

Ref: Radiographics (2007); 27:173–187.

44 (a)
There is a wide differential diagnosis for the 'Erlenmeyer flask' deformity. This includes hypophosphatasia, rheumatoid arthritis, leukaemia, achondroplasia, sickle cell disease, thalassaemia, rickets and Down's syndrome.

Ref: Radiology Review Manual, 6th Ed, p. 11.

45 (c)
The changes in the feet are characteristic of psoriatic arthropathy with soft tissue swelling and erosive changes leading to a 'pencil-in-cup' deformity. When seen, the changes at the interphalangeal joint of the great toe are pathognomonic. The SI joints are involved in 40% of cases and involvement can be either uni- or bi-lateral. As with Reiter's syndrome, a large bulky paravertebral area of ossification ('floating osteophyte') is often seen.

Ref: Radiology Review Manual, 6th Ed, p. 149.

46 (e)
The exact appearance of Paget's disease depends on which phase it is in (active, mixed or quiescent). It may be complicated by malignant degeneration, fracture or neurological entrapment. 'Hair-on-end' appearance is seen in thalassaemia, hereditary spherocytosis and sickle cell disease amongst others.

Ref: Radiology Review Manual, 6th Ed, p. 145.

47 (c)
A subdural haematoma can cross the dural reflections, including the falx, and therefore cross the midline.

Ref: Radiology Review Manual, 6th Ed, p. 327.

48 (e)
Other differential diagnoses include sickle cell, thalassaemia, congenital syphilis and acromegaly.

49 (a)
Although many expansile lesions can extend to involve both vertebral bodies and posterior elements, the commonly described lesions that preferentially affect the posterior elements are ABC, osteoblastoma, and metastases. EG commonly involves the vertebral body and only rarely involves the posterior elements. Other lesions such as haemangiomata, GCT and myeloma typically affect the vertebral bodies.

Ref: Radiology Review Manual, 6th Ed, p. 189.

50 (a)
This is the 'trough' sign also known as a 'reverse Hill-Sachs' lesion and is caused by contact against the posterior glenoid labrum during posterior dislocation.

Ref: Radiology Review Manual, 6th Ed, p. 70.

51 (b)

Classification	Scapholunate angle	Capitolunate angle
Normal	30–60°	≤ 20°
Scapholunate dissociation	> 60°	≤ 20°
Volar intercalated segment instability	< 30°	> 20°
Dorsal intercalated segment instability	> 60°	> 20°

Ref: Musculoskeletal Imaging: the Requisites, 3rd Ed, p. 353.

52 (c)
This is the characteristic patient age and site of GCT, where the unfused physis acts as a barrier to spread of the lesion. After fusion, extension to within 1cm of the articular surface is the commonest pattern, although transarticular spread has been reported. It can have either a 'soap bubble' like appearance or, as described here, a uniform lytic appearance. 10% present with pathological fractures.

Ref: Radiology Review Manual, 6th Ed, p. 95.

53 (d)
Osteochondritis dissecans is the fragmentation and sometimes separation of a portion of the articular surface usually seen in adolescent males. It is most commonly related to repetitive microtrauma although associations with other conditions such as Osgood-Schlatter's and Scheuerman's disease have been reported. It is most common in the medial femoral condyle although the humerus, capitellum and talus may be involved. It is bilateral in 10–20%.

Ref: Radiology Review Manual, 6th Ed, p. 135.

54 (b)
The carpal angle is formed by two tangential lines, the first drawn between the proximal scaphoid and lunate, and the second between the triquetrum and lunate. It has a normal range of 130–137 ^{o} in the adult and normal ranges have been derived for children of different ages. Down's syndrome is associated with an increased carpal angle (>139°) along with other conditions such as arthrogryposis.

Ref: Fundamentals of Hand and Wrist Imaging, 1st Ed, p. 166.

55 (b)
Hereditary multiple exostoses (also known as diaphyseal aclasia) is an autosomal dominant condition characterised by multiple exostoses. Malignant transformation to chondrosarcoma occurs in 1–5%.

Ref: Ophanet J Rare Dis (2008); 3:3.

56 (b)
Gout is polyarticular in 10% of cases. The soft tissue components have characteristic appearances and may calcify. Bilateral olecranan bursal effusions are considered pathognomonic.

Ref: Curr Opin Rheumatol (2009); 21(2): 124–31

57 (b)
The joints are rarely involved in bone sarcoidosis. Other musculoskeletal features include the presence of paravertebral soft tissue masses, osteolytic lesions of the skull and well defined cystic bone lesions.

Ref: Radiographics (2003); 23(6):1389–99.

58 (a)
The underlying condition described is tuberous sclerosis. The associated bone cysts most commonly affect the small bones of the hand. Other skeletal features include sclerotic bone islands which most commonly affect the calvarium (in 45% of cases) and also the pelvis and long bones.

Ref: Radiology Review Manual, 6th Ed, p. 333.

59 (e)
SAPHO syndrome (synovitis, acne, pustulosis, hyperostosis and osteitis) is a rare inflammatory bone disorder that is associated with skin manifestations. The associated hyperostosis is frequently located at the points of the bone where tendons attach, and the SCJs are the commonest site affected (70-90%). The patient is the wrong age for options (b) and (d); osteomyelitis is the main differential, but the patient is systemically well and the other features support a diagnosis of SAPHO.

Ref: Radiology Review Manual, 6th Ed, p. 160.

60 (e)
Type I (6%) is a pure wedge shaped cleavage fracture. Type II (25%) is a mixed cleavage and median compression fracture. Type III (36%) is a pure compression (depression) fracture. Type IV (10%) is a medial comminuted plateau fracture. Type VI (20%) is a transverse/oblique fracture separating the metaphysis from the diaphysis. Type V fractures are the rarest.

Ref: Radiographics (2009); 29: 585–97.

61 (b)
McCune-Albright syndrome is a form of fibrous dysplasia. It is seen in 10% of cases. Radiologically, it is characterised by a polyostotic, unilateral pattern of involvement. The skull is commonly involved. A champagne glass appearance of the pelvis is seen in achondroplasia.

Ref: Radiology Review Manual, 6th Ed, p. 79.

62 (c)
In rheumatoid arthritis, the changes classically affect the MCP and PIP joints but spare the DIP joints.

Ref: Radiology Review Manual, 6th Ed, p. 155.

63 (d)
Sickle cell disease is characterised radiologically by marrow hyperplasia. This leads to a decrease in the density of the skull with diploic widening, with widening of the medullary space. There is usually cortical thinning, along with changes related to infarction such as the 'bone-in-bone' appearance or osteonecrosis.

Ref: Radiographics (2007); 27:1005–21.

64 (c)
Spondylolisthesis is graded from I-IV with each grade corresponding to 25% of displacement.

Ref: Radiology Review Manual, 6th Ed, p. 224.

65 (b)
Morton's neuroma is actually a peri-neural fibrosis entrapping a plantar digital nerve. It is most commonly found in the 3rd/ 4th intermetatarsal space. The fibrous nature of the lesion accounts for the described MR findings. The 'click' which can be heard or palpated on examination is known as 'Mulder's' sign.

Ref: Radiology Review Manual, 6th Ed, p. 122.

66 (a)
These are the typical findings of myositis ossificans. Although in the acute stages, it can be confused with other entities, as it matures and calcifies, it can be discriminated from osteosarcomas by the pattern of peripheral calcification and from parosteal sarcomas by the lack of a connecting stalk to the cortex.

Ref: Radiology Review Manual, 6th Ed, p. 127.

67 (c)
Serial radiographs are required for full assessment of the joint replacement. As a minimum the British Orthopaedic Association suggest post-operative radiographs, then check radiographs at 1 year, 5 years and every subsequent 5 years. Other signs include progressive radiolucency at the cement bone interface, the presence of well-defined lucencies at the interface which may suggest granulomatous disease and acetabular migration. A degree of subsidence of the femoral component is considered normal and either progressive change or an absolute value of greater than 10 mm is abnormal.

Ref: Clin Rad (2009); 64: 961–71.

68 (b)
Melorheostosis is thought to be caused by a gene mutation. The characteristic plain film findings of 'candle wax dripping' is described. It tends to be monostoic, and is more common in the lower limbs with at least two bones involved. Rib, spine and skull involvement has also been reported. It can cause severe pain due to encroachment of bone onto nerves and blood vessels (which can also lead to skin fibrosis). Limb length discrepancy or contractures can result.

Ref: **BJR (1991); 64:***60–62.*

69 (e)
The onset is 24-72 hours after trauma (the chest radiograph may be normal up to 72 hours). The radiographic appearance can be similar to pulmonary oedema, however, the heart size is normal.

Ref: Aids to Radiological Differential Diagnosis, 4th Ed, p. 163.

70 (a)
Pseudomonas is the commonest responsible organism in drug users. *S. aureus* is the commonest responsible organism in non-diabetics. Diabetic patients typically have multiple responsible organisms. Plain films can be normal for up to 2 weeks. The earliest sign is soft tissue swelling. Other signs include osteolysis, endosteal erosion, and the formation of an involucrum, followed by a sequestrum.

Ref: Radiology Review Manual, 6th Ed, p. 138.

71 (d)
MFH is the commonest primary malignant soft tissue tumour of later life. It presents as a painless progressively enlarging mass. Calcification is seen in up to 20%. Cortical erosion of adjacent bone is a suggestive feature.

Ref: Radiology Review Manual 6th Ed, p. 80.

72 (a)
These are the classic radiographic findings of osteomalacia. Other causes relate to interference with vitamin D metabolism such as previous partial gastrectomy, or decreased calcium deposition in bone such as in bisphosphonate treatment in Paget's disease.

Ref: Radiology Review Manual, 6th Ed, p. 4.

73 (e)
Other causes include gout, myeloma, osteomyelitis and previous trauma.

Ref: RITI 2_035 Differential diagnosis of ACJ erosion.

74 (c)
A Jefferson fracture involves both the anterior and posterior arches, and may be either unilateral or (more usually) bilateral.

Ref: Musculoskeletal Imaging: the Requisites, 3rd Ed, p. 167.

75 (d)
The main differential diagnosis for epiphyseal lesions would be GCT. However, these typically arise in a slightly older age group and only cross the physis once it has fused. Chondrosarcomas occur in an older age group (median age 45 years) and chondromyxoid fibromas are rare (usually but not exclusively metaphyseal) cartilaginous tumours arising from the cortex.

Ref: Fundamentals of Skeletal Radiology, 3rd Ed, p. 24.

Gastro-intestinal Mock Paper Questions

1 **A 13 year old boy is undergoing his final course of chemotherapy for lymphoma. He presents to the clinic with a fever and acute right iliac fossa pain. Contrast-enhanced CT shows enhancement and circumferential thickening of the caecal wall, appendix and terminal ileum with surrounding fat stranding and free fluid.**

What is the likely diagnosis?

(a) Appendicitis
(b) Lymphomatous infiltration
(c) *Mycobacterium avium-intracellulare*
(d) Sclerosing mesenteritis
(e) Typhlitis

2 **A 42 year old woman presents with acute right upper quadrant pain and abdominal distension. She has a 1-week history of dark urine, particularly in the mornings, and is found to have pancytopaenia.**

What is the most likely diagnosis?

(a) Acute cholecystitis
(b) Acute pyelonephritis
(c) Budd-Chiari syndrome
(d) Ruptured renal cell carcinoma
(e) Infectious mononucleosis

3 **An MRI liver report reads: "There is a hyperintense lesion on T2-weighted imaging, which is hypointense on T1-weighted images. Following administration of *i.v.* Gadolinium, there is peripheral nodular enhancement in the arterial phase with progressive enhancement on the portal venous and delayed phases."**

What is the most likely diagnosis?

(a) Haemangioma
(b) Cyst
(c) Focal nodular hyperplasia
(d) Hepatocellular adenoma
(e) Hepatocellular carcinoma

4 **A 58 year old lady undergoes a CT of the abdomen and pelvis which identifies a 4 cm cyst within the pancreas. Endoscopic US-FNA shows a unilocular cyst and yields fluid with high amylase and lipase but low CEA antigen levels.**

What is the diagnosis?

(a) Serous cystadenoma
(b) Mucinous cystadenoma
(c) Intraductal papillary mucinous neoplasm
(d) Mucinous cystadenocarcinoma
(e) Pseudocyst

5 **You are asked to review a follow-up CT for a patient with a metastatic melanoma in a clinical trial. There is a single deposit within the liver which measured 10 cm on the initial study and now measures 6 cm.**

How should you classify the response by RECIST criteria?

(a) Complete Response
(b) Complete Response Unconfirmed
(c) Partial Response
(d) Stable Disease
(e) Progressive Disease

6 **A 40 year old man presents with acute left iliac fossa pain. He is afebrile and the WCC is normal. CT demonstrates a 2.5 cm ovoid lesion with surrounding fat stranding arising from the anterior wall of the sigmoid colon. The lesion enhances peripherally and has a central attenuation of –50 HU. There is no associated thickening of the colonic wall.**

What is the most likely diagnosis?

(a) Diverticulitis
(b) Epiploic appendagitis
(c) Mesenteric panniculitis
(d) Omental infarct
(e) Sclerosing mesenteritis

7 A 42 year old woman undergoes a barium swallow. This shows hold up of contrast medium in the lower oesophagus which resolves completely when the patient is given a cup of hot water.

What is the most likely diagnosis?

(a) Oesophageal varices
(b) Diffuse oesophageal spasm
(c) Presbyoesophagus
(d) Primary achalasia
(e) Intramural diverticulosis

8 Regarding pancreas divisum, which of the following statements is true?

(a) The dorsal pancreas drains via the major papilla
(b) Pancreatic drainage is *via* the duct of Santorini
(c) The dorsal and ventral pancreas drain via the same channel
(d) The common bile duct and dorsal pancreas drain via the same channel
(e) The major papilla lies proximal to the minor papilla

9 A 57 year old man presents with diarrhoea and is noted to have elevated ACTH levels. A small bowel enema demonstrates no ulceration or strictures but there is sharp angulation of loops of distal ileum.

What is the most likely diagnosis?

(a) Cushing's disease
(b) Cushing's syndrome
(c) Crohn's disease
(d) Desmoid tumour
(e) Carcinoid

10 Which of the following polyposis syndromes is not associated with malignancy?

(a) Gardner's syndrome
(b) Cronkhite Canada syndrome
(c) Turcot's syndrome
(d) Cowden's disease
(e) Peutz-Jegher's disease

11 A 51 year old lady with recurrent episodes of central abdominal pain undergoes a CT study. This is reported to show diffuse enlargement of the pancreas with a peripancreatic 'halo'.

What is the most likely diagnosis?

(a) Intraductal papillary mucinous neoplasm
(b) Autoimmune pancreatitis
(c) Chronic pancreatitis
(d) Primary pancreatic lymphoma
(e) Acute pancreatitis

12 Which of the following is not considered to be a risk factor for the development of cholangiocarcinoma?

(a) Tobacco smoking
(b) Heavy alcohol consumption
(c) Hepatitis C virus
(d) Polyvinyl chloride exposure
(e) Caroli disease

13 A 33 year old woman undergoes an MRI study to characterise a 4 cm focal liver lesion found incidentally on US. The lesion is isointense to liver on T1 and T2-weighted images, enhances homogeneously and avidly in the arterial phase and is isointense in the portal venous and delayed phases. 1 hour after the administration of contrast medium (Gd-Bopta), the lesion is hyperintense to liver.

What is the most likely diagnosis?

(a) Haemangioma
(b) Focal nodular hyperplasia
(c) Hepatocellular adenoma
(d) Fibrolamellar hepatocellular carcinoma
(e) Metastasis

14 A 52 year woman with a history of atrial fibrillation and rheumatoid arthritis presents with right-sided renal colic. On the unenhanced CT study there is diffuse low density in the liver.

Which of the following might account for this appearance?

(a) Amyloidosis
(b) Amiodarone therapy
(c) Haemochromatosis
(d) Haemosiderosis
(e) Wilson's disease

15 What is the most common site for actinomycosis infection within the abdomen?

(a) Appendix
(b) Liver
(c) Spleen
(d) Terminal Ileum
(e) Jejunum

16 A 47-year old man presents with atypical RIF pain; a CT abdomen is requested to rule out appendicitis. No cause for abdominal pain is identified. The only finding of note is an 8 mm low-attenuation lesion within the left lobe of the liver. The lesion lies inferior to the portal vein and lateral to the left hepatic vein.

What segment of the liver is the lesion in?

(a) Segment I
(b) Segment II
(c) Segment III
(d) Segment IV-A
(e) Segment IV-B

17 A 46 year old man presents with dysphagia and weight loss. He is noted to have hyperkeratosis of the palms and soles. Barium swallow shows a malignant stricture of the mid oesophagus.

What is the most likely underlying diagnosis?

(a) Dermatomyositis
(b) Epidermolysis bullosa
(c) Pemphigus vulgaris
(d) Scleroderma
(e) Tylosis

18 A patient undergoes local staging of rectal carcinoma by MRI. The report concludes that there is "a circumferential tumour extending beyond the muscularis layer which is 1 mm away from the mesorectal fascia."

How might this also be expressed?

(a) T3 disease threatening the circumferential resection margin
(b) T3 disease involving the circumferential resection margin
(c) T4 disease threatening the circumferential resection margin
(d) T4 disease involving the circumferential resection margin
(e) None of the above

19 A patient is referred for chemo-embolisation of a hepatocellular carcinoma in the right lobe of the liver. The initial angiogram demonstrates that the lesion is supplied from the superior mesenteric artery.

What proportion of patients have an arterial supply to liver from the SMA?

(a) 7%
(b) 14%
(c) 17%
(d) 21%
(e) 25%

20 Which of the following conditions does not predispose patients to gastric volvulus?

(a) Hiatus hernia
(b) Phrenic nerve palsy
(c) Previous sigmoid volvulus
(d) Diaphragmatic eventration
(e) Splenic abnormalities

21 A patient with a primary oesophageal tumour undergoes a PET-CT study using ^{18}FDG before and after receiving 1 course of chemotherapy.

In order to achieve a partial response, by how much does the standardised uptake value (SUV) need to fall between these 2 studies?
(a) 10%
(b) 15%
(c) 20%
(d) 25%
(e) 50%

22 A 47 year old woman undergoes a barium swallow. It is reported to show a diverticulum in the mid-oesophagus.

What is the most likely aetiology?
(a) Structural defect
(b) Pulsion
(c) Traction
(d) Reflux
(e) Achalasia

23 In the assessment of small bowel disease, for which of the following criteria is MRI superior to other imaging modalities?

(a) Shorter imaging time
(b) Better depiction of early disease
(c) Superior spatial resolution
(d) Better mucosal detail
(e) Superior tissue contrast

24 A 52 year old lady undergoes liver transplantation for autoimmune liver disease. 6 months later, she presents with deranged liver function and an MRCP demonstrates a non-anastamotic stricture.

What is the most common aetiology of non-anastamotic strictures in this group?

(a) Ischaemia
(b) Rejection
(c) Recurrent autoimmune liver disease
(d) Biliary cast syndrome
(e) Post-transplantation lymphoproliferative disease

25 A 48 year old man undergoes a CT colonography study which identifies a single polyp measuring 11 mm in diameter.

What is the likelihood that this polyp will contain a focus of carcinoma?

(a) 0.1%
(b) 0.8%
(c) 2.6%
(d) 6.6%
(e) 12.3%

26 A 56 year old woman is referred for an US of the liver which shows a solitary 3 cm hypoechoic lesion. US contrast is given which demonstrates the lesion to be hyporeflective with rim enhancement. The rim enhancement fades in the portal venous phase and the lesion becomes increasingly hyporeflective and well-defined.

What is the most likely diagnosis?

(a) Cyst
(b) Haemangioma
(c) Focal nodular hyperplasia
(d) Hepatocellular carcinoma
(e) Metastasis

27 A 47 year old man with multifocal hepatocellular carcinoma and chronic liver disease is referred for consideration of liver transplantation.

Which of the following would be considered for transplantation in the UK?

(a) 2 lesions measuring 5 cm or less
(b) 2 lesions measuring 4 cm or less
(c) 3 lesions measuring 3 cm or less
(d) 4 lesions measuring 2 cm or less
(e) 5 lesions measuring 2 cm or less

28 Which of the following techniques is not used to reduce patient dose during abdominal CT?

(a) Dual energy CT
(b) Reduced mAs
(c) Increased kV
(d) Iterative reconstruction
(e) Automatic exposure control

29 A 47 year old man attends for a barium swallow. This shows a lacelike pattern in the lower oesophagus above a lax lower oesophageal sphincter.

What is the most likely diagnosis?

(a) Barrett's oesophagus
(b) Oesophageal varices
(c) Oesophageal carcinoma
(d) Oesophageal candidiasis
(e) Normal oesophageal mucosa

30 You are asked to supervise a CT enterography study for inflammatory bowel disease which has been protocolled for a single 'enteric phase'.

Approximately how long after the commencement of the *i.v.* injection of contrast medium should the study be acquired?

(a) 20 secs
(b) 45 secs
(c) 70 secs
(d) 100 secs
(e) 180 secs

31 Which of the following is not a recognised complication of partial gastrectomy?

(a) Bezoar
(b) Gastric carcinoma
(c) Fistula formation
(d) Gastric lymphoma
(e) Marginal ulceration

32 A 47 year old lady with right upper quadrant pain undergoes an US. This demonstrates gallbladder calculi and focal thickening of the wall at the fundus of the gallbladder. The patient undergoes an MRCP to further evaluate this which shows multiple foci of high signal within the wall of the GB on the T2-weighted images in addition to the calculi.

What is the most likely diagnosis?
(a) Acute cholecystitis
(b) Chronic cholecystitis
(c) Gallbladder carcinoma
(d) Adenomyomatosis
(e) Xanthogranulomatous cholecystitis

33 In patients with AIDS, which portion of the GI tract is most commonly affected by cytomegalovirus infection?

(a) Oesophagus
(b) Stomach
(c) Jejunum
(d) Ileum
(e) Colon

34 A 53 year old lady undergoes a small bowel enema study. This shows delayed transit with a marked increase in the number of mucosal folds.

What is the most likely diagnosis?
(a) Systemic sclerosis
(b) Whipple's disease
(c) Intestinal lymphangectasia
(d) Eosinophilic gastroenteritis
(e) Mastocytosis

35 Which of the following primary tumours is least likely to metastasize to the small bowel?

(a) Bronchus
(b) Thyroid
(c) Melanoma
(d) Renal cell carcinoma
(e) Breast

36 A 67 year old lady is referred for staging of an anal carcinoma. On MRI, the tumour measures 5.5 cm in diameter and invades the internal sphincter, but not the external sphincter.

What is the T-stage of the tumour?
(a) T1
(b) T2
(c) T3
(d) T4
(e) T5

37 Which of the following imaging features is more suggestive of a diagnosis of Ulcerative colitis rather than Crohn's colitis?

(a) Multiple anal fistulae
(b) Aphthoid ulceration
(c) Enlarged lymph nodes
(d) Entero-enteric fistulae
(e) Granularity

38 A 35 year old man undergoes an abdominal US. The report reads: "The liver has a coarse echotexture and there appear to be multiple areas of saccular dilatation of the intrahepatic bile ducts, but no strictures. The CBD is normal. The spleen measures 16 cm. Note is also made of bilateral renal cysts."

What is the most likely diagnosis?
(a) Primary sclerosing cholangitis
(b) Primary biliary cirrhosis
(c) AIDS cholangiopathy
(d) Caroli's disease
(e) Polycystic liver disease

39 A 28 year old patient is referred to the radiology department for abdominal imaging following extensive neck surgery to remove a medullary thyroid cancer and hyperplastic parathyroid glands.

What, in particular, would you look for in this patient?

(a) Pancreatic islet cell tumour
(b) Gastrointestinal stromal tumour
(c) Adrenal cortical tumour
(d) Gastrointestinal ganglioneuroma
(e) Adrenal medullary tumour

40 What is the most common site of colonic lipomas?

(a) Caecum
(b) Transverse colon
(c) Descending colon|
(d) Sigmoid colon
(e) Rectum

41 You are referred a patient with a history of previous left hepatectomy. What liver segments will have been resected?

(a) I & II
(b) II & III
(c) I, II &III
(d) II, III & IV
(e) I, II, III & IV

42 A 42 year old man undergoes a CT of the abdomen which demonstrates the presence of a 4 cm diameter cystic lesion in the pancreas. Further evaluation with endoscopic US demonstrated that the lesion comprises innumerable small cysts each less than 15 mm in diameter.

What is the most likely diagnosis?

(a) Serous cystadenoma
(b) Pseudocyst
(c) Intraductal papillary mucinous neoplasm
(d) Mucinous cystadenoma
(e) Mucinous cystadenocarcinoma

43 A 56 year old woman who has undergone previous surgery is referred to nuclear medicine for a gastric emptying study. The patient ingests radio-labelled fruit juice, bread and scrambled egg. The gastric emptying curves demonstrate the liquid phase to have a T½ of 10 minutes and the solid phase to have a T½ of 20 minutes.

How would you interpret these findings?

(a) Normal gastric emptying
(b) Dumping syndrome
(c) Gastric stasis
(d) Previous vagotomy
(e) Gastric outlet obstruction

44 What volume of haemorrhage, approximately, would be required to give a positive result on at scintigraphy with radio-labelled red blood cells?

(a) 5 ml
(b) 25 ml
(c) 50 ml
(d) 100 ml
(e) 200 ml

45 A patient with multiple medical conditions is referred for the further investigation of a neuroendocrine tumour with ^{123}I-mIBG.

Which of the following drug classes do not affect mIBG uptake?

(a) Opioids
(b) Tricyclic antidepressants
(c) Calcium channel blockers
(d) Non-steroidal anti-inflammatory drugs
(e) Angiotensin converting enzyme inhibitors

46 With regard to non-alcoholic steato-hepatitis (NASH), which of the following statements is not true?

(a) It is seen in up to 30% of the population
(b) Diabetes mellitus is a risk factor
(c) Up to 15% of patients progress
(d) Is associated with hepatic fibrosis
(e) May resolve with dietary modifications alone

47 A 32 year old man with weight loss is referred for a barium follow through. This is reported to show mild jejunal dilatation. There is a reduction in the number of jejunal folds, an increase in the ileal folds, but only very slight fold thickening.

What is the most likely diagnosis?

(a) Whipple's disease
(b) Coeliac disease
(c) Eosinophilic enteritis
(d) Scleroderma
(e) Lymphangectasia

48 Amyloid deposition in the smooth muscle of the small bowel would most likely present with which of the following?

(a) Pseudo-obstruction
(b) Volvulus
(c) Bleeding
(d) Pain
(e) Watery diarrhoea

49 A 56 year old lady with upper abdominal pain is referred for a CT of the abdomen and pelvis. This shows an abnormal loop of small bowel passing between the portal vein and IVC.

What type of internal hernia is this?

(a) Foramen of Winslow
(b) Left paraduodenal
(c) Transmesenteric
(d) Right paraduodenal
(e) Inter-sigmoid

50 A 45 year old female patient undergoes simultaneous pancreas and kidney transplantation. A Doppler US of the pancreatic graft 1 week later shows a normal systolic flow but complete reversal of diastolic blood flow in the artery.

What is the most likely diagnosis?
(a) Arterial thrombosis
(b) Acute rejection
(c) Acute pancreatitis
(d) Venous thrombosis
(e) Arterio-venous shunt

51 What is the most common cause for small bowel intussusception in adults?

(a) Meckel's diverticulum
(b) Lymphoma
(c) Crohn's disease
(d) Gastrointestinal stromal tumour
(e) Polypoid tumour

52 A 39 year old man is referred for an MRI examination of an anal fistula. This demonstrates a fluid track extending from the perineum on the right, running medial to the external anal sphincter throughout its course and entering the anus at the 6 o'clock position.

How should you report this?
(a) Horseshoe fistula
(b) Extrasphincteric fistula
(c) Transphincteric fistula
(d) Suprasphincteric fistula
(e) Intersphincteric fistula

53 A 46 year old man presents with vomiting, epigastric pain, ankle swelling, poor appetite, and weight loss. OGD shows marked enlargement of the proximal rugal folds and ulceration. A subsequent barium follow-through examination shows dilution of barium in the stomach and thickening of folds within the small intestine.

What is the most likely diagnosis?

(a) Carney syndrome
(b) *Helicobacter pylori* infection
(c) Ménétrier's disease
(d) Pernicious anaemia
(e) VIPoma

54 A 56 year old lady with jaundice undergoes an MRCP. This demonstrates a gallstone impacted in the neck of the gallbladder. The gallbladder wall is thickened and there is intrahepatic duct dilatation due to the gall bladder compressing the common bile duct.

What is the diagnosis?

(a) Caroli's disease
(b) Klatskin syndrome
(c) Choledocholithiasis
(d) Mirizzi syndrome
(e) Cholangitis

55 Which of the following conditions is not associated with *Helicobacter pylori* colonisation?

(a) Oesophageal cancer
(b) Gastric ulcer
(c) Gastric carcinoma
(d) MALT lymphoma
(e) Duodenal ulcer

56 A 67 year old man presents with abdominal pain, weight loss, fever and diarrhoea. The small bowel enema demonstrates discrete ulcers, both circumferential and longitudinal, with mucosal fold thickening.

Which of the following conditions is most likely?

(a) Actinomycosis
(b) Tuberculosis
(c) Giardiasis
(d) Yersiniosis
(e) Strongyloidiasis

57 According to the RCR's 'Making the best use of clinical radiology services', for which of the following indications is an abdominal radiograph given the recommendation 'Indicated'?

(a) Acute GI bleeding
(b) Ingested coin
(c) Chronic pancreatitis
(d) Palpable mass
(e) Constipation

58 A 48 year old man with diabetes mellitus and abnormal liver function undergoes an MRI of the liver. The liver parenchyma has a smooth contour and is relatively hypointense on the T1-weighted image and hypointense to muscle on the T2-weighted image.

What is the most likely diagnosis?

(a) Acute hepatitis
(b) Fatty liver
(c) Haemochromatosis
(d) Autoimmune liver disease
(e) Wilson's disease

59 A previously well 56 year old man presents with right upper quadrant pain and tenderness associated with nausea and vomiting. A liver US demonstrates the presence of a large cyst containing a number of smaller cysts with a honeycomb appearance.

What is the most likely diagnosis?

(a) Cystadenoma
(b) Cholangiocarcinoma
(c) Hydatid cyst
(d) Hepatocellular carcinoma
(e) Caroli disease

60 Which of the following is not a recognised association of polycystic liver disease?

(a) Non-Hodgkin lymphoma
(b) Haemorrhage
(c) Portal hypertension
(d) Infection
(e) Polycystic kidney disease

61 A 46 year old woman is diagnosed with HIV cholangiopathy.

What is the most likely causative organism?

(a) Cryptosporidium
(b) Clonorchis
(c) Ascaris
(d) E. coli
(e) Fasciola hepatis

62 A pregnant lady presents with severe right iliac fossa pain. The surgical team request an MRI to evaluate the appendix.

What imaging sequence is best for depicting the appendix?

(a) T1
(b) T2
(c) STIR
(d) FLAIR
(e) DWI

63 Which of the following conditions is not associated with nodular regenerative hyperplasia?

(a) Polycythaemia rubra vera
(b) Rheumatoid arthritis
(c) Cirrhosis
(d) Systemic lupus erythematosus
(e) Non-Hodgkin's lymphoma

64 A 78 year old man with long history of constipation presents with severe acute abdominal pain. A supine abdominal radiograph demonstrates a dilated loop of bowel extending from the pelvis and overlying the liver, reaching to the level of the D9 vertebra. The descending colon is markedly distended.

What is the diagnosis?
(a) Giant diverticulum
(b) Megacolon
(c) Pseudo-obstruction
(d) Diverticulitis
(e) Sigmoid volvulus

65 With regard to pseudomembranous colitis, which of the following is not true?

(a) Ascites is seen in 1/3 of cases
(b) The organism is usually confined to the mucosa
(c) It is associated with the use of proton pump inhibitors
(d) Skip lesions indicate co-infection or underlying Crohn's disease
(e) It causes megacolon more frequently than ulcerative colitis

66 Following solid organ transplantation, post-transplantation lymphoproliferative disorder most commonly affects which of the following organs?

(a) Lungs
(b) Liver
(c) Spleen
(d) Kidneys
(e) Bowel

67 **A 78 year old lady presents to A&E with small bowel obstruction. A CT study demonstrates the transition point to be a loop of small bowel lying immediately behind the pectineus muscle.**

What is the diagnosis?
(a) Perineal hernia
(b) Sciatic hernia
(c) Inferior lumbar triangle hernia
(d) Femoral hernia
(e) Obturator hernia

68 **Which of the following extra-intestinal manifestations of inflammatory bowel disease is seen more commonly with ulcerative colitis rather than Crohn's disease?**

(a) Iritis
(b) Gallstones
(c) Sacroiliitis
(d) Nephrolithiasis
(e) Erythema nodosum

69 **With regard to diverticular disease, which of the following statements is true?**

(a) The rectum is involved in approximately 5% cases
(b) Localised right colonic disease is seen in 20% cases
(c) Giant diverticula most commonly arise from the caecum
(d) NSAIDs increase the risk of perforation
(e) Haemorrhage is most commonly due to sigmoid disease

70 **In abdominal imaging with 3T MRI, parallel imaging is commonly used to reduce aliasing and susceptibility artefacts.**

Which of the following is not a feature of parallel imaging?
(a) Increased signal-to-noise ratio
(b) Reduced acquisition time
(c) Increased homogeneity of signal across the field of view
(d) Improved contrast on T1-weighted images
(e) Reduced T2 blurring

71 A 45 year old man is referred for abdominal imaging with a history of watery diarrhoea, hypokalaemia and achlorhydria. CT imaging demonstrates a 4 cm diameter lesion within the pancreas which demonstrates uptake of ^{111}In-pentetreotide at scintigraphy.

What is the most likely diagnosis?

(a) Insulinoma
(b) Gastrinoma
(c) Glucagonoma
(d) VIPoma
(e) Somatostatinoma

72 With regard to squamous cell carcinoma of the oesophagus, which of the following statements is not true?

(a) It is associated with alcohol ingestion
(b) It most commonly occurs in the middle third of the oesophagus
(c) It is more common in Afro-Carribean population
(d) It is associated with smoking
(e) It is more common in women

73 A patient undergoing an endoscopic US examination is found to have a lesion within the muscularis propria layer of the stomach wall.

What is the most likely diagnosis?

(a) Adenocarcinoma
(b) Lipoma
(c) Gastro-intestinal stromal tumour
(d) Peritoneal metastasis
(e) Varices

74 An otherwise well 35 year old man undergoes an US of the liver which shows a heterogeneous echotexture. Subsequent CT and MRI images demonstrate that the liver is normal in size and has a smooth contour, but that there are innumerable tiny lesions throughout measuring less than 5 mm in diameter. These are predominantly cystic in nature, although a small solid component is present, and return a high signal on T2-weighted images.

What is the most likely diagnosis?

(a) Polycystic liver disease
(b) Metastases
(c) Caroli disease
(d) Biliary hamartomas
(e) Primary sclerosing cholangitis

75 A 47 year old man undergoes a CT of the abdomen and pelvis for suspected renal colic. Other than a previous road traffic accident, the patient has no medical history. Incidentally, the radiologist finds a number of lesions throughout the abdominal cavity of uncertain aetiology. The patient subsequently undergoes a ^{99m}Tc-sulphur colloid study and the lesions show tracer uptake.

What is the most likely diagnosis?

(a) Peritoneal metastases
(b) Tuberculosis
(c) Sarcoidosis
(d) Splenosis
(e) Mesothelioma

Gastro-intestinal Mock Paper Answers

1 (e)
Typhlitis (neutropaenic colitis) represents acute inflammation of the caecum, appendix and occasionally terminal ileum. The aetiology is unknown, but profound neutropaenia appears to be universal. Mucosal injury from cytotoxic drugs during chemotherapy is thought to play an important role; infection may be involved (*e.g.* CMV). Lymphomatous deposits would be expected to produce a more eccentric thickening.

Ref: Radiology Review Manual, 6th Ed, p. 872–3.

2 (c)
The patient has classical features of underlying paroxysmal nocturnal haemoglobinuria (PNH), which predisposes to Budd-Chiari syndrome. Budd-Chiari syndrome presents with these symptoms; the severity of the initial liver disease is variable depending upon the extent of venous occlusion.

Ref: Radiographics (1997); 17:263–5

3 (a)
These are characteristic findings of a haemangioma. A cyst will not enhance; FNH and adenoma are benign hypervascular lesions that equilibrate in the portal phase. HCC is hypervascular with washout on delayed imaging; the liver is usually cirrhotic.

Ref: Semin Ultrasound CT MR (2005); 26:116–31.

4 (e)
These are typical findings; there may or may not be a clear history of pancreatitis. An elevated CEA >200 ng/ml is an indicator of malignancy.

Ref: Clin Rad (2007); 62:1142–53.

5 (c)
A reduction of >30%, falling short of a complete response, constitutes a partial response.

Ref: European Journal of Cancer 2009;45:228–247

6 (b)
Epiploic appendages are peritoneal fat outpouchings that arise from the serosal surface of the colon, attached by vascular stalks (supplied by 1-2 small end-arteries and a draining vein). They contain adipose tissue and vessels, and measure up to 5 cm (typically 1–2 cm). Epiploic appendagitis is inflammation secondary to torsion or venous occlusion. The most common location is anterior to the sigmoid colon, there is surrounding fat stranding, and a low-density (fat) centre is seen; associated colon thickening is rare. Omental infarction can appear similar, but lacks the hyperdense ring enhancement and is more typically seen as an oval soft-tissue mass in the right lower quadrant, deep to the anterior abdominal muscles.

Ref: AJR (2004)*; 183:1303–1307.*

7 (d)
Patients often report that hot drinks provide relief in achalasia. On imaging, the sphincter relaxes and the oesophagus is seen to clear.

Ref: Diagnostic Radiology, 5th Ed, p. 621.

8 (b)
Dorsal and ventral pancreas drain separately in to the duodenum *via* the minor and major papillae respectively.

Ref: Radiographics (2009); 29:1003–26.

9 (e)
Carcinoid syndrome commonly presents with non-specific symptoms, with obstruction, bleeding pain or diarrhoea all seen. A polypoid nodule may be seen in the wall of the bowel but the desmoplastic reaction in the adjacent mesentery causes sharp angulation of bowel loops.

Ref: Radiographics (2007); 1:237–257.

10 (b)
Cronkhite Canada syndrome is a rare non-familial condition with multiple hamartomatous polyps resulting in a protein-losing enteropathy. It is seen most commonly in Japan and the underlying cause remains unclear.

Ref: Cronkhite-Canada syndrome: eMedicine.

11 (b)
This is a typical clinical presentation and characteristic imaging finding. The diagnosis needs to be confirmed histopathologically and then treated with corticosteroids, unlike other forms of pancreatitis. Relapse is well documented. Patients may progress to develop biliary complications, atrophy and chronic symptoms.

Ref: Radiology (2009); 250:118–129.

12 (a)
Tobacco smoking is not associated with cholangiocarcinoma, but there are a large number of other associations, including viral agents (HIV, HBV, EBV), liver flukes, heptolithiasis, primary sclerosing cholangitis and biliary anomalies.

Ref: Radiographics (2009); 29:683-700.

13 (b)
These imaging features are characteristic of FNH. FNH is a benign tumour thought to represent a hyperplastic response to a pre-existing arterial malformation. It is most commonly seen in women and has no malignant potential. A central scar may be seen which shows delayed enhancement.

Ref: Radiographics (2009); 29: 385–402.

14 (a)
The most common cause of diffuse low attenuation is fatty infiltration; amyloidosis is another due to amyloid deposition. Amyloidosis can be a primary condition, or secondary to chronic infectious, chronic inflammatory disease (*e.g.* rheumatoid arthritis), or multiple myeloma. Answers (b) – (d) increase copper/iron deposition within the liver, which will lead to increased liver density on a pre-contrast CT.

Ref: Radiology Review Manual, 6th Ed, p. 319.

15 (a)
Caused by *Actinomycoces israelii*, this is a rare condition which clinically mimics an appendix abscess. Sinus tracks, fistulae and a mass may all be seen at imaging. Risk factors include previous abdominal surgery, GI perforation, diabetes mellitus and steroid therapy.

Ref: Diagnostic Radiology, 5th Ed, p. 671.

16 (c)
The Couinaud classification divides the liver into 8 functionally independent segments, each with its own blood supply and biliary drainage. The portal vein divides the liver into superior and inferior segments. The middle hepatic vein divides the left (segments I-IV) and right lobes (segments V-VIII). The right hepatic vein divides the right lobe into anterior (V and VIII) and posterior (VI and VII) segments. The left hepatic vein divides the left lobe into medial (segments IV-A and IV-B) and lateral part (segments II and III); segment I is the caudate lobe, situated posteriorly.

17 (e)
Tylosis is an autosomal dominant inherited disorder characterized by thickening (hyperkeratosis) of the palms and soles, oral leukoplakia, and SCC of the oesophagus (in 95% by 70 yrs). Epidermolysis bullosa has a high association with SCC of the skin, there are rare case reports of associated oesophageal cancer. Pemphigus has a rare paraneoplastic form, typically associated with lymphoma. Dermatomyositis has a high association with various internal malignancies, in such cases it is thought to be a 'paraneoplastic' phenomenon, indicating the presence of cancer. Scleroderma results in oesophageal dysmotility, predisposing to reflux and increasing the risk of oesophageal cancer.

18 (a)
Extension through the muscularis layer in to the mesorectal fat without invasion of other structures is T3 disease. Surgeons operating on rectal cancer perform a total mesorectal excision (TME) and remove the mesorectum en bloc. At least 3 mm clearance is required on MRI to confidently predict that the circumferential margin will be negative following TME. Neo-adjuvant chemo/ radiotherapy is usually given to patients in this instance.

19 (e)
14% of patients have an accessory right hepatic artery, 7% have a replaced right hepatic artery and 4% have a totally replaced hepatic artery arising from the SMA.

20 (c)
Other predisposing factors include gastric distension and traumatic diaphragmatic hernia. It is more commonly seen in the elderly and presents with acute upper GI obstruction and wretching without producing vomitus. It is important to assess the patient for signs of ischaemia on cross-sectional imaging as this is a surgical emergency.

Ref: Diagnostic Radiology, 5th Ed, p. 639–40.

21 (b)
The EORTC define a partial response as a 15% reduction at 1 cycle or 25% reduction at 2 or more cycles. Progressive disease is a 15% increase after 1 cycle or 25% after 2 or more cycles.

Ref: Eur J Cancer (1999); 35:1773–1782.

22 (c)
In the upper oesophagus, a pharyngeal pouch may be seen as a structural defect. In the mid-oesophagus, traction from adjacent mediastinal or pulmonary fibrosis is most common, whereas pulsion causes lower-third diverticula.

Ref: Surg Clin North Am (2005); 85:495–503.

23 (e)
Small bowel enema has the best resolution and better depicts early disease. CT is the fastest study to perform. MRI has superior tissue contrast.

24 (a)
Ischaemia is the underlying cause in approximately 50% of cases; the bile ducts are supplied by the hepatic artery and their blood supply is inevitably disrupted to some extent during transplantation. Evaluation of the hepatic arterial supply to the graft is crucial as thrombosis usually requires re-transplantation in the adult population.

Ref: US of Abdominal Transplantation, p. 90–104.

25 (c)
The likelihood of there being advanced neoplasia (high grade dysplasia or >25% villous adenoma) or malignancy in a polyp is, respectively, 1.7% and <0.1% for a polyp <5 mm, 6.6% and 0.2% for a polyp measuring 6-9 mm, and 30.6% and 2.6% for a polyp measuring 1 cm or more.

Ref: Gastroenterology (2008); 135:1100–5.

26 (e)
These are the characteristic features of a hypovascular metastasis. Lesions enhance in a fashion similar to that seen on CT or MRI.

Ref: Contrast-Enhanced US in Clinical Practice, p. 7–17.

27 (c)
Transplantation is considered in patients with 1 lesion <5 cm or up to 3 lesions measuring 3 cm or less, the 'Milan Criteria'.

Ref: NEJM (1996); 334:693–699.

28 (c)
Increasing the kV will increase patient dose. Automatic exposure control modulates the mAs delivered in real time and reduces the dose to the patient. Dual energy CT alternates two energy sources and has the result of reducing dose.

Ref: Radiologic Clinics of North America (2009); 47(1):27–40.

29 (a)
Barrett's oesophagus is dysplasia of the lower oesophageal mucosa as a consequence of chronic gastro-oesophageal reflux disease. It is a premalignant condition and patients are usually enrolled in a surveillance programme.

Ref: R-ITI 3_002. The Gastro-Oeosophageal Junction, Hiatus Hernia and Reflux Disease.

30 (b)
This optimises mural enhancement. By contrast, in the evaluation of small bowel neoplasia or obscure GI bleeding, an unenhanced, arterial and portal venous study are usually used. Neutral oral contrast agents are usually favoured, although positive agents may have a role when intravenous contrast medium is contraindicated.

Ref: Radiologic Clinics of North America (2009); 47(1):117–132.

31 (d)
Partial gastrectomy was previously a common operation for the treatment of peptic ulcer disease, often in association with a vagotomy.

Ref: Diagnostic Radiology, 5th Ed, p. 642–4.

32 (d)
Adenomyomatosis of the gall bladder is characterised by deep, branching invaginations into the thickened GB wall. Seen in approximately 8% GB specimens, and associated with gallstones (90% cases), it is more common in women and often presents with RUQ pain. There are both diffuse and focal forms. The 'string of beads' sign in the GB wall is the hallmark of the disease on MRI and is said to be highly specific in differentiating it from carcinoma.

Ref: Radiographics (2008); 28:135–155.

33 (e)
CMV is one of the most common causes of enteric disease in AIDS patients, usually affecting those with a CD4 count <100. The colon is the most commonly affected site, followed by the small bowel, oesophagus and stomach.

Ref: Radiographics (1995); 15:1155–1178.

34 (a)
The 'wire-sprung' or 'hidebound' appearances are characteristic. Dilatation of the duodenum and jejunum, decreased peristalsis and sacculations (pseudodiverticulae) are also features. The remaining conditions cause a non-specific thickening of the mucosal folds.

Ref: Diagnostic Radiology, 5th Ed, p. 674–5.

35 (b)
The remaining are the commonest tumours to have blood-borne metastases to the small bowel. Direct invasion may be seen from the prostate, uterus, ovary, colon or kidney; lymphatic spread is less common but may be seen from caecum to terminal ileum.

Ref: Diagnostic Radiology, 5th Ed, p. 670.

36 (c)
Lesions <2 cm are T1, 2–5 cm are T2 and >5 cm are T3. T4 lesions are those invading adjacent organs. There is no T5 category. Depth of invasion is irrelevant with the exception of T4 disease.

Ref: TNM Atlas, p. 114-121.

37 (e)
The granular appearance on barium enema is typical. UC is typically contiguous from the rectum and appears symmetrical. In chronic disease, fibro-fatty proliferation is seen in the mesorectum and there is submucosal fat deposition.

Ref: Diagnostic Radiology, 5th Ed, p. 695.

38 (d)
These are the typical findings at US or MRI. Complications include biliary stasis, cholangitis and abscesses. The coarse echotexture would be in keeping with hepatic fibrosis (not a feature of polycystic disease), whilst PSC and AIDS cholangiopathy have thickening of the bile ducts with strictures. Caroli's disease is associated with renal cysts and medullary sponge kidney.

Ref: Ultrasound: The Requisites, p. 55–72.

39 (e)
The patient has 2/3 components of MEN Type IIA; adrenal medullary tumour being the 3rd component. MEN Type I comprises parathyroid adenoma/ hyperplasia, pancreatic islet cell tumours and pituitary adenoma. MEN Type IIB comprises medullary thyroid carcinoma, adrenal medullary tumour and a variety of mucosal and cutaneous neurogenic lesions.

Ref: Diagnostic Radiology, 5th Ed, p. 1713.

40 (a)
Lipomas are relatively common sub-mucosal lesions in the GI tract, seen in 4.4% of patients at autopsy, and may be solitary or multiple. In the colon, 45% of these are seen in the caecum.

Ref: Radiographics (2007); 27:1039–54.

41 (b)
These segments are also referred to as the left lateral lobe. Resection of Segment IV also is termed an extended left hepatectomy. Resection of V, VI, VII and VIII is a right hepatectomy; an extended right hepatectomy includes segment IV also. The caudate lobe is usually only resected during liver transplantation.

42 (a)
This is the typical appearance of this benign cystic lesion, formerly referred to as a microcystic tumour. Mucinous tumours tend to produce larger cysts and IPMN may extend along the main or side pancreatic ducts. A pseudocyst is often unilocular but may contain debris.

Ref: Clin Rad (2007); 62:1142–53.

43 (b)
The T½ for both of these phases is abnormally low indicating rapid transit of liquid and solid components; dumping syndrome may be seen following gastric surgery. Normal rates of emptying are T½ <30 minutes for liquids, and 30-120 minutes for solid food. Vagotomy leads to rapid gastric emptying and delayed solid emptying. Gastric stasis will result in delayed transit of solid and liquid components.

Ref: R-ITI 7g_002. Gastric emptying.

44 (c)
Approximately 50 ml, which is similar to the volume required to give malaena. Nuclear medicine techniques are unlikely to be of value when GI bleeding is only detected by chemical tests, *e.g.* faecal occult blood.

Ref: R-ITI 7g_003. Gastrointestinal bleeding.

45 (d)
Tramadol, antipsychotics, phenothiazines, butyrophenones, salbutamol, amiodarone and cocaine may also interfere with MIBG uptake.

Ref: R-ITI 7o_011. Neuroendocrine imaging with mIBG and somatostatin receptor scintigraphy (SRS).

46 (a)
Hepatic steatosis is seen in this proportion of the population; of these, 6-8% progress to NASH, where there is inflammation of the hepatocytes and abnormal liver function.

Ref: R-ITI 3_114. Liver: Cirrhosis and NASH.

47 (b)
This appearance, known as jejunisation of the ileum, is typical of coeliac disease. There is an associated increase in the frequency of both epithelial tumours and NHL in patients with coeliac disease.

Ref: R-ITI 3_055a. Small bowel session 1: Diffuse and multi-system diseases of the small bowel.

48 (a)
Pain, bleeding or diarrhoea might be seen with deposition in the bowel wall. Volvulus is not a feature of amyloidosis. Both primary and secondary amyloidosis may affect the bowel, as well as other organs.

Ref: R-ITI 3_055a. Small bowel session 1: Diffuse and multi-system diseases of the small bowel.

49 (a)
The loop of bowel passes through the foramen of Winslow in to the lesser sac. Left paraduodenal hernias pass through a defect in the descending mesocolon and lie to the left of the 4th part of the duodenum; the rarer right paraduodenal hernia passes behind the SMA and is associated with malrotation. Transmesenteric hernias are commoner following surgery.

Ref: R-ITI 3_062 Small bowel session 2: Structural and Vascular Abnormalities of the Small Bowel. Small Bowel Infections.

50 (d)
This is the effect of the entire blood supply to the graft passing back and forth through the artery and is well recognised in pancreatic or renal transplantation. This requires prompt intervention and may result in graft loss.

Ref: US of Abdominal Transplantation, p. 24–7.

51 (e)
Polypoid tumours are the most common cause for small bowel intussusceptions in adults and these may have one of a number of histopathological diagnoses. Crohn's disease does not cause an intussusception but the other conditions can on occasion.

Ref: R-ITI. 3_060. Small bowel obstruction.

52 (e)
There are 4 types of fistula (b) – (e), with the intersphincteric type the only one that does not pass through the external sphincter (hence it is always medial to it). If a fistula extends around both sides of the anal canal, this is termed a horseshoe extension.

Ref: R-ITI 3_071. Endoanal Ultrasound and Anal/Rectal MRI (Non-Malignant) Fistula Disease.

53 (c)
Ménétrier's disease (giant hypertrophic gastritis) results in marked thickening of the gastric mucosal folds, typically in the proximal half of the stomach. The gastric mucosa secretes copious mucus (dilution of barium), which results in a protein-losing enteropathy (leading to SB fold thickening). There is associated achlorhydria which can lead to ulceration.

Ref: Primer of Diagnostic Imaging, 4th Ed, p. 170.

54 (d)
This is Mirizzi syndrome. The inflamed gallbladder compresses the CBD to result in obstructive jaundice. Patients often have a low insertion of the cystic duct in the common bile duct.

55 (a)
Oesophageal carcinoma rates have been increasing as *H. pylori* colonisation rates have fallen. A protective effect against some conditions has been postulated but this is highly controversial.

Ref: Clin Microbiol Rev (2006); 19(3):449–90.

56 (b)
Lesions are often multiple, and stricture formation is also commonly seen. When the terminal ileum is involved, a rigid and gaping ileocaecal valve may be seen. Cross-sectional imaging may show low attenuation lymph nodes (due to caseous liquefaction), ascites and peritoneal nodules.

Ref: Diagnostic Radiology, 5th Ed, p. 670–1.

57 (c)
The AXR may show calcification, but is of little value in excluding this diagnosis. Ingested foreign bodies should only have abdominal radiographs if they may be dangerous *e.g.* battery. Constipation is only an indication in specific circumstances.

Ref: Making the best use of clinical radiology services, 6th Ed, RCR.

58 (c)
The low signal within the liver parenchyma on T2-weighted images is due to the susceptibility artefact from iron overload. Patients with haemochromatosis deposit iron within the skin, heart, liver and pancreas. This degree of iron within the liver can be quantified using MRI.

Ref: Semin Ultrasound CT MR (2005); 26:116–31.

59 (c)
Hydatid infection is caused by Echinococcus multilocularis, and may give rise to a number of appearances at US with cysts being uni- or multi-loculated, thin or thick-walled, with or without calcification. The appearance described here is referred to as daughter cysts. Cystadenoma gives rise to a large unilocular cyst or septated cyst. Caroli disease is due to duct abnormalities; hepatocellular carcinoma and cholangiocarcinoma are solid lesions.

Ref: AJR (1985); 145:639–648.

60 (a)
Polycystic liver disease is a hereditary condition that may or may not be associated with polycystic kidney disease. There is no malignant potential within the cysts but complications may arise from the sheer size of the cysts, and therapeutic interventions. Aspiration, fenestration and enucleation may provide short term relief, but some cases will require repeated therapy or transplantation.

Ref: Radiographics (2006); 26:1655–68.

61 (a)
HIV (or AIDS) cholangiopathy is due to opportunistic infection, most commonly with Cryptospordium, in patients with established HIV infection. Radiological features include duct wall thickening, strictures and duct dilatation.

Ref: Diagnostic Radiology, 5th Ed, p. 778–9.

62 (b)
T2 weighted images best depict the appendix, but a STIR sequence is sensitive for indentifying an inflamed and oedematous appendix. MRI has a sensitivity, specificity and accuracy of over 90% for the diagnosis of acute appendicitis.

Ref: Radiographics (2007); 27:1419–31.

63 (c)
NRH is diffuse nodularity of the liver produced by regenerative nodules in the absence of hepatic fibrosis. Although a rare entity, it is commonly associated with portal hypertension (50% cases).

Ref: European Radiology (2000); 10(Supp 2); S179-80.

64 (e)
These are the classical radiological features of sigmoid volvulus on the plain abdominal film. The sigmoid is prone to twisting as it has a short mesentery and when it does so, it rotates anti-clockwise and may become ischaemic. It is seen more commonly in the elderly with constipation, in those with high fibre diets, and in children. Decompression alone will lead to representation in 50% within 2 years.

Ref: Can Assoc Radiol J (2004); 55:297-303.

65 (d)
Clostridium difficile, the organism which causes pseudomembranous colitis, acts through the release of endotoxins which produce diarrhoea and abdominal pain. The use of PPIs increases the survival of vegetative matter in the stomach and is strongly associated with this condition. The colon may be affected from the rectum to the caecum in a variety of patterns.

Ref: Radiology (2006); 240:623–38.

66 (b)
The liver is affected most frequently, with involvement seen in up to 45% of liver transplant PTLDs, 40% of pancreas transplant PTLDs, 23% of heart transplant PTLDs and 10% of lung transplant PTLDs.

Ref: Radiographics (2009); 29:981–1002.

67 (e)
The pectineus muscle is the anterior border of the obturator canal, with the obturator externus the posterior margin. Bowel is commonly obstructed with this type of hernia, often seen in elderly patients.

Ref: R-ITI 3_009. Abdominal wall hernia.

68 (c)
Crohn's disease is more commonly associated with a peripheral, migratory, non-deforming seronegative arthropathy.

Ref: http://www.gastroresource.com/GITextbook/en/chapter10

69 (d)
Rectal involvement is rare, with localised right colonic disease seen in around 5% of cases whilst sigmoid disease accounts for 80%. Giant diverticulae most commonly arise in the sigmoid colon, but bleeding is more common from the right colon. Glucocorticoids also increase the risk of perforation.

Ref: R-ITI 3_073. Colon: Diverticular disease of the colon.

70 (a)
Parallel imaging has a number of advantages, but reduces the signal-to-noise ratio. Abdominal imaging at 3.0T brings a number of challenges which are more difficult to overcome than in neurological or musculoskeletal imaging.

Ref: Radiographics (2007); 27:1433–44

71 (d)
These are the characteristic clinical features (Verner-Morrison syndrome) associated with these uncommon tumours. 90% of tumours are intrapancreatic and they measure 2–7 cm at diagnosis. Extrapancreatic lesions are usually benign, but 50% of pancreatic lesions are malignant. Lesions also take up ^{123}I-VIP.

Ref: Diagnostic Radiology, 5th Ed, p. 1719–22.

72 (e)
It is most commonly seen (50% cases) in the middle third, between the aortic arch and the inferior pulmonary vein. Smoking and alcohol are the major risk factors and appear to have a synergistic effect in increasing incidence. It is more commonly seen in men.

Ref: R-ITI 3_024. Oesophagus: Tumours of the oesophagus 1.

73 (c)
GIST, leiomyoma and leiomyosarcoma arise in this level. Adenocarcinoma arises within the mucosa, lipoma within the submucosa and metastases are seen at the serosal surface. Varices may be in the submucosa or extrinsic to the stomach.

Ref: R-ITI. 3_059. Gastro-intestinal stromal tumours (hollow organ and mesentery).

74 (d)
These are the typical appearances of biliary hamartomas (von Meyenberg complexes), a benign abnormality of the ductal plate which may be misinterpreted as metastases.

Ref: Diagnostic Radiology, 5th Ed, p. 744–6.

75 (d)
Splenosis represents the heterotopic autotransplantation of splenic tissue that usually follows traumatic rupture of the spleen. The diagnosis may also be made with ^{99m}Tc-labelled heat denatured erythrocytes or MRI following administration of iron-oxide particles.

Ref: Diagnostic Radiology, 5th Ed, p. 1768–9.

Genito-urinary, Adrenal, Obstetrics & Gynaecology and Breast Mock Paper Questions

1 **A 52 year old man presents with loin pain and microscopic haematuria. KUB reveals no abnormality. A CT KUB demonstrates a 7 mm mid-ureteric calculus.**

What is the most likely composition of the calculus?

(a) Calcium phosphate
(b) Calcium oxalate
(c) Urate
(d) Xanthine
(e) Cystine

2 **A 63 year old lady is discovered to have a 3 cm adenocarcinoma of the right lung. Staging CT reveals a unilateral, well-defined, round 12 mm adrenal lesion. A further CT characterization study reveals the lesion has Hounsfield value of + 20 on the unenhanced study. Enhancement is uniform, with delayed images demonstrating 65% washout of contrast medium.**

What is the likeliest diagnosis?

(a) Metastasis from lung carcinoma
(b) Adrenocortical adenoma
(c) Adrenal haemorrhage
(d) Adrenocortical carcinoma
(e) Adrenocortical hyperplasia

3 **A 40 year old man presents with a scrotal mass. US shows a smooth, round, well defined thin walled 2 cm hypoechoic lesion in the epididymal head. The lesion contains low level echoes which move on close examination.**

The most likely diagnosis is?

(a) Epididymal cyst
(b) Spermatocoele
(c) Adenomatoid tumour
(d) Papillary cystadenoma
(e) Haemangioma

4 A 46 year-old woman presents with abdominal pain, dysuria and abdominal distension. A plain AXR is performed, which shows air within the right ureter and renal pelvis.

Which of the following is the least likely aetiology?
(a) Caecal tumour
(b) Urinary tract infection with Clostridium spp.
(c) Meckel's diverticulum
(d) Pelvic actinomycosis
(e) Small bowel MALT

5 A frail 72 year old diabetic woman has serum creatinine measurements which are persistently at the upper end of the normal range. A nuclear medicine clearance scan is requested for a more accurate estimate of glomerular filtration rate.

Which of the following tracers would be most appropriate?
(a) ^{51}Cr-EDTA
(b) ^{99m}Tc-DMSA
(c) ^{99m}Tc-Glucoheptonate
(d) ^{99m}Tc-HIDA
(e) ^{99m}Tc-MAG3

6 A 34 year old man presents with gradual onset bilateral loin pain. Ultrasound demonstrates multiple bilateral renal cystic masses.

Which of the following would not support a diagnosis of Von-Hippel Lindau?
(a) Contrast enhancement on CT of more than 20 HU
(b) Raised urinary catecholamines
(c) Multiple pancreatic cysts
(d) Cutaneous angiofibromas
(e) Cerebellar haemangioblastomas on brain MRI

7 A 60 year old man with a prostate specific antigen of 15 ng/ml and a smooth feeling prostate on digital rectal examination is referred for prostate biopsy.

Which of the following statements is incorrect?

(a) A transperineal rather than transrectal approach is possible
(b) Urinary retention is a common complication
(c) Both peripheral and transitional zones should be sampled
(d) A negative biopsy does not exclude prostate cancer
(e) Prophylactic antibiotics should be given routinely

8 A 52 year old man is referred for a renal US as part of an investigation for proteinuria. US shows a 2 cm round, well-defined right upper pole cystic lesion. At CT, the lesion demonstrates internal hairline-thin septae and barely perceptible enhancement after the administration of intravenous contrast medium.

Which of the following statements is true?

(a) This is a Bosniak IV lesion
(b) This lesion should be surgically excised
(c) This lesion should be followed-up
(d) This is a Bosniak I lesion
(e) Bosniak classification can be defined on US

9 A 55 year old female patient presents with a history of unilateral breast pain. 11 years earlier she had undergone breast augmentation for cosmetic reasons. Her sister has recently been diagnosed with breast cancer and she is concerned she may also have breast cancer.

Which of the following statements is true?

(a) Most implants fail at 5 years
(b) MRI is the initial investigation of choice
(c) Screening mammography is contraindicated
(d) The linguine sign is indicative of rupture on US
(e) Most implants are placed in the retroglandular region

10 A 45 year old man with a childhood history of orchidopexy for undescended testis presents with a painless mass in his right hemiscrotum. US shows a discrete uniform hypoechoic mass confined within the tunica albuginea. MRI shows the lesion is of uniformly low signal intensity on T2W. Serum αFP is normal and β-HCG is elevated.

What is the likeliest diagnosis?

(a) Teratoma
(b) Yolk sac tumour
(c) Seminoma
(d) Embryonal cell carcinoma
(e) Lymphoma

11 A 62 year old woman presents with a solitary palpable breast lump. Mammography does not demonstrate any microcalcification within the mass. US demonstrates an irregular solid mass which casts a posterior acoustic shadow.

Which of the following techniques is most appropriate for obtaining tissue diagnosis?

(a) Ultrasound guided core biopsy
(b) Ultrasound guided FNA
(c) Stereotactic guided core biopsy
(d) Stereotactic vacuum assisted biopsy
(e) MRI guided biopsy

12 A 2 month old presents with vomiting and diarrhoea present from the neonatal period. On examination abdominal distension with hepatosplenomegaly is noted. CT demonstrates significantly enlarged adrenal glands which maintain their normal shape and have extensive punctuate calcification bilaterally. Small bowel wall thickening is also noted.

What is the likeliest diagnosis?

(a) Waterhouse-Friedrichsen syndrome
(b) Wolman disease
(c) Neuroblastoma
(d) Tuberculosis
(e) Phaeochromocytoma

13 Which of the following are not radiological signs of renal artery stenosis?

(a) Delayed appearance of contrast material on IVU
(b) Notching of proximal ureter on IVU
(c) Spectral broadening and flow reversal on Duplex US
(d) Decreased density of contrast material on IVU
(e) Tardus/ parvus waveform on Duplex US

14 A 50 year old woman is found to have multiple, round, well defined filling defects in her left ureter on IVU.

Which of the following is the least likely diagnosis?

(a) Emphysematous ureteritis
(b) Ureteritis cystica
(c) Malakoplakia
(d) Leukoplakia
(e) Cervical carcinoma

15 A 16 year old boy presents with a history of headaches, abdominal pain, palpitations and sweating. CT examination shows bilateral well defined adrenal lesions, each measuring approximately 2 cm, which enhance avidly with intravenous contrast medium. MRI shows the lesions to be hyperintense to spleen on T2W with no change in signal on opposed phase T1W. Angiography shows a 'spoke-wheel' like appearance of both lesions.

What is the likeliest diagnosis?

(a) Bilateral phaeochromocytoma
(b) Adrenocortical carcinoma with contralateral metastasis
(c) Adrenal hyperplasia
(d) Li-Fraumeni syndrome
(e) Bilateral hyperfunctioning adrenocortical adenomas

16 A 63 year old man with a history of renal calculi presents with a 4 month history of unilateral flank pain, weight loss and fever. Renal US shows loss of cortico-medullary differentiation, with hypoechoic dilated calyces with an echogenic rim and multiple hypoechoic masses with low level internal echoes replacing much of the renal parenchyma. CT confirms a 1 cm calculus in the renal pelvis and multiple low attenuation masses within the kidney. Angiography shows displacement of segmental arteries around an avascular masses.

What is the likeliest diagnosis?

(a) Candida pyelonephritis
(b) Renal sarcoma
(c) Chronic renal infarction
(d) Multilocular renal cell carcinoma
(e) Xanthogranulomatous pyelonephritis

17 A 50 year old metformin-controlled diabetic man presents with renal colic. His serum creatinine is 90 µmol/L. Initial CT KUB is equivocal and the decision is made to administer *i.v.* contrast medium.

Which of the following statements is incorrect?

(a) Contrast induced nephropathy (CIN) is usually transient
(b) The single most important risk factor for CIN is pre-test GFR
(c) High osmolar contrast media are more nephrotoxic than low osmolar contrast media
(d) The patient should stop his metformin for 48 hours after the examination
(e) The patient should be well hydrated prior to the examination

18 A 38 year old man presents with an infected, hydronephrotic kidney secondary to an impacted 9 mm distal ureteric calculus. The decision is made to proceed to percutaneous nephrostomy.

Which of the following sites would be best approached for initial puncture?

(a) Renal pelvis
(b) Anterior approach to upper pole calyx
(c) Posterior approach to upper pole calyx
(d) Anterior approach to lower pole calyx
(e) Posterior approach to lower pole calyx

19 A 48 year old man presents with urinary frequency, urgency and dysuria. A cystogram demonstrates superior and anterior displacement of the bladder with a 'teardrop' appearance. IVU shows medial displacement of the distal ureters with mild bilateral hydronephrosis.

What is the likeliest diagnosis?

(a) Liposarcoma
(b) Lipoblastoma
(c) Pelvic lipomatosis
(d) Hibernoma
(e) Teratoma

20 A 28 year old lady presents with PV bleeding and right-sided lower abdominal pain. Serum β-HCG is elevated. Transabdominal US does not show an intrauterine pregnancy.

What is the likeliest site of an ectopic pregnancy?

(a) Right ovary
(b) Tubal ampulla
(c) Tubal isthmus
(d) Pouch of Douglas
(e) Cervix

21 A 30 year old woman presents with chronic pelvic pain and dyspareunia. PV examination reveals tenderness in the right adnexa. Pelvic US shows a 4 cm cystic lesion arising from the right ovary with diffuse homogeneous low-level internal echoes and echogenic wall foci.

What is the likeliest diagnosis?

(a) Haemorrhagic ovarian cyst
(b) Endometrioma
(c) Dermoid
(d) Cystadenocarcinoma
(e) Tubo-ovarian abscess

22 Regarding traumatic urethral injury, which of the following statements is true?

(a) It occurs in 1% of all pelvic fractures
(b) The posterior urethra is more commonly injured than the anterior
(c) It is equally common in males and females
(d) It is associated with bladder rupture in 50% of cases
(e) At urethrography, the AP view provides most information

23 A 50 year old woman develops microscopic haematuria and is referred for an IVU. This demonstrates bilateral bulbous cavitation of the papillae with streaks of contrast material extending from the fornix parallel to the axis of the papillae and diminished density of the nephrogram. In addition, small filling defects are seen in the renal calyces.

Which of the following is most likely to account for these findings?

(a) Sickle cell disease
(b) Analgesic nephropathy
(c) Renal vein thrombosis
(d) Christmas disease
(e) Hepatic cirrhosis

24 A 35 year old man presents with night sweats and weight loss. CT examination shows multiple enlarged lymph nodes in the thorax and abdomen with homogeneous, ill defined masses in the kidney. A diagnosis of renal lymphoma is suspected.

Which of the following statements is incorrect?

(a) Renal involvement is more common in NHL than Hodgkin's disease
(b) Primary renal lymphoma is less common than secondary renal lymphoma
(c) It is more commonly bilateral than unilateral
(d) Enhanced through transmission is commonly seen on US
(e) Avid enhancement after contrast medium administration is seen on CT

25 A 30 year old woman presents with a history of hypertension and headache. She undergoes renal angiography which demonstrates alternating areas of stenosis and ectasia in the distal third of both main renal arteries.

What is the likeliest diagnosis?

(a) Atherosclerosis
(b) Takayasu's arteritis
(c) Polyarteritis nodosa
(d) Fibromuscular dysplasia
(e) Buerger's disease

26 A 30 year old woman presents to the emergency department hypotensive and unwell. CT shows retroperitoneal blood which is arising from a 6 cm renal mass. The mass is well defined and on unenhanced imaging has a mean density of –5 HU.

What is the most likely diagnosis?

(a) Renal oncocytoma
(b) Renal cell carcinoma
(c) Renal angiomyolipoma
(d) Renal liposarcoma
(e) Renal lipoma

27 A 32 year old woman presents with dysmenorrhoea and menorrhagia. MRI confirms the presence of a large fibroid.

Which of the following statements is true regarding uterine fibroid embolisation (UFE)?

(a) Uterine artery is usually embolised on one side
(b) The uterine artery is a branch of the posterior division of the internal iliac artery
(c) An 8 Fr catheter should be used to catheterize the uterine artery
(d) Embolisation is best achieved with coils
(e) UFE is generally not preferred for pedunculated fibroids

28 Regarding the practical use of Hyoscine-N-butylbromide as a smooth muscle relaxant in imaging of the pelvis, which of the following statements is true?

(a) The dose is 2 mg given intravenously
(b) A history of angina is a contraindication
(c) It is contraindicated in patients with porphyria
(d) Open angle glaucoma is a contraindication
(e) The patient should not drive him/herself home

29 A 28 year old woman is referred for investigations for infertility. HSG and MRI demonstrate normal fundal contour but no division of the uterine horns and a single uterine canal with a saddle shaped fundus.

What is the most likely diagnosis?

(a) Arcuate uterus
(b) Septate uterus
(c) Bicornuate uterus
(d) Uterus didelphys
(e) Unicornuate uterus

30 A 63 year old man is diagnosed with prostate cancer on needle biopsy. Staging MRI shows a solitary low signal intensity lesion on T2W extending from the right peripheral zone into the seminal vesicle on that side. No abnormal local lymph nodes are seen. Bone scintigraphy is unremarkable.

What is the TNM staging of this cancer?

(a) T1c N0 M0
(b) T2c N0 M0
(c) T3a N0 M0
(d) T3b N0 M0
(e) T4a N0 M0

31 A 73 year old woman is referred to the post-menopausal bleed fast track clinic where she undergoes a transvaginal US.

Which of the following statements is incorrect?

(a) Endometrial measurement should be of both opposed endometrial layers
(b) The normal endometrial thickness measurement should be less than 5 mm
(c) If she is taking HRT, normal endometrial thickness can be up to 20 mm
(d) Normal measurement limits can be increased by 1–2 mm in obese patients
(e) Biopsy/D+C is advisable if she is not on HRT and has an endometrial thickness of >8 mm

32 A 26 year old man is involved in an RTA, and falls from his motorcycle at 60 mph. On arrival in the emergency department he is alert and mobile with a blood pressure of 115/72 and a pulse rate of 60/min. He complains of mild discomfort over his left lower ribcage. A urine sample demonstrates rose coloured urine.

Which of the following is the most appropriate next step?

(a) Renal ultrasound
(b) Admit for observation and image should he deteriorate
(c) Contrast enhanced CT of the abdomen
(d) IVU
(e) Renal angiography

33 Regarding breast MRI techniques, which of the following is incorrect?

(a) The patient should be prone
(b) The phase encoding direction should be in the anterior to posterior plane
(c) Reducing the field of view improves the in plane resolution
(d) Chemical shift artefact can be reduced by increasing the bandwidth per pixel of the imaging sequence
(e) Wrap-around artefact can be reduced by increasing the number of sampling points in the phase encoding direction

34 An otherwise normal baby is found to have an impalpable right testis at birth. At 6 months he undergoes an US to confirm the presence of an undescended testis.

What is the most likely location for such a testis?
(a) Inguinal canal
(b) Pubic tubercle
(c) Immediately inferior to the right kidney
(d) Contralateral hemiscrotum
(e) Perineum

35 A 26 year old woman who has a Mirena IUCD in situ presents with intermittent lower abdominal pain.

Which of the following statements is correct?
(a) 3T MRI is contraindicated
(b) Mirena IUCDs are better visualised than copper IUCDs on transabdominal US
(c) Threads of a lost coil are not visible on ultrasound
(d) IUCDs increase the risk of ectopic pregnancy
(e) The Mirena is commonly used for the treatment of dysfunctional uterine bleeding

36 A 30 year old woman with a previous history of pelvic inflammatory disease is undergoing investigations for infertility.

With regards to assessment of tubal patency, which of the following statements is correct?

(a) Gadolinium enhanced MRI is the investigation of choice
(b) Normal fallopian tubes are visible on pelvic US
(c) Hysterosalpingography should be performed in the first half of the menstrual cycle
(d) Hysterosalpingo contrast sonography is as good as laparoscopy and dye instillation
(e) Iodine based contrast is used for hysterosalpingo contrast sonography

37 A 34 year old woman with 2 previous unremarkable vaginal deliveries presents with a history of pelvic pain. TV US shows diffuse heterogeneous myometrial echotexture with multiple tiny myometrial cystic lesions and poor definition of the junctional zone. MRI shows an indistinct diffuse predominantly low signal intensity lesion with small foci of increased signal intensity on T2W along with diffuse widening of the junctional zone on T2W.

What is the most likely diagnosis?

(a) Adenomyosis
(b) Leiomyoma
(c) Endometrial carcinoma
(d) Muscular hypertrophy
(e) Myometrial contraction

38 A 35 year old man is involved in a high speed RTA and sustains a Malgaigne's type pelvic fracture. A small urethral catheter is successfully passed in the emergency department. The patient subsequently develops dark haematuria.

Which of the following statements is true?

(a) The haematuria is most likely to be related to catheter trauma
(b) 70% of patients with pelvic fractures have a bladder rupture
(c) At cystography, widening of the fat planes of obturator internus on the control film suggests intraperitoneal rupture
(d) Extraperitoneal rupture accounts for 40% of traumatic bladder injuries
(e) 10% of ruptures can only be detected after emptying the bladder of contrast medium at cystography

39 A 23 year old woman presents with abdominal pain. Her β-HCG test is positive and her LMP was 6 weeks ago. An US scan is arranged.

Which of the following features suggest a pseudogestational sac rather than a true gestational sac?

(a) A well defined complete decidual reaction of greater than 2 mm
(b) Location of the lesion within the fundus
(c) A round or oval appearance
(d) The lack of a double decidual sign
(e) Eccentricity of the lesion relative to the endometrium

40 A 54 year old man presents with microscopic haematuria. CT shows a 3 cm renal mass containing flecks of calcification and which demonstrates heterogeneous enhancement with *i.v.* contrast medium.

What is the likeliest diagnosis?

(a) Oncocytoma
(b) Angiomyolipoma
(c) Lymphoma
(d) Transitional cell carcinoma
(e) Renal cell carcinoma

41 Regarding the anatomy of the normal kidney, which of the following statements is true?

(a) The renal arteries typically have three divisions
(b) The column of Bertin is isoechoic to renal cortex
(c) The column of Bertin represents the fusion of the embryological anterior and posterior kidneys
(d) The right renal artery typically arises at the level of the L3 intervertebral disc
(e) The left renal artery is usually longer and lower than the left

42 A 72 year old man is referred to breast clinic with a unilateral painless breast lump. He has no significant past medical history and is not on any medication.

Which of the following statements is true?
(a) Unilateral swelling makes gynaecomastia unlikely
(b) Gynaecomastia is a risk factor for breast cancer
(c) Male breast cancer presents as earlier stage disease than female breast cancer
(d) Male breast cancer is usually oestrogen receptor positive
(e) Microcalcification in male breast cancer is common

43 With regards to ^{99m}Tc-DTPA in renal imaging, which of the following statements is incorrect?

(a) It has a rapid extravascular, extracellular distribution
(b) It is cleared mainly by tubular secretion
(c) It undergoes 5–10% plasma protein binding
(d) Good post test hydration and frequent voiding reduce radiation dose
(e) It is useful in providing information relating to GFR

44 A 40 year old man undergoes a scrotal ultrasound as part of his investigations for infertility. US shows multiple hypoechoic serpiginous tubular structures with slow flow within them, superior and lateral to the left testicle.

Which of the following statements is false?

(a) Renal US should also be performed
(b) This lesion can be treated with embolisation *via* a RIJ vein approach
(c) This lesion can be treated with laparoscopic surgery
(d) Treatment does not improve sperm quality
(e) Coil embolisation is preferred to particulate embolisation

45 During a routine antenatal ultrasound performed at 11 weeks gestation, the nuchal skin thickness is measured at 5 mm.

Which of the following is not part of the differential?

(a) Normal variation
(b) Noonan's syndrome
(c) Zellwegger syndrome
(d) Klippel-Feil syndrome
(e) Fragile X syndrome

46 With regards to nuclear imaging of the scrotum in cases of suspected torsion which of the following statements is false?

(a) ^{99m}Tc-Pertechnetate is the radioisotope of choice
(b) A peripheral rim of increased activity with a central photopaenic zone is seen in delayed or missed torsion
(c) An area of increased activity extending from the iliac vessels to the scrotum is seen in torsion
(d) Torsion of the hydatid of morgagni is seen as a photopaenic defect
(e) It should not be performed in children under the age of 2 years

47 Antenatal ultrasound at 22 weeks shows thick walled oedematous freely floating bowel loops outside the foetal abdomen. A 2 cm defect in the anterior abdominal wall is seen to the right of a normally inserted umbilical cord. Polyhydramnios but no foetal ascites is noted. No other congenital abnormality can be detected at this stage.

What is the likely diagnosis?

(a) Gastroschisis
(b) Omphalocoele
(c) Limb-body wall complex
(d) Amniotic band syndrome
(e) Ectopia cordis

48 A 70 kg, 55 year old man undergoes a CT KUB for suspected ureteric colic. Reviewing the study, with the patient on the table, an opacity is identified on the side of the pain which lies approximately 5 cm from the VUJ, however it is difficult to be certain whether or not the opacity lies within the ureter.

Which of the following is the next best step?

(a) Repeat unenhanced examination with the patient prone
(b) Repeat examination post *i.v.* contrast medium, acquiring at 50s post administration
(c) Repeat examination post *i.v.* contrast medium, acquiring at 100s post administration
(d) Repeat unenhanced examination in 24 hours
(e) Repeat examination with post *i.v.* contrast medium, acquiring at 300s post administration

49 A 32 year old male is found to have a complete duplex ureteric system on the left side at IVU.

Which of the following statements is incorrect?

(a) The upper moiety ureter is more prone to obstruction
(b) Enuresis is less likely in female patients
(c) The lower moiety ureter is more prone to reflux
(d) The upper moiety ureter inserts inferior and medial to the lower moiety ureter
(e) The ‘drooping lily’ sign may be seen on his IVU

50 **A 38 year old woman presents with a palpable breast mass. On mammography it is 3 cm, lobulated, well defined with a halo appearance around it. It contains central popcorn calcification. On US it has a length to depth ratio of 1.5:1 and is slightly compressible.**

What is the likely diagnosis?

(a) Fibrocystic disease
(b) Sclerosing adenosis
(c) Fibroadenoma
(d) Lymphoma
(e) Phyllodes tumour

51 **A 2 year old presents with pain and abdominal swelling. US shows an 8 cm hyperechoic poorly defined mass in the retroperitoneum, crossing the midline, with areas of acoustic shadowing within it. CT demonstrates the presence of retroperitoneal adenopathy and encasement of the IVC.**

What is the likely diagnosis?

(a) Wilm's tumour
(b) Rhabdomyosarcoma
(c) Renal cell carcinoma
(d) Neuroblastoma
(e) Polycystic kidney disease

52 **A 54 year old woman presents with a painful discharging nipple. Clinical examination suggests a small lump. Mammogram shows coarse, smooth bordered rod shaped calcifications in the subareolar area. However, no discrete mass could be identified on magnified views. On MRI dilated tubular structures containing high signal intensity material on T1W and T2W are seen, with no enhancement following *i.v.* gadolinium.**

What is the likely diagnosis?

(a) Paget's disease
(b) Lymphoma
(c) Nipple adenoma
(d) Duct ectasia
(e) Subareolar carcinoma

53 A 56 year old woman is found to have a 1.2 cm lesion in the right adrenal gland on CT KUB during an examination for renal colic. MRI characterisation suggests that the lesion is a metastasis.

Which of the following sites is the most likely primary?

(a) Ovary
(b) Melanoma
(c) Breast
(d) Lung
(e) Thyroid

54 With regards to normal ovarian anatomy on US, which of the following statements is false?

(a) Normal ovarian volume in a woman of reproductive age is up to 12 mls
(b) Normal ovarian volume in a postmenopausal woman is up to 4 mls
(c) The broad ligament contains the round ligaments within it
(d) Resistance to flow on Doppler imaging of the ovary is greatest in the luteal phase of the menstrual cycle
(e) The ovarian ligaments are not normally seen

55 A 30 week pregnant 23 year old lady with a history of previous Caesarian section is found to have extension of her placenta through the uterine scar. She undergoes an MRI study which shows extension of the placenta in to the bladder wall.

What is the diagnosis?

(a) Placenta accreta
(b) Choriocarcinoma
(c) Placenta percreta
(d) Endometriosis
(e) Placenta increta

56 **A 50 year old man presents with chronic dull flank pain. US shows normal sized kidneys with mild prominence of their calyces. IVU shows ureterectasis above L4, medial displacement of the ureters bilaterally in their middle thirds and subsequent distal tapering. CT shows a retroperitoneal periaortic mass of attenuation similar to muscle.**

What is the most likely diagnosis?

(a) Retroperitoneal fibrosis
(b) Lymphoma
(c) Liposarcoma
(d) Leiomyoma
(e) Amyloid

57 **A 52 year old woman presents with a suprapubic mass. CT shows a 6 cm mass lying anterosuperior to the bladder extending along the course of the urachus. The mass demonstrates heterogeneous enhancement and has peripheral stippled psammomatous calcifications within it.**

Which of the following is the likeliest histological subtype?

(a) Transitional cell carcinoma
(b) Papillary cell carcinoma
(c) Adenocarcinoma
(d) Squamous cell carcinoma
(e) Teratoma

58 **A 50 year old recent immigrant from Tanzania presents with a history of vague flank pain. CT KUB shows coarse calcification in a thickened bladder wall with extension of the calcification into the walls of the distal ureters.**

What is the most likely diagnosis?

(a) Tuberculosis
(b) Transitional cell carcinoma
(c) Schistosomiasis
(d) Lymphoma
(e) Histoplasmosis

59 A 60 year old diabetic woman presents with a history of recurrent coliform UTIs. CT urogram shows multiple smooth dome shaped filling defects within the bladder and both distal ureters. At ureteroscopy the lesions have a yellow appearance and biopsy demonstrates the presence of Michaelis-Gutmann bodies.

What is the likely diagnosis?

(a) Polureteritis cystica
(b) Actinomycosis
(c) Squamous cell carcinoma
(d) Malakoplakia
(e) Leukoplakia

60 Which of the following structures are mullerian duct remnants?

(a) Hydatid of Morgagni
(b) Epididymis
(c) Vas deferens
(d) Ejaculatory duct
(e) Tunica albuginea

61 A 3 year old child born to an HIV positive mother is found to have bilateral enlarged kidneys on ultrasound.

Which of the following conditions is least likely?

(a) ADPKD
(b) Obstructive pelvic mass
(c) HIV nephropathy
(d) Medullary cystic disease
(e) Lymphoma

62 A male infant is found to have multiple bladder diverticulae along with other congenital abnormalities.

Which of the following conditions is least likely?

(a) William's syndrome
(b) Menke's kinky hair syndrome
(c) Eagle-Barrett syndrome
(d) Diamond-Blackfan syndrome
(e) Meckel-Gruber syndrome

63 A 50 year old woman presents with vague left sided abdominal pain. KUB demonstrates no renal tract calcification but an enlarged left renal outline is noted.

Which of the following is not part of the differential diagnosis?

(a) Cervical carcinoma
(b) Nephrotic syndrome
(c) Pyelonephritis
(d) Congenital duplication
(e) Renal artery dissection

64 A 50 year old man undergoes an IVU for suspected ureteric colic. No abnormality is found other than a right ureter which swings medially at the level of L3/L4.

Which of the following is the likeliest diagnosis?

(a) Para-aortic lymphadenopathy
(b) Neurofibroma
(c) Retrocaval ureter
(d) Pelvic lipomatosis
(e) Aortic aneurysm

65 A 25 year old woman presents with a 6 month history of debilitating right loin pain. IVU and arteriography show a vascular impression on the superior infundibulum with secondary dilatation of the upper pole calyx.

Which of the following is the likeliest diagnosis?

(a) Fraley's syndrome
(b) Cavernous haemangioma
(c) Bartter syndrome
(d) Bardet-Biedel syndrome
(e) Alport syndrome

66 A 58 year old man is found to have a midline prostatic cystic lesion on MRI.

Which of the following is not part of the differential diagnosis?

(a) Prostate carcinoma
(b) Recent TURP
(c) Utricular cyst
(d) Posterior urethral diverticulum
(e) Ejaculatory duct cyst

67 With regards to fallopian tube recanalisation, which of the following statements is incorrect?

(a) It is used in cases of infertility associated with proximal tubal obstruction
(b) It cannot be employed after reversal of sterilization surgery
(c) Technical success is achieved in 80-90%
(d) It is associated with increased rates of ectopic pregnancy
(e) Salpingitis isthmica nodosa is a contraindication

68 A 30 year old woman who is 10 weeks pregnant presents with bleeding and lower abdominal pain. US shows an endometrial thickness of 8 mm but gross distortion of its normal midline position by heterogeneous material, with no definite sac identified.

What is the likely diagnosis?

(a) Complete miscarriage
(b) Incomplete miscarriage
(c) Delayed miscarriage
(d) Intrauterine haematoma
(e) Ectopic pregnancy

69 A 30 year old man is involved in a high speed RTA. At contrast enhanced CT, he is noted to have a laceration in the upper pole of his right kidney extending through the corticomedullary junction into the collecting system with extravasation and surrounding haematoma.

According to the American Association for the Surgery of Trauma guidelines, how would you categorise this injury?

(a) Grade I
(b) Grade II
(c) Grade III
(d) Grade IV
(e) Grade V

70 A 55 year old man presents with a vague longstanding history of scrotal discomfort. US shows a right sided lesion, predominantly composed of branching cystic structures lying immediately posterior to the mediastinum. At MRI, the lesion is hypointense on T1W and isointense on T2W.

Which of the following is the likeliest diagnosis?

(a) Sertoli cell tumour
(b) Intratesticular varicocoele
(c) Intratesticular tubular ectasia
(d) Congenital cystic dysplasia
(e) Teratoma

71 A 63 year old man with an elevated PSA is diagnosed with prostate cancer following needle biopsy. He undergoes an MRI examination to help stage his disease.

Which of the following sequences would be most helpful in identifying location and local extent of the tumour?

(a) T1 Weighted
(b) T1 Weighted with intravenous gadolinium
(c) T2 Weighted
(d) Fat suppressed T1
(e) Fat suppressed T2

72 A 69 year old woman presents with PV bleeding. US shows a normal sized uterus with an AP endometrial bilayer thickness of 16 mm. The maximally thickened endometrium is predominantly echogenic with scattered hypoechoic areas within it. At MRI a lesion of lower signal intensity than surrounding endometrium but higher signal intensity than myometrium on T2W is seen.

Which of the following is the likeliest diagnosis?

(a) Adenomatous hyperplasia
(b) Submucosal leiomyoma
(c) Endometritis
(d) Endometrial carcinoma
(e) Benign endometrial hyperplasia

73 A 31 year old male presents with a painless lump of the testicle. He is referred for an US, which demonstrates a well circumscribed encapsulated lesion measuring 2 cm in diameter, containing alternating hypo/ hyperechoic layers. There is no flow on Doppler imaging.

What is the likely diagnosis?

(a) Choriocarcinoma
(b) Epidermoid
(c) Lymphoma
(d) Seminoma
(e) Yolk sac tumour

74 With regards to the UK national breast screening programme, which of the following statements is incorrect?

(a) All women aged between 50 and 70 are invited to attend
(b) The current detection rate is approximately 16 cancers per 1000 women screened
(c) 2 views are obtained as standard in all rounds
(d) It is recommended that readers should report at least 5,000 screening mammograms/year
(e) Women are invited to return at 3 year intervals

75 A 35 year old man undergoes renal transplantation. On the 1st post operative day he becomes oliguric. Doppler ultrasound shows an enlarged, generally hypoechoic graft with diffusely diminished cortical perfusion, decreased systolic rise time and a plateau like reversal of diastolic flow.

Which of the following is the likeliest diagnosis?

(a) Normal day 1 post transplant changes
(b) Renal allograft necrosis
(c) Renal vein thrombosis
(d) Renal artery stenosis
(e) Arteriovenous fistula

Genito-urinary, Adrenal, Obstetrics & Gynaecology and Breast Mock Paper Answers

1 (c)
Although both xanthine and urate stones are radiolucent, urate stones are much more common. Cystine stones are mildly opaque. Calcium oxalate and calcium phosphate stones are radio-opaque

Ref: Radiology Review Manual, 6th Ed, p. 989.

2 (b)
Greater than 60% washout on delayed post contrast imaging is highly specific and sensitive for adenoma as opposed to metastases. Lipid poor adenomas may have a density of greater than 10 HU. Adrenocortical carcinoma typically exhibits peripheral, nodular enhancement.

Ref: Radiology Review Manual, 6th Ed, p. 918–21.

3 (b)
Epididymal cysts and spermatocoeles are common benign cystic lesions of the epididymis. They can be differentiated by the presence of low level echoes in spermatocoeles, which move on careful examination. Occasionally, spermatocoeles contain crystallised material which can give the initial impression that the lesion is hyperechoic.

Ref: Clin Rad (2008); 63(8):929–38.

4 (e)
The finding of air within the right ureter and pelvis implies either a colovesical fistula, or UTI by a gas-producing organism. Diverticulitis is the commonest cause of a colovesical fistula (of which Meckel's diverticulum can be a rare cause). Colorectal tumour, Crohn's disease, ulcerative colitis, previous radiotherapy, and pelvic infection/ infective colitis are other causes. Lymphoma typically encases bowel and blood vessel and is unlikely to cause fistulation.

Ref: Fundamentals of Diagnostic Radiology, 2nd Ed, p. 904.

5 (a)
GFR is a commonly accepted standard measure of renal function. It can be measured by tracers that are cleared exclusively by glomerular filtration, the most common being ^{51}Cr-EDTA (the standard radiopharmaceutical in Europe) and ^{99m}Tc-DTPA (more common in the USA).

Ref: British nuclear medicine society guidelines: http://www.bnmsonline.co.uk/dmdocuments/gfrguidelinesv5.2.pdf

6 (d)
VHL is associated with CNS, haemangioblastomas, retinal angiomas, pancreatic cysts and carcinomas and phaeochromocytoma. In the kidney it is associated with the presence of RCC and multiple cysts. The renal cell tumours are usually of the clear cell type, and have a variable appearance depending on the degree of soft tissue involvement. Cutaneous angiofibromas are seen in tuberous sclerosis.

Ref: Clin Rad (2009); 64:589–99.

7 (b)
Prostate biopsy is performed usually *via* a transrectal route for patients with an elevated (age-specific) PSA, or an abnormal DRE. Complications include haematuria (frequent and usually transient), PR bleeding, infection and retention (uncommon). A negative initial biopsy does not exclude cancer and repeat biopsy (sometimes with extended core protocols) may be required.

Ref: RITI 4_017 TRUS guided biopsy of the prostate gland.

8 (c)
The Bosniak classification is a CT classification of cystic renal lesions. Bosniak I are simple cysts, Bosniak II are minimally complicated cysts. Bosniak IIf (lesions that should be followed-up) have hairline thin septae and subtle wall enhancement or are intrarenal lesions >3 cm with high density content. Bosniak III cysts are complicated lesions with irregular thickened septae, measurable enhancement and coarse irregular calcification. These should be treated surgically. Bosniak IV lesions are clearly malignant with a large necrotic component, irregular wall thickening and solid enhancing elements.

Ref: Radiology Review Manual, 6th Ed, p. 961.

9 (e)
The typical lifespan of an implant is 10 years. Standard triple assessment remains the initial investigative of choice even with implants *in situ*. The linguine sign is a sign of rupture on MRI. 75% of implants are placed in the retroglandular region. 25% are placed in the sub-pectoral region.

Ref: RITI 4a_009 Radiological assessment of women with breast implants.

10 (c)
Seminoma presents in a slightly older age group than the non-seminomatous germ cell tumours. It has the highest rate of association with undescended testis. Lymphoma typically has a more diffuse infiltrative pattern and is the commonest bilateral tumour.

Ref: Radiology Review Manual, 6th Ed, p. 978.

11 (a)
US-guided core biopsy remains the first choice diagnostic test. FNA is helpful for evaluating lesions with fluid components. Stereotactic biopsy is useful for lesions with areas of microcalcification. Vacuum assisted biopsy, whether by US or stereotactic technique helps obtain larger samples but at present its cost means that it is not used as first line. MRI guided biopsy is reserved for equivocal lesions that cannot be clearly identified on US.

Ref: RITI 4a_014 Breast Intervention.

12 (b)
Wolman disease is a rare autosomal recessive lipidosis with accumulation of cholesterol and triglycerides in various tissues presenting in the neonatal period with malabsorption, failure to thrive and hepatosplenomegaly. The classic imaging finding is bilateral enlarged adrenal glands which maintain their normal shape and have extensive punctuate calcification throughout.

Ref: Radiology Review Manual, 6th Ed, p. 993.

13 (d)
An increase in density of contrast material is seen on IVU due to relative increased water reabsorption. Other IVU signs include delayed washout of contrast medium and lack of distension of the collecting system. US findings include peak Renal artery:Aortic velocity >3.5, absence of blood flow during diastole, no detectable Doppler signal in a visualized renal artery, loss of early systolic peak and a resistive index <0.56.

Ref: Radiology Review Manual, 6th Ed, p. 956–7.

14 (a)
The differential diagnosis for ureteric filling defects also includes TCC and radiolucent calculi. Emphysematous ureteritis typically causes streak like filling defects on IVU.

Ref: Radiology Review Manual, 6th Ed, p. 952.

15 (a)
The imaging features of Phaeochromocytoma in addition to those described also include uptake of $^{131}I/^{123}I$– MIBG on nuclear imaging. This can be useful when a primary adrenal lesion cannot be identified on CT or MRI in the context of high clinical suspicion (*e.g.* Raised urinary VMA). Phaeochromocytomas have the 'rule of 10s': 10% bilateral/multiple, 10% malignant, 10% familial, and 10% extra-adrenal. Hyperfunctioning adrenocortical adenomas tend to be unilateral with contralateral atrophy. Li-Fraumeni syndrome resulting from the loss of the p53 tumour suppressor gene results in multiple neoplasms including adrenocortical carcinoma. These demonstrate heterogeneous contrast enhancement with a well circumscribed rim on CT.

Ref: Radiology Review Manual, 6th Ed, p. 919–21 & 943.

16 (e)
XGP is a chronic granulomatous infection in chronic renal obstruction with progressive macrophage infiltration of the renal parenchyma. Fungal renal infections can cause pyelonephritis with fungal balls. Renal sarcoma typically presents with an infiltrative and expansile mass. Mutilocular RCC is a type of a cystic RCC.

Ref: Radiology Review Manual, 6th Ed, p. 953.

17 (d)
If the serum creatinine is within the normal range, or the estimated GFR is >60 ml/min, then metformin need not be stopped. If these are abnormal then discussion with the clinical team is required.

Ref: RCR- Standards for iodinated intravascular contrast agent administration to adult patients 2005 (updated 2009).

18 (e)
The upper pole is best avoided due to the risk of pneumothorax. Renal pelvis punctures increase the risk of vascular damage and persistent urine leaks. Generally, anterior punctures are regarded as unfavourable as there is a risk of damage to anterior structures such as bowel, liver or spleen

Ref: Interventional Radiology: A survival guide, 2nd Ed, p. 281.

19 (c)
A ‘teardrop’ or ‘pear’ shaped bladder on cystography is the classic finding of pelvic lipomatosis. CT shows symmetrical abundant intra-pelvic fat. Lipoblastomas are rare soft tissue neoplasms derived from foetal adipose tissue, seen in children. Hibernomas are rare benign, soft tissue tumours composed of brown fat, that present in adult as a firm, painless, slowly growing mass.

Ref: Radiographics (2009); 29: 261–90.

20 (b)
95% of ectopic pregnancies are tubal, with ampullary pregnancies accounting for 80% of these. Abdominal, ovarian, and cervical pregnancies are extremely rare. In 5% of cases the pelvic US is normal.

Ref: Radiology Review Manual, 6th Ed, p. 1036.

21 (b)
The classic features of an endometrioma are described, others include wall nodularity, a fluid-fluid level and acoustic enhancement. A haemorrhagic ovarian cyst or a tubo-ovarian abscess would present more acutely. A dermoid may have similar appearances but would usually have fat and/or calcium within. A cystic ovarian tumour is in the differential and typically appears as a multilocular cyst with large associated soft tissue component mass, sometimes with papillary excrescences into the cysts.

Ref: Radiology Review Manual, 6th Ed, p. 1040.

22 (b)
Urethral trauma is common in the presence of pelvic fractures (up to 24%) and typically presents with haematuria, meatal blood, perineal swelling or a high riding prostate on DRE in men and labial oedema, vaginal bleeding or urinary leak PR in women. It is more common in men and the posterior urethra, particularly the distal membranous urethra is most commonly injured. It is associated with bladder rupture in 20%. At urethrography, if the patient is able, a right or left anterior oblique view is commonly employed.

Ref: Radiographics (2008); 28:1631–43.

23 (b)
These are the IVU signs of papillary necrosis. There is a wide differential diagnosis for these appearances including diabetes mellitus, SCD, obstructive uropathy, and pyelonephritis. Overall, diabetes is the most common cause, but analgesic nephropathy is particularly common in middle-aged females.

Ref: Radiographics (2006); 26:1827–36.

24 (e)
Renal lymphoma typically occurs in B-Cell non-Hodgkin's lymphoma, where it is the second most common organ involved after the haematopoietic and reticulo-endothelial systems. Primary renal lymphoma is uncommon as the normal kidney does not contain significant amounts of lymphoid tissue. Intra-renal lymphoma appears as an ill-defined, homogeneous mass on CT which enhance poorly relative to the surrounding parenchyma.

Ref: Radiographics (2006); 26:1151–68.

25 (d)
Overall, the commonest cause of renal artery stenosis is atherosclerosis, but FMD accounts for up to 30% of all cases, and is commoner in young patients. It typically affects the mid and distal portion of the artery and a 'string of beads' appearance is often seen.

Ref: Radiology Review Manual, 6th Ed, p. 957.

26 (c)
Renal AML is a benign tumour containing fat, smooth muscle and thick-walled blood vessels. They can bleed (50-60% of AMLs > 4cm bleed spontaneously), and can cause haemorrhagic shock (Wunderlich syndrome). Fat on non-contrast CT in the absence of calcification is virtually diagnostic. They can be associated with tuberous sclerosis (in 80% of TS patients), VHL, and NF.

Ref: Radiology Review Manual, 6th Ed, p. 922.

27 (e)
Bilateral uterine artery embolisation with particulate (PVA or microspheres) are required for satisfactory treatment. A 4Fr catheter is a suitable size to reach the uterine artery. The uterine artery is a branch of the anterior division of the IIA. Pedunculated fibroids may necrose their stalk and fall into the uterine or abdominal cavity, therefore UFE is not the treatment of choice.

Ref: Interventional Radiology: A survival guide. 2nd Ed, p. 206.

28 (c)
Buscopan is a commonly used short acting (up to 1 hour) anti-muscarinic drug. The dose is 20 mg *i.v.*. A history of allergy should be explored. All patients should be warned that in the event of painful, blurred vision, medical attention should be sought. Stable cardiac disease is not an absolute contraindication. Porphyria and closed angle glaucoma are contraindications.

Ref: Clin Rad (2008); 63(7): 739–43.

29 (a)
Arcuate uterus is the most common uterine anomaly associated with reproductive failure. Uterus didelphys is a duplication defect with 2 vaginas, 2 cervices and 2 uterine horns. Bicornuate and unicornuate abnormalities demonstrate an abnormal fundal contour.

Ref: Radiographics (2006); 26:419–31.

30 (d)
T1c cancers are impalpable tumours detected on needle biopsy. T2c tumours are intra-capsular but involve both lobes. T3a cancers are extra-capsular without other organ involvement. T3b cancers involve the seminal vesicles. T4 cancers have direct extension into adjacent organs other than the seminal vesicles.

Ref: TNM Atlas, 5th Ed, 2005.

31 (c)
HRT can increase the normal thickness of the post-menopausal endometrium up to 15 mm (depending on the HRT). Measurements should be of bi-layer thickness. For post-menopausal women not on HRT, 5 mm is the upper limit of normal.

Ref: Radiology Review Manual, 6th Ed, p. 1024.

32 (c)
With a high velocity injury and frank haematuria, CT is the investigation of choice. 25% of patients with frank haematuria and blunt trauma have a significant renal injury. Normotensive patients with microscopic haematuria have a significant renal injury in <0.2%.

Ref: RITI 4c_059 – Guidelines in uroradiology.

33 (b)
Blood flow, cardiac, respiratory and patient motion all cause 'ghosting' artifact in the phase encoding direction. If the phase encoding direction is incorrectly set in the anterior to posterior plane, large amounts of breast tissue will be obscured.

Ref: Radiographics (2007); 27: s131–45.

34 (a)
The inguinal canal is the commonest site for an undescended testis, although it can lie anywhere along its embryological passage from kidney to scrotum. Ectopic testes can be found in the femoral canal, perineum, contralateral hemiscrotum or prepubic space. Localisation is important as, if present, there is a greatly increased risk of malignancy.

Ref: Office urology – The clinicians guide, 1st Ed.

35 (e)
The Mirena is a polyethylene IUCD and is well seen on MRI. Metal IUCDs are not a contraindication to 1.5T MRI examination although safety in a 3T machine has not been fully evaluated. Threads of a lost coil can ball up to form an echogenic mass on ultrasound. IUCDs do not increase the risk of ectopic pregnancy *per se*, but a higher percentage of ectopic pregnancies are seen in patients with IUCDs as endometrial implantation is restricted. The Mirena is commonly used for treatment of dysfunctional uterine bleeding with success rates of up to 70%.

Ref: RITI 4b_007 Intrauterine contraceptive devices.

36 (c)
Laparoscopy and blue dye instillation (with spillage of dye into the peritoneal cavity indicating patency) is the gold standard, but requires a general anaesthetic. MRI and standard pelvic US do not clearly demonstrate the fallopian tubes. HSG provides an accurate indication of tubal patency but employs ionizing radiation. It should therefore be performed in the first half of the menstrual cycle to avoid irradiating a patient with possible early pregnancy. Hysterosalpingo-Contrast-Sonography uses microbubbles to demonstrate the fallopian tubes and has the advantage of not using ionizing radiation or requiring anaesthesia but is less accurate than the other methods.

Ref: RITI 4b_023 HyCoSy and hysterosonography.

37 (a)
Adenomyosis is a term relating to benign invasion of the myometrium by endometrium. It can exist in either focal or diffuse forms. The diffuse form is characterised by junctional zone widening. Dilated cystic glands or haemorrhagic foci can be seen within the myometrium in 40% of diffuse cases.

Ref: Radiology Review Manual, 6th Ed, p. 1028.

38 (e)
High velocity trauma with a significant pelvic fracture means that bladder injury must be excluded. 70% of traumatic bladder ruptures are associated with pelvic fracture. On control film at cystography, widening of the fat planes of obturator internus along with a homogeneous soft tissue density and displacement of ileal loops suggest extraperitoneal rupture. Overall, extraperitoneal ruptures account for 80% of ruptures. 10% of ruptures are detected on post micturition imaging only.

Ref: Clin Rad (2008); 63:1361–71.

39 (d)
The double decidual sign is useful in determining a true gestational sac particularly after 5 weeks gestation. It comprises two hyperechoic rings separated by the hypoechoic apposed endometrial walls. It has a PPV for pregnancy of 98%.

Ref: RITI 4b_004 Ultrasound assessment of the first trimester of pregnancy.

40 (e)
RCC is by far the commonest malignant renal tumour. 10% of these tumours calcify.

Ref: Primer of Diagnostic Imaging, 4th Ed, p. 291.

41 (b)
The column of Bertin is an area of focal cortical hyperplasia, typically seen between the upper and interpolar region. It has the imaging characteristic of renal cortex. Its main clinical significance is that it can be mistaken for a renal tumour. Both renal arteries usually have two divisions. The renal arteries typically arise at the L1/L2 level. The right renal artery is usually longer and lower than the left.

Ref: Clinically Oriented Anatomy, 5th Ed, p. 311.

42 (d)
Male breast cancer represents 0.5% of all breast cancers. Gynaecomastia for which there is a wide differential (including physiological, endocrine, neoplastic and drug related causes) may be unilateral and asymmetrical. Male breast cancer presents at a later stage than female breast cancer and at an older age. It is usually ER positive and unlike in female breast cancer, microcalcification is relatively uncommon.

Ref: RITI module 4a_011 Male breast disease.

43 (b)
It is mainly cleared by glomerular filtration hence its utility as a GFR agent. It is useful in assessing the degree of obstructive uropathy. ^{99m}Tc-MAG3 is cleared by tubular secretion and is the agent of choice in patients with renal insufficiency as it is not GFR dependent.

Ref: Primer of Diagnostic Imaging, 4th Ed, p. 939.

44 (d)
This is a left sided varicocoele. An obstructing left renal lesion should be excluded. Sperm quality is improved in up to 53% of patients. The commonest approach for embolisation is *via* the right CFV vein but the RIJ jugular may also be used.

Ref: Interventional Radiology: A survival guide. 2nd Ed, p. 204.

45 (e)
The nuchal skin thickness should measure up to 3 mm at 9–13 weeks, up to 5 mm at 14–19 weeks and up to 6mm at 19–24 weeks. Although rare (<1%) normal variation is observed. Other causes of nuchal skin thickening include Turners and Downs syndromes.

Ref: Radiology Review Manual, 6th Ed, p. 1003.

46 (d)
Torsion of the hydatid cannot be identified on scintigraphy as the structure is too small to be accurately defined. An area of increased activity extending from the iliac vessels to the scrotum can sometimes indicate increased perfusion to the scrotum *via* the pudendal vessels (nubbin sign).

Ref: Primer of Diagnostic Imaging, 4th Ed, p. 942.

47 (a)
This can be differentiated from omphalocoele by its location (right paraumbilical as opposed to midline), lack of covering membrane and relatively small defect size. It is also less commonly associated with other congenital defects. It is difficult to reliably diagnose this condition until at least 20 weeks gestation.

Ref: Radiology Review Manual, 6th Ed, p. 1044.

48 (e)
Although exact techniques vary from department to department, the principles remain the same. In this situation, an excretory phase image is required to determine whether or not the opacity is in the ureter. This phase begins at 240 secs post contrast administration. The nephrographic phase (80–120 secs) provides homogeneous enhancement of the parenchyma and is best for identifying parenchymal lesions. Turning the patient prone can be useful in delineating VUJ calculi and is performed routinely in some centres.

Ref: Radiographics (2004); 24:e20.

49 (b)
In men the upper moiety ureter always inserts proximal to the external urethral sphincter, thus enuresis is less likely. By way of contrast, in females the upper moiety ureter commonly inserts distal to the sphincter, making enuresis more likely. The drooping lily sign refers to an obstructed upper moiety ureter displacing the lower ureter inferiorly on IVU.

Ref: RITI 4c_018 Imaging of suspected hydronephrosis and obstruction.

50 (c)
Popcorn calcification with a halo around a well defined compressible lesion in a pre-menopausal woman is typical of fibroadenoma.

Ref: RITI 4c_011 Benign breast disease.

51 (d)
Neuroblastoma is the commonest solid abdominal mass in infants. It is characterised by difficulty in defining it separately from the kidney, the presence of coarse stippled calcification and the fact it crosses the midline. It may arise from any site within the sympathetic neural chain.

Ref: Radiology Review Manual, 6th Ed, p. 941.

52 (d)
Stasis of intraductal secretions leads to dilatation and inspissation of material within the subareolar ducts which can calcify. The diagnosis is much more likely if it is bilateral.

Ref: Radiographics (2007); 27: s57–67.

53 (d)
Lung is the most common site (40%) followed by breast (20%). Other sites include kidney, pancreas and colon.

Ref: Radiology Review Manual, 6th Ed, p. 936.

54 (d)
Highest resistance to flow on Doppler is seen on days 1–8 of the menstrual cycle, gradually reducing with follicular development until day 21.

Ref: RITI 4b_002 Normal gynaecological anatomy – Vagina and ovaries.

55 (c)
In a normal pregnancy, the placenta is adherent to the endometrial lining. Penetration beyond this is abnormal and is categorised according to depth of invasion. In *placenta accreta* there is superficial invasion of the myometrium by the placental villi, whereas deep invasion of the myometrium is termed *placenta increta.* Extension of the placental tissue to the peritoneum, often in to the adjacent organs, is termed *placenta percreta.* The incidence of abnormal placental implantation ranges from 1 in 533 to 1 in 2,500, with both foetal and maternal mortality associated, due to haemorrhagic complications.

Ref: European Radiology (2007); 17:1647-9.

56 (a)
Retroperitoneal fibrosis may be primary (2/3 of cases) where it may be associated with fibrosis in other organ systems, or secondary to drugs, radiation therapy or a desmoplastic reaction to local tumours.

Ref: Radiology Review Manual, 6th Ed, p. 970.

57 (c)
Urachal carcinoma is a relatively rare tumour characterized by a midline suprapubic mass that may or may not invade the bladder. 10% lie at the umbilical end. Peripheral curved or stippled calcifications are pathognomonic of the mucinous adenocarcinoma subtype which may be complicated by pseudomyxoma peritonei.

Ref: Radiology Review Manual, 6th Ed, p. 985.

58 (c)
Although schistosomiasis is rare in the west, it is the commonest cause of mural calcification worldwide. TB causes calcification relatively rarely. TCC can cause mural calcification but this is usually thin curvilinear calcification outlining a normal sized bladder.

Ref: Radiology Review Manual, 6th Ed, p. 972.

59 (d)
A rare condition characterised by altered host response to infection (*E. coli* in 94%) at the macrophage level. It is multifocal in 75% and bilateral in 50%. Renal involvement is less common, is usually unilateral, and is characterised by diffuse renal enlargement with displacement and distortion of the pelvi-calyceal system.

Ref: Radiology Review Manual, 6th Ed, p. 933.

60 (a)
The mullerian duct degenerates at around 6 weeks in the male due to production of mullerian inhibiting factor by Sertoli cells, its remnants form the appendix testis and the utricle.

Ref: Radiology Review Manual, 6th Ed, p. 908.

61 (d)
Medullary cystic disease appears either as a juvenile (rapidly progressive) or as an infantile form. It is characterised by the presence of bilateral small kidneys with numerous small cortico-medullary cysts which give an appearance of increased parenchymal echogenicity, with loss of the corticomedullary junction. Although rare, ADPKD can present in this age group.

Ref: Radiology Review Manual, 6th Ed, p. 934.

62 (e)
Meckel-Gruber syndrome is a cause of multiple renal cortical cysts but is invariably fatal at birth due to a combination of lung hypoplasia and renal failure.

Ref: Radiology Review Manual, 6th Ed, p. 923.

63 (e)
Renal artery dissection causes the affected kidney to decrease in size due to arterial insufficiency. Ureteric obstruction with hydronephrosis can be a presenting feature of cervical cancer.

64 (c)
Retrocaval ureter is due to a rare embryological failure of IVC formation with persistence of the right posterior cardinal vein and failure of the right supracardinal system to develop. It may be asymptomatic or cause varying degrees of proximal hydroureter.

Ref: JK-Practitioner (2005); 12(1): 24–5.

65 (a)
Fraley's syndrome is rare, comprising superior infundibular narrowing due to a crossing vessel causing significant loin pain. It is more common in young women and on the right side. If symptomatic surgery is indicated.

Ref: Eur Radiol (2000); 38(4): 410–4.

66 (a)
Other causes include mullerian duct cyst and vas deferens cyst.

Ref: Abdom imaging (1995); 20:70–1.

67 (b)
Although primarily used in cases of proximal tubal obstruction, it can be used to treat mid tubal obstructions after reversal of sterilisation surgery.

Ref: RITI 1c_046 – Treatment of female subfertility.

68 (b)
This condition can be asymptomatic and the typical findings on US are those of an expanded endometrial cavity packed with blood and the products of conception.

Ref: RITI 4b_005 Early pregnancy problems.

69 (d)
Grade I refers to contusion or non-expanding subcapsular haematoma and is the commonest type. Grade II refers a laceration less than 1 cm deep without extravasation. Grade III describes a laceration more than 1 cm deep without extravasation. Grade IV refers to the above or alternatively to a segmental renal artery or vein injury with contained haematoma. Grade V refers to a shattered kidney or to renal pedicle injury.

Ref: Radiology Review Manual, 6th Ed, p. 981.

70 (c)
Dilatation of the rete testis is due to blockage of the efferent ductules. It is usually bilateral and lies in the region of the mediastinum. Most testicular tumours are of low signal intensity on T2W.

71 (c)
T2 weighted imaging clearly depicts the distinction between the peripheral zone and the remainder of the gland. Tumours are seen as foci of low signal on T2. Haemorrhage from recent biopsy can cause confusion. Fat suppression and intravenous gadolinium is not necessary.

Ref: RITI 4c_013 MRI of the urinary tract.

72 (d)
Other features to suggest malignancy include a resistive index of <0.7, disruption of the junctional zone or other evidence of myometrial invasion.

Ref: Radiology Review Manual, 6th Ed, p. 1039.

73 (b)
The classic US 'onion-skin' appearance of an epidermoid cyst of the testis is described. These are benign teratomas containing ectodermal components. The alternating hypo/ hyperechoic layers are due to compact keratin layers contrasted with loosely arranged desquamated squamous cells.

Ref: Radiology review manual, 6th Ed, p. 977.

74 (b)
The current detection rate is approximately 6 cancers per 1000 women screened. At the moment the age range for selection is 50–70 years although plans exist to expand the age range from 47–73 years.

Ref: Quality assurance guidelines for breast screening radiology NHSBSP publication 59 (January 2005).

75 (c)
Renal/iliac vein thrombosis occurs in up to 5% of cases. If it occurs in the immediate post-operative period it is usually due to endothelial injury at the anastomosis site or extrinsic compression. An absence of venous flow can also be observed with Doppler US.

Ref: Radiology (1989); 170: 557–8.

Paediatrics Mock Paper Questions

1 In a neonate with respiratory distress, which of the following CXR findings are more indicative of a diagnosis of meconium aspiration over hyaline membrane disease?

(a) Air bronchograms
(b) Ground glass changes
(c) Humeral heads not ossified
(d) Hyperinflation
(e) No pleural fluid

2 You are asked by one of the junior paediatric medical doctors to review the chest and abdominal radiographs taken on patients from the neonatal unit.

Which of the following lines is inappropriately sited and needs repositioning?

(a) Endotracheal tube with its tip seen 1.5 cm above the carina
(b) Left arm PICC line with its tip at the level of the left brachio-cephalic vein
(c) Nasogastric tube with its tip sited below the diaphragm
(d) UAC with its tip located at the level of the aortic arch
(e) UVC with its tip at the junction of the IVC/right atrium

3 A neonate presents with vomiting, choking and drooling of secretions. An 8 Fr NG feeding tube cannot be passed into the stomach.

What is the most likely diagnosis?

(a) Oesophageal agenesis with no distal oesophageal bud and no tracheal fistula
(b) Oesophageal atresia with a distal oesophageal bud, but no tracheal fistula
(c) Oesophageal atresia with a proximal tracheal fistula
(d) Oesophageal atresia with a distal tracheal fistula
(e) Oesophageal atresia with both proximal and distal tracheal fistula

4 **Regarding congenital lobar emphysema.**

Which lobe is most commonly affected?

(a) Left lower lobe
(b) Left upper lobe
(c) Right middle lobe
(d) Right lower lobe
(e) Right upper lobe

5 **A 2 year old child presents with an acute history of coughing and wheezing. On examination, there is reduced air entry on the right side.**

Which single CXR view would you advise to maximise the chances of confirming the suspected diagnosis?

(a) Expiratory film
(b) Left lateral decubitus film
(c) PA erect film
(d) Prone film
(e) Supine film

6 **You are asked to perform a barium follow-through examination in an infant; you discuss with the senior radiographer ways to reduce dose to the patient. The following are suggested, but which will actually increase patient dose?**

(a) Begin with cones open and close to required FOV, rather than opening closed cones
(b) Keep the image intensifier as close to the child as possible
(c) Removal of the grid
(d) Use of an over-couch fluoroscopy unit, rather than under-couch fluoroscopy
(e) Using pulsed-fluoroscopy, rather than continuous-fluoroscopy

7 **Regarding fluoroscopically guided reduction for the treatment of intussusception in children.**

Which of the following is an advantage of hydrostatic barium over air reduction?

(a) It produces smaller tears if perforation occurs
(b) It is easier to confirm reduction across the ileo-caecal valve
(c) It is faster, thus less radiation dose
(d) It results in less contamination of the abdominal cavity if perforation occurs
(e) It delivers higher intracolic pressures

8 **A 3 year old boy with a Wilm's tumour undergoes CT examination to aid staging. The CT shows a large mass arising from the right kidney, with liver lesions, vertebral lesions, and enlarged hilar lymph nodes.**

Based on these findings, the stage is?

(a) Stage I
(b) Stage II
(c) Stage III
(d) Stage IV
(e) Stage V

9 **A neonate presents with a visible mass within the left flank. US confirms a solid intra-renal lesion.**

What is the likeliest tumour?

(a) Mesoblastic nephroma
(b) Multicystic dysplastic kidney
(c) Nephroblastomatosis
(d) Neuroblastoma
(e) Wilm's tumour

10 A screening antenatal US shows an abdominal wall defect. The differential diagnosis is between gastroschisis and omphalocoele.

Which additional feature confirms the diagnosis of gastroschisis?

(a) Associated herniation of the liver
(b) Central herniation into the umbilical cord
(c) Involvement of all 3 layers of the abdominal wall
(d) Multiple associated anomalies
(e) The presence of a covering membrane

11 A cranial US is performed in a pre-term neonate. There is hyperechoic material within the ventricles consistent with recent haemorrhage, but the ventricles are not dilated.

How would you grade this germinal matrix bleed?

(a) Grade I
(b) Grade II
(c) Grade III
(d) Grade IV
(e) Grade V

12 What is the commonest presenting symptom of Wilm's tumour?

(a) Abdominal pain
(b) Haematuria
(c) Hypertension
(d) Palpable abdominal mass
(e) Weight loss

13 A 2 year old girl presents with fatigue, loss of appetite and fever. A CXR done as part of a septic screen shows a centrally placed mass with loss of the right paratracheal stripe, and subtle splaying of the ribs. The hilar structures and right heart border are clearly seen.

What is the most likely diagnosis?

(a) Germ cell tumour
(b) Hodgkin's Disease
(c) Leukaemia
(d) Neuroblastoma
(e) Non-Hodgkin's Lymphoma

14 A 4 week old boy presents with a history of non-bilious vomiting and failure-to-thrive, but clinical examination is normal.

Which of the following US features confirm the diagnosis of pyloric stenosis?

(a) Hyperechoic pyloric muscle
(b) Pyloric canal length of 13 mm
(c) Pyloric muscle wall thickness of 4 mm
(d) Reduced peristaltic waves within the antrum
(e) Transverse pyloric canal diameter of 10 mm

15 Which of the following is most commonly associated with cystic fibrosis?

(a) Low sodium concentration in sweat
(b) Meconium plug syndrome
(c) Pectus excavatum
(d) Pneumothorax
(e) Situs inversus

16 Regarding a skeletal survey for the investigation of suspected non-accidental injury.

Which of the following radiographic views is classed as a 'supplementary view' rather than a 'standard view'?

(a) Abdomen (including pelvis and hips)
(b) AP Chest
(c) DP Hands
(d) Oblique ribs
(e) Towne's

17 A 12 year old boy falls off his bike onto his outstretched right hand. Radiographs of his wrist show a fracture through the radial growth plate and epiphysis, with an intact metaphysis.

Which Salter-Harris type of epiphyseal plate injury does this represent?

(a) Type I
(b) Type II
(c) Type III
(d) Type IV
(e) Type V

18 A young child presents in great distress with breathing difficulties.

Which of the following would be more typical of croup rather than epiglottitis?

(a) The child is 1 year old at presentation
(b) Predominantly supraglottic involvement
(c) The child is febrile
(d) Associated dysphagia
(e) Increased stridor when placed supine

19 Antenatal US shows bilateral renal pelvis dilation. A micturating cysto-urethrogram is performed. On the right side there is reflux of contrast into the ureter, renal pelvis and calyces but no dilatation. On left side there is mild/moderate dilatation of the ureter, renal pelvis and calyces with minimal blunting of the fornices.

What is the correct grading of the patient's vesico-ureteric reflux?

(a) Right grade 0, left grade I
(b) Right grade I, left grade II
(c) Right grade II, left grade III
(d) Right grade III, left grade IV
(e) Right grade IV, left grade V

20 A 4 year old boy presents following a recent history of a fever, cervical lymphadenopathy, and a rash around both elbows and conjunctivitis.

What is the most likely diagnosis?

(a) Fibromuscular dysplasia
(b) Giant cell arteritis
(c) Henoch Schonlein purpura
(d) Kawasaki's disease
(e) Takayasu's disease

21 Which of the following is not a cause of secondary craniosynostosis?

(a) Crouzon's syndrome
(b) Hypothyroidism
(c) Previous shunt procedures
(d) Rickets
(e) Thalassaemia

22 An active 13 year old boy complains of acute pain in the right hip following a game of football. An AP pelvis x-ray shows an irregular bone fragment below the right inferior pubic ramus.

What muscle has been avulsed?

(a) Adductor magnus
(b) Iliopsoas
(c) Pectineus
(d) Rectus femoris
(e) Vastus medialis

23 A skeletal survey is performed on a 2 year old at high risk for NAI.

Which of the following findings would be the most specific for NAI?

(a) Fracture of the middle third of the clavicle
(b) Greenstick fracture of the radius
(c) Linear fracture of the parietal bone
(d) Spiral fracture of the tibia
(e) Scapula fracture

24 Which of the following eponymous osteochondroses, common in the paediatric population, is incorrectly described?

(a) Blount – proximal medial tibial epiphysis
(b) Frieberg's – metatarsal head
(c) Kohler's – scaphoid
(d) Perthe's – femoral head
(e) Sever's – calcaneal apophysis

25 An 18 month old boy presents with fever and intractable watery diarrhoea and is found to be hypertensive. On examination there is a palpable mass in the left side of the abdomen. US and subsequent CT examination reveal a mass superior to the left kidney which is noted to contain hypoechoic areas on US and low attenuation areas on CT.

What is the most likely diagnosis?

(a) Adrenocortical carcinoma
(b) Adrenal haemorrhage
(c) Neuroblastoma
(d) Tuberculosis
(e) Wilm's tumour

26 A 14 year old boy presents with a head injury following an RTA. A junior SpR reviews the unenhanced-CT head examination and is happy there is no sign of trauma, however, they are concerned by an area of calcification.

At which of the following sites would calcification be considered abnormal, requiring further investigation?

(a) Basal ganglia
(b) Choroid plexus
(c) Dura
(d) Pineal gland
(e) Pituitary gland

27 Radiation protection is of particular concern in children.

Which of the following is not true?

(a) Deterministic effects are more common in children
(b) Failure to modify parameters (*e.g.* CT) for children increases dose
(c) Children's organs are more radiosensitive compared to adults
(d) Children's organs receive a higher dose per examination compared to adults
(e) There is the potential for multiple non-diagnostic exposures in an uncooperative child

28 A 2 day old ex-premature boy on the neonatal unit with suspected necrotising enterocolitis has deteriorated, and the clinical team are worried about perforation.

Which investigation should you recommend?

(a) Cross-table lateral AXR
(b) Erect CXR
(c) Left-side down decubitus AXR
(d) Right-side down decubitus AXR
(e) Supine AXR

29 A neonate is noted to be jaundiced. Investigations are subsequently requested by the clinicians.

Which of the following results is most supportive of the diagnosis of neonatal hepatitis over biliary atresia?

(a) Blood tests reveal a conjugated bilirubinaemia
(b) HIDA scintigraphy shows rapid hepatic tracer accumulation
(c) HIDA scintigraphy shows visualisation of tracer in bowel at 12 hours
(d) US shows no intra-hepatic duct dilatation
(e) US cannot visualise the gallbladder

30 Regarding enteric duplication cysts, which of the following is true?

(a) They are most commonly located in duodenum
(b) The majority communicate with the lumen
(c) There is usually calcification within the wall
(d) The majority are located on the anti-mesenteric side
(e) The capsule contains two walls

31 An 8 year old girl is examined by her GP and is noted to be short for her age and pale. An X-ray is performed to assess bone age, which reveals the predicted bone age to be 6 years, and shows dense bands within the metaphyses of the metacarpals.

What is the most likely diagnosis?
(a) Congenital adrenal hyperplasia
(b) Hypervitaminosis-D
(c) Lead poisoning
(d) Polyostotic fibrous dysplasia
(e) Turner's syndrome

32 A 3 year old presents with a persistent cough that has not responded to antibiotics. CXR demonstrates a triangular shaped-mass medially at the left lung base. CT is arranged for further investigation.

What feature favours a diagnosis of intra- over extra-pulmonary sequestration?
(a) Air seen within lesion
(b) Communication with the bronchial tree
(c) Multiple associated anomalies
(d) Systemic venous drainage
(e) Systemic arterial supply

33 A neonate is cyanosed. A CXR is performed which shows slight cardiac enlargement and oligaemia of the pulmonary vasculature.

Which of the following is the most likely diagnosis?
(a) Single ventricle
(b) Total anomalous pulmonary venous connection
(c) Transposition of the great arteries
(d) Tricuspid atresia
(e) Truncus arteriosus

34 A 2 day old baby born to a diabetic mother presents with abdominal distension, never having opened the bowels. Water-soluble enema demonstrates a collapsed descending colon to the splenic flexure, with dilated proximal colon and small bowel. Following the study, copious amount of meconium are immediately passed.

What is the most likely diagnosis?

(a) Hirschsprung's disease
(b) Ileal atresia
(c) Imperforate anus (high malformation type)
(d) Meconium ileus
(e) Meconium plug syndrome

35 What is the commonest presenting feature of a Meckel's diverticulum?

(a) Obstruction
(b) Perforation
(c) Diverticulitis
(d) Volvulus
(e) Bleeding

36 A neonate is found to have a left kidney measuring 5.4 cm, right kidney 4.3 cm. A subsequent IVU demonstrates a complete duplication of the left kidney. The patient returns for follow-up IVU late in childhood.

Which of the following signs would be unexpected?

(a) Concave upper border of the left kidney
(b) Increased number of calyces in the left kidney compared to the right
(c) Obstruction of the ectopic ureter
(d) Upper pole (ectopic) ureter inserting more inferior and medially
(e) Filling defect inferiorly within the bladder

37 Which of the following features is not a typical finding of the normal infant thymus on CXR?

(a) Wavy inferior margin
(b) Change in size on inspiratory/ expiratory films
(c) No mass effect
(d) Convex lateral borders
(e) Homogeneous density

38 A 20 week antenatal US shows multiple cysts within the left kidney. These vary in size and are randomly arranged. The parenchyma is difficult to demonstrate and the left renal pelvis cannot be identified. No other anomalies are identified.

What is the most likely diagnosis?
(a) Autosomal dominant polycystic kidney disease
(b) Autosomal recessive polycystic kidney disease
(c) Meckel-Gruber syndrome
(d) Multicystic dysplastic kidney
(e) Multilocular cystic nephroma

39 A 6 year old child is a passenger in an RTA. The cervical spine cannot be clinically cleared and C-spine films are requested.

Which of the following findings are trauma-related rather than a normal variant?
(a) Anterior subluxation of C2 on C3
(b) Anterior wedging of the C3 vertebral body
(c) Atlanto-dens interval of 5 mm
(d) Lucent line in C3 spinous process
(e) Prevertebral space of 8 mm anterior to C3

40 A 7 year old boy falls on his outstretched hand. He has pain around the right elbow. X-rays show elevated anterior and posterior fat pads. The capitellum, radial head and trochlea ossification centres are clearly seen, no fracture line is identified.

Which of the following is most likely diagnosis?

(a) Avulsion of the medial epicondyle
(b) Avulsion of the lateral epicondyle
(c) Occult radial head fracture
(d) Occult supracondylar fracture
(e) Normal

41 Which of the following is not a risk factor for neonatal renal vein thrombosis?

(a) Birth trauma
(b) Dehydration
(c) Diabetic mother
(d) Right adrenal haemorrhage
(e) Sepsis

42 A 20 week antenatal US shows the femur length to be at the lower limit of normal. A follow-up study at 27 weeks, shows the femur to be below the normal 95th centile, but the tibia is of normal length.

What is the correct categorisation of this skeletal dysplasia?

(a) Acromelic
(b) Mesomelic
(c) Metromelic
(d) Micromelic
(e) Rhizomelic

43 Which of the following conditions occurs more frequently in post-maturity rather than pre-term neonates?

(a) Germinal matrix haemorrhage
(b) Meconium aspiration
(c) Necrotizing entero-colitis
(d) Periventricular haemorrhage
(e) Respiratory distress syndrome

44 A 3 month old boy presents with irritability, failure to thrive and an unexplained swelling over his right shin. Skeletal survey reveals periosteal bone thickening in the diaphysis of the right tibia with associated soft tissue swelling. Similar findings are seen in the right clavicle and the left mandible.

What is the most likely diagnosis?
(a) Caffey's disease
(b) Hypervitaminosis A
(c) Non-accidental injury
(d) Rickets
(e) Scurvy

45 CXR shows asymmetrical density, with the right hemithorax more translucent that the left and there is noted to be normal and symmetrical pulmonary vascularity. Inspiratory/ expiratory films show symmetrical size changes of the hemithoraces.

What is the most likely diagnosis?
(a) Congenital lobar emphysema
(b) Large pneumatocoele
(c) Pneumothorax
(d) Poland's syndrome
(e) Pulmonary artery hypoplasia

46 A neonate with complex congenital heart disease has been referred for a cardiac MRI in order to obtain more precise anatomical and function information.

Which of the following factors is the most problematic for MR imaging in this age group?
(a) Breath holding cannot be achieved
(b) Imaging takes over 1 hour
(c) The size of the coronary vessels
(d) Neonates cannot lie still
(e) Neonates have slow heart rates

47 An 18 month old, ambulatory girl presents with irritability and genu varum. On examination there is delayed dentition. Knee x-rays show bilateral widening of the epiphyseal plates with irregularity of the metaphyses, and course medullary trabelculation.

What is the most likely diagnosis?

(a) Blount disease
(b) Neurofibromatosis
(c) Osteogenesis imperfecta
(d) Rickets
(e) Scurvy

48 Regarding antenatal foetal imaging, which of the following is false?

(a) Intravenous gadolinium use enables better cardiac assessment in MR imaging
(b) MR imaging should be avoided before 18 weeks
(c) MR imaging is better than US for evaluating CNS abnormalities
(d) US-guided amniocentesis is usually performed at 15-16 weeks
(e) US to assess foetal growth uses Crown-Rump length at 6-12 wks

49 A 4 week old ex-premature baby has a witnessed seizure. A cranial US is performed which shows cystic structures bilaterally, adjacent to the trigone of the lateral ventricles.

Which of the following favours a diagnosis of chronic periventricular leukomalacia over porencephaly?

(a) Anechoic cysts
(b) Persistence of cysts on follow-up US
(c) Septated cysts
(d) Symmetrical distribution
(e) Watershed territory distribution

50 A 2 week old baby presents with bilious vomiting. The surgical team request an upper GI Barium study looking for malrotation.

Which of the following is the expected normal position of the duodenojejunal junction on the frontal view, making malrotation unlikely?

(a) Above the level of duodenal bulb, to the left of spine
(b) Above the level of duodenal bulb, to the right of spine
(c) At the level of duodenal bulb, to the right of spine
(d) Below the level of duodenal bulb, to the left of spine
(e) Below level of duodenal bulb, to right of spine

51 In a neonate with Tetralogy of Fallot, which of the following findings would not be expected at echocardiography?

(a) Atrial septal defect
(b) Aorta over-riding the interventricular septum
(c) Obstructed right ventricular outflow tract
(d) Right ventricular hypertrophy
(e) Ventricular septal defect

52 A 1 day old neonate has bile-stained vomiting. An AXR shows a dilated gas-filled stomach with air also within the duodenal bulb. No bowel gas seen distally.

Which of the following is the more likely cause of these appearances?

(a) Annular pancreas
(b) Duodenal stenosis
(c) Meconium ileus
(d) Mid-gut volvulus
(e) Pyloric stenosis

53. Regarding rhabdomyosarcoma in the paediatric population.

What is the most likely site of origin?

(a) Extremities
(b) Genito-urinary system
(c) Head and neck
(d) Orbits
(e) Retroperitoneal

54 Regarding nuclear medicine studies and the investigation of pathology in the paediatric population.

Which of the following investigations and tracers are least likely to be used?

(a) ^{99m}Tc-DMSA for dynamic renal study
(b) ^{99m}Tc-HIDA for biliary atresia
(c) ^{99m}Tc-MDP for osteomyelitis
(d) ^{99m}Tc-MIBG for neuroblastoma staging
(e) ^{99m}Tc-Pertechnatate for testicular torsion

55 A 2 year old child is seen by her GP following recurrent chest infections. A CXR is performed and the thymus can be seen to extend down to the diaphragm.

Which of the following is the least likely cause?

(a) Cushing's disease
(b) Recovery from illness
(c) DiGeorge syndrome
(d) Hyperthyroidism
(e) Normal

56 Regarding the diagnosis of Hodgkin's disease in paediatric patients.

Which of the following is not true?

(a) It is associated with EBV infection
(b) Breast cancer is a late iatrogenic complication
(c) It is commoner than NHL
(d) Nodular sclerosing Hodgkin's disease is commonest sub-type
(e) Reed-Sternberg cells are pathognomonic

57 A 28 week antenatal US scan shows absence of the septum pellucidum and a radial array pattern of the medial cerebral sulci. The ventricles are abnormal, with a dilated, elevated 3rd ventricle, disproportionate enlargement of the occipital horns and small, widely separated frontal horns.

Which of the following is not associated with this condition?
(a) Chiari II malformation
(b) Dandy-Walker syndrome
(c) Encephalocoele
(d) Interhemispheric arachnoid cyst
(e) Lobar holoprosencephaly

58 A term day 1 baby has a seizure on the neonatal unit. Cranial US shows hyperechoic periventricular areas. A subsequent CT shows multiple punctuate calcifications in a symmetrical periventricular distribution.

Which congenital infection is the most likely cause of these appearances?
(a) CMV
(b) Herpes simplex
(c) HIV
(d) Rubella
(e) Toxoplasmosis

59 A neonate has multiple apnoeic episodes, bradycardia, difficulty in swallowing, and increased tone in the upper limbs. Cranial US shows hydrocephalus and absence of the corpus callosum. An MRI scan is performed which shows a small posterior fossa.

Which feature makes Chiari III rather than Chiari II malformation the likely diagnosis?
(a) Agenesis of the corpus callosum
(b) Encephalocoele
(c) Klippel-Feil anomaly
(d) Myelomeningocoele
(e) Syringohydromyelia

60 A neonate is noted to have an enlarged head. Trans-cranial US confirms symmetrical dilation of the ventricles consistent with hydrocephalus.

Which of the following is true regarding congenital hydrocephalus?

(a) Aqueduct stenosis is the commonest cause
(b) It can be readily seen at the 12 week antenatal US
(c) It is more commonly associated with intra- rather than extra-cranial anomalies
(d) Most germinal matrix haemorrhage-related hydrocephalus requires shunting
(e) US is the most sensitive modality for identifying the cause

61 A 6 hour old term baby delivered by Caesarian section has increased respiratory rate with intercostal recession. CXR shows prominent vascular markings, Kerley B lines and small bilateral pleural effusions. There is full resolution of symptoms and CXR findings after 2 days.

What is the most likely diagnosis?

(a) Hyaline membrane disease
(b) Meconium aspiration
(c) Neonatal pneumonia
(d) Transient tachypnoea of the newborn
(e) Tricuspid atresia

62 A 10 year old boy presents with right hip pain, there is no history of trauma. Only an AP film has been performed and the epiphysis is aligned on this view.

What feature would make the diagnosis of early slipped upper femoral epiphysis more likely diagnosis than Perthe's disease?

(a) Bilateral changes
(b) Fragmented epiphysis
(c) Reduced epiphysis height
(d) Subchondral fissure
(e) Widened growth plate

63 A 6 year old boy presents with worsening left knee pain, but no history of trauma. X-ray reveals a 1.5 cm lytic, oval lesion in the proximal tibial metaphysis. There is a surrounding rim of sclerosis with a lucent channel extending towards the growth plate.

What is the most likely diagnosis?

(a) Brodie abscess
(b) Chondroblastoma
(c) Ewing's sarcoma
(d) Osteoid osteoma
(e) Multiple myeloma

64 Regarding developmental dysplasia of the hips in a neonate.

Which of the following is not a recognised risk factor?

(a) Breech delivery
(b) Duodenal atresia
(c) Family history
(d) Female sex
(e) Prune-belly syndrome

65 A neonate presents at 48 hours with abdominal distension, bilious vomiting, and failure to pass meconium. The AXR shows multiple dilated loops of bowel, with a 'soap bubble' appearance in the RIF. Water soluble enema confirms microcolon and meconium is subsequently passed.

What is the most likely underlying condition?

(a) Cystic fibrosis
(b) Duodenal atresia
(c) Hirschsprung's disease
(d) Maternal diabetes
(e) Pancreatic duct atresia

66 A neonate with a history of intra-uterine growth retardation has a bilateral deformity of the knees. X-rays reveal a dense femoral diaphysis, with alternating lucent/ dense lines extending longitudinally through the metaphysis, but no periosteal reaction.

What is the most likely diagnosis?
(a) Achondroplasia
(b) Rickets
(c) Rubella
(d) Scurvy
(e) Syphilis

67 A 2 year old boy presents with rectal bleeding. He is not obviously in discomfort, there are no signs of obstruction and the AXR is normal. A Meckel's diverticulum is suspected and a nuclear medicine study is arranged.

Which of these pharmaceuticals should be avoided prior to image acquisition?
(a) Cimetidine
(b) Glucagon
(c) Pentagastrin
(d) Perchlorate
(e) Pertechnetate

68 A 14 day old neonate born at 32 weeks has been treated for respiratory distress syndrome and has remained on a ventilator. Increasing ventilatory pressures have been required. The CXR shows overinflated lungs, black 'streaks' running in the line of the bronchi but a normal heart size.

What is the most likely diagnosis?
(a) Broncho-pulmonary dysplasia
(b) Patent ductus arteriosus
(c) Pulmonary haemorrhage
(d) Pulmonary interstitial emphysema
(e) Wilson Mikity Syndrome

69 What is the most common cause of renal artery stenosis in a child?

(a) Fibromuscular dysplasia
(b) Middle aortic syndrome
(c) Neurofibromatosis
(d) Takayasu's arteritis
(e) William's syndrome

70 A 6 year old boy presents with a 2 day history of limp and right hip/ anterior thigh pain. He has a low-grade fever and the ESR is 30 mm/hr. An US is requested to help differentiate transient synovitis (TS) from septic arthritis.

Which of the following is true?
(a) Capsular distension of 2 mm diagnoses an effusion
(b) Definitive US features can exclude septic arthritis
(c) Synovial membrane thickening favours a diagnosis of TS
(d) US is more sensitive than hip X-Ray for detecting Perthe's disease
(e) US is performed with the hip in internal rotation

71 Regarding fluoroscopically-guided air reduction for the treatment of intussusception in a child.

Which of the following is most likely to predict a successful outcome?
(a) 24 hour history of symptoms
(b) Intussusception seen in the sigmoid colon on US
(c) US demonstrates fluid in the lumen around the intussusceptum
(d) US shows blood flow in the intussusceptum
(e) The child is aged > 12 months

72 A 4 year old boy falls off a climbing frame onto his back. On examination there is tenderness in the lumbosacral spine. X-rays reveal no fracture, but the lateral films demonstrate a 'bone-in-bone' appearance of a vertebra body.

Which of the following is not a cause for this appearance?

(a) Gaucher's disease
(b) Hyperparathyroidism
(c) Normal
(d) Osteopetrosis
(e) Thalassaemia

73 A 2 year old boy is below the 5th centile for height. On examination there is irregular dentition. CXR reveals resorption of the lateral ends of the clavicles and dense vertebral bodies. Lateral skull x-ray reveals an obtuse angle to the mandible and multiple Wormian bones.

What is the likely diagnosis?

(a) Fluorosis
(b) Melorheostosis
(c) Osteopetrosis
(d) Osteopoikilosis
(e) Pyknodysostosis

74 Which of the following fracture types is the most commonly seen as a presentation of non-accidental injury?

(a) Diaphyseal fracture
(b) Fracture of outer third clavicle
(c) Metaphyseal fracture
(d) Scapular fracture
(e) Spinous process fracture

75 A 4 day old boy has abdominal distension and has not opened his bowels. A contrast enema shows a narrow rectum and dilated descending colon. AXR after 24 hours shows contrast medium within the descending colon.

What is the most likely diagnosis?

(a) Hirschsprung's disease
(b) Ileal atresia
(c) Imperforate anus (high malformation type)
(d) Meconium ileus
(e) Meconium plug syndrome

Paediatrics Mock Paper Answers

1 (d)
In HMD the lungs are hypoinflated due to surfactant deficiency and hypoaeration (unless the patient is intubated). In meconium aspiration the lungs may be of normal volume, but are typically hyperinflated due to air trapping. The other findings are non-specific and may be present in both conditions.

Ref: Primer of Diagnostic Imaging, 4th Ed, p. 835–6.

2 (d)
ET tubes should be positioned 1–1.5 cm above the carina. UACs should be sited above the renal arteries between T6-10, or alternatively between L3-5; a position within the aortic arch is too high. PICC lines should lie in a central vein, beyond the subclavian vein ideally at the SVC/ RA junction, but a position in the branchiocephalic vein is also acceptable.

Ref: Diagnostic Radiology, 5th Ed, p. 1463.

3 (d)
The most common type of oesophageal atresia is that associated with a distal tracheal fistula (type C in the Gross classification, and referred to as 'N' shape), which accounts for 75–80% of cases. Pure atresia occurs in 10%, TOF in 10% (type E, and referred to as 'H' shape); other forms are rare. Oesophageal atresia with no distal oesophageal bud is very rare and is not classified within the Gross system.

Ref: Radiology Review Manual, 6th Ed, p. 817.

4 (b)
The most commonly affected lobes, in order of decreasing frequency are: LUL (42-42%), RML (32-35%), RUL (20%). Two or more lobes are only affected in 5% of cases.

Ref: Radiology Review Manual, 6th Ed, p. 486.

5 (a)
The triad of cough, wheeze and reduced air entry in a child of appropriate age (6 months–4 years) is classic for an inhaled foreign body. Most are radiolucent, paired inspiratory/ expiratory CXRs are the most sensitive, however, the child may not cooperate. Lateral decubitus views may show air trapping, but the abnormal lung should be dependent. Fluoroscopy can show air-trapping dynamically, CT can also be considered prior to bronchoscopy.

Ref: Clin Rad (2004); 59(7):609–15.

6 (a)
Beginning fluoroscopy with the cones closed then opening to the desired field size will help reduce dose. Grid removal will lower dose, however, in larger children, a grid may be needed to produce images of adequate quality. Patient dose is lower with an over-couch table (staff dose will be higher).

Ref: R-ITI 5_001 – The effects of radiation on children and dose reduction.

7 (b)
Fluoroscopy has the 'rule of 3s': 3 feet above the table (pressure 120 mmHg), a maximum of 3 attempts with 3 mins/ attempt and 3 mins between attempts. Air reduction is now used in most centres and answers (a), (c), (d) and (e) list its advantages. The only disadvantage of air reduction is confirmation of reduction across the ileo-caecal valve, especially when gas is present in the ileum. Although there is also a small risk of tension pneumoperitoneum with air reduction, any potential peritoneal 'spill' following perforation will be less than with barium reduction.

Ref: R-ITI 5_047 - Paediatric Intussusception.

8 (d)
Stage I: tumour limited to the kidney. Stage II: extension into the perinephric space +/-vessel invasion. Stage III: LNs in the abdomen or pelvis, or peritoneal invasion. Stage IV: haematogeneous spread to lung/ liver/ brain/ bone, or to LNs outside the abdomen or pelvis. Stage V: bilateral renal tumours at diagnosis.

Ref: Radiology Review Manual, 6th Ed, p. 902–3.

9 (a)
Mesoblastic nephroma is the most common solid intrarenal mass in the neonate. 90% present within the 1st year (most by 3 months). It is benign, but there is a risk of sarcomatous degeneration. Wilm's tumour is commoner in older infants; neuroblastoma is the commonest *abdominal* malignancy in neonates.

Ref: Primer of Diagnostic Imaging, 4th Ed, p. 866–8.

10 (c)
Gastroschisis is a defect involving all 3 layers of the abdominal wall, and is located to the right side of the cord in 90% of cases. There is normal insertion of the umbilical cord, and a lower incidence of associated anomalies. Omphalocoele is herniation of intra-abdominal contents into the base of the umbilical cord, any organs may herniate, but liver herniation is typical +/- bowel. Omphalocoeles have a covering membrane.

Ref: Primer of Diagnostic Imaging, 4th Ed, p. 789–90.

11 (b)
Grade I: subependymal haemorrhage, Grade II: intraventricular haemorrhage, no ventricular dilation (10% mortality), Grade III: intraventricular hemorrhage with ventricular dilation (20% mortality), Grade IV: intraparenchymal haemorrhage (>50% mortality). There is no Grade V.

Ref: Primer of Diagnostic Imaging, 4th Ed, p. 890.

12 (d)
The commonest presenting features of Wilm's tumour are: palpable mass (90%; 12 cm is the mean diameter at diagnosis), hypertension (50%), pain (35%), anorexia (15%), fever (15%) and haematuria (5%).

Ref: Primer of Diagnostic Imaging, 4th Ed, p. 865.

13 (d)
Pyrexia of unknown origin has a malignant aetiology in 10% of cases (*e.g.* leukaemia, lymphoma, neuroblastoma, hepatoma, or sarcoma in children). A posterior mediastinal mass is described, lymphoma/ leukaemia can present like this, but they are classically in the anterior mediastinum; in this case the most likely diagnosis is neuroblastoma.

Ref: Aids to Radiological Differential Diagnosis, 4th Ed, p. 180–5.

14 (c)
Pyloric stenosis can be diagnosed clinically. US diagnostic criteria include: pyloric volume > 1.4 cm^3, pyloric muscle wall thickness > 3 mm, pyloric canal length > 17 mm, pyloric transverse diameter > 13 mm when the pyloric channel is closed. In pyloric stenosis, a hypoechoic ring of hypertrophied muscle around the inner echogenic mucosa produces the 'target sign'. Peristaltic waves are increased and hyperdynamic in an attempt to overcome the obstruction.

Ref: Radiology Review Manual, 6th Ed, p. 842–3.

15 (d)
Pneumothorax is common and may be recurrent, due to rupture of bulla/blebs. Kartagener's syndrome is associated with situs inversus. Sweat has *high* sodium and chloride levels. Meconium ileus, not meconium plug syndrome, is associated. Like asthma, CF is associated with pectus carinatum.

Ref: Radiology Review Manual, 6th Ed, p. 488-9 & R-ITI 5_026 – Cystic Fibrosis.

16 (e)
There are 20 'standard views': AP chest, AXR (to include pelvis and hips), lateral C-spine, lateral T/L-spine, single AP and lateral skull, and bilateral views of the humeri, forearms, femurs, tibias/ fibulas, hands, feet and oblique rib views. Supplemental views include: Towne's (if suspected occipital injury), coned views of the relevant joint (metaphyseal injury) and lateral views of a relevant long bone (diaphyseal fracture).

Ref: Clin Rad (2008); 63(6):651-6.

17 (c)
The Salter-Harris classification applies to fractures that involve the grow plate in growing children (peak = 12 years). There are 5 main types, the mnemonic '**SALTR**' aids memory: I: **S**lipped, II: **A**bove (above growth plate, through metaphysis), III: **B**elow (below growth plate, through epiphysis), IV: **T**hrough (through all 3 elements), V: **R**ammed (compressed fracture of the growth plate).

Ref: Radiology Review Manual, 6th Ed, p. 84.

18 (a)
Croup is characterised by oedema of the glottis and subglottis, producing a 'steeple shaped' laryngeal airway on AP radiograph. It is not typically associated with either fever or dysphagia. Epiglottitis occurs in older children.

Ref: Neuroradiology: the requisites, 2nd Ed, p. 671.

19 ([illegible])
Grade I – reflux into ureter. Grade II – reflux into the ureter/ pelvis/ calyces; no dilatation. Grade III – moderate dilatation with minimal blunting of the fornices. Grade IV – moderate ureteral tortuosity and obliteration of the fornices. Grade V – gross dilatation with tortuous ureter.

Ref: Primer of Diagnostic Imaging, 4th Ed, p. 864.

20 (d)
Kawaski's disease is an idiopathic acute febrile, multisystem vasculitis. It is usually self-limiting, with peak presentation at 1–2 years. Complications include coronary artery aneurysms, myocarditis, and acute MI. Treatment is with aspirin and gamma globulins.

Ref: Radiology Review Manual, 6th Ed, p. 642.

21 (b)
Craniosynostosis is the premature closure of the sutures, which may be primary (idiopathic) or secondary. Secondary causes include: metabolic (rickets, hypercalcaemia, hyperthyroidism, hypervitaminosis D), haematological (thalassaemia, SCD), and bone dysplasias (achondroplasia, metaphyseal dysplasia). It is also associated with syndromes (Crouzon, Apert, Treacher-Collins), and can occur following shunt surgery for hydrocephalus.

Ref: Radiology Review Manual, 6th Ed, p. 178.

22 (a)
Avulsion injuries to the pelvis are common in active adolescents, injury results from sudden traction of a muscle on an apophysis. The commonest is the adductor/ hamstrings insertion onto the ischial tuberosity of the inferior pubic ramus. Other pelvic avulsions include ASIS (sartorius muscle), AIIS (rectus femoris) and the lesser trochanter (iliopsoas). Pectineus originates from the superior pubic ramus.

Ref: Diagnostic Radiology, 5th Ed, p. 1615–6.

23 (e)
The following fractures have high specificity for NAI: outer 1/3 clavicle, metaphyseal, posterior ribs, scapula, spinous processes, sternal, and depressed fractures of the occiput. Moderate specificity: multiple fractures, fractures of differing ages, spiral fractures humerus, digital injury in non-mobile child. Fractures that occur frequently but have a relatively low specificity for NAI are answers (a) – (d) and single diaphyseal fractures.

Ref: Diagnostic Radiology, 5th Ed, p. 1623.

24 (c)
Kohler's disease affects the navicular bone, Preiser's disease is osteochondrosis of the scaphoid. Other common paediatric osteochondroses include: Panner's disease (humeral head), Osgood-Schlatter disease (tibial tubercle), and Scheuermann's disease (vertebral apophysis).

Ref: Primer of Diagnostic Imaging, 4th Ed, p. 476

25 (c)
Although some of the imaging features may overlap between these conditions, the history is highly suggestive of neuroblastoma. Intractable diarrhoea is secondary to elevated levels of VIP. Hypertension suggests the presence of increased catecholamine (VMA and HVA) production.

Ref: Diagnostic Radiology, 5th Ed, p.1647.

26 (e)
Pathological calcification is present in 1.6% of children; examples include pituitary fossa, mamillary bodies, habenular commissure, corpus callosum and tectal plate. Calcification within the intrasellar or parasellar region raises the possibility of a craniopharyngioma. All 'normal' sites of intracranial calcification increase in frequency with age, and include pineal (< 1 cm), choroid plexus, dural (may also be due to haemorrhage). There are numerous causes of basal ganglia calcification, but idiopathic is seen as a normal variant.

Ref: R-ITI 5_105 – Intracranial Calcification.

27 (a)
Deterministic effects are extremely rare in children. Stochastic effects are of greater concern, principally the chance of developing future cancers.

Ref: R-ITI 5_001 – The effects of radiation on children and dose reduction.

28 (c)
Left-side down decubitus is the optimal view, it allows air to rise to the right lateral abdomen, which can then be seen between the liver edge and the abdominal wall; with right-side down films it is harder to detect free air due to presence of stomach/ splenic flexure. An erect CXR is likely to be impractical in a ventilated neonate. Signs on supine AXRs are often subtle (football sign, Rigler's sign, or air around the falciform ligament). In a cross-table lateral it will be hard to differentiate free air and distended bowel (both rise centrally).

Ref: R-ITI 5_044 - Necrotising Enterocolitis – NEC.

29 (c)
Both conditions have conjugated hyperbilirubinaemia. The findings of a normal (> 1.5 cm) or enlarged gallbladder supports neonatal hepatitis, however, either finding can be present in BA as the GB can appear normal if the atresia is distal (in 20%). There is no intrahepatic duct dilatation in BA due to panductal sclerosis. In HIDA scintigraphy BA has good hepatic visualisation within 5 mins, but no excretion into the bowel, and no tracer uptake seen by 24 hours; in neonatal hepatitis there is slow and reduced uptake of the tracer by the liver, but bowel activity is seen by 24 hours.

Ref: Radiology Review Manual, 6th Ed, p. 709–10 & Primer of Diagnostic Imaging, 4th Ed, p. 852.

30 (e)
Duplication cysts can be located anywhere along the GI tract, the most common location is the terminal ileum, followed by oesophagus, duodenum, colon, jejunum and stomach. They represent 15% of paediatric abdominal masses, and may be detected on antenatal US. Small bowel cysts are usually located on the mesenteric side of the bowel, oesophageal ones are typically intra-luminal. The cysts have a double capsule made of the bowel wall and mucosa, they are typically non-communicating and calcification is rare.

Ref: Radiology Review Manual, 6th Ed, p. 824.

31 (c)
The patient has delayed skeletal maturity and dense metaphyseal bands, lead-poisoning fits both these criteria. Now rare, but it may occur with neglect or pica syndrome. Options (a) and (d) produce precocious puberty, (b) can produce dense metaphyseal lines, but skeletal maturation is not affected, (e) is associated with delayed maturity only.

Ref: Radiology Review Manual, 6th Ed, p. 3.

32 (a)
Intralobar type is within the lung, sharing its pleura; it may be of airless, or air-containing, cystic type, and presents late in childhood/adulthood with recurrent infections or haemoptysis. Arterial supply is systemic, drainage is to the pulmonary vein in 95% and there is a low association with other anomalies. Extrapulmonary sequestration presents in neonates, is located outside the lung with its own pleura, has a systemic arterial supply, and drainage is to the systemic circulation. In 65% there are associated anomalies and it is 'always' airless (unless there is a communication with the GI tract).

Ref: Primer of Diagnostic Imaging, 4th Ed, p. 830 & Radiology Review Manual, 6th Ed, p.479–80.

33 (d)
The list given is that of the '5 Ts' of cyanotic heart disease with *increased* pulmonary vasculature. The differential diagnosis for cyanosis and pulmonary oligaemia is tricuspid atresia, Tetralogy of Fallot, Ebstein's anomaly and pulmonary atresia. In tricuspid atresia there will only be increased pulmonary flow if there is an associated VSD but no pulmonary stenosis (a frequent association); the majority have reduced pulmonary blood flow.

Ref: Primer of Diagnostic Imaging, 4th Ed, p. 119–20.

34 (e)
Meconium plug syndrome results from colonic inertia with subsequent inspissation of meconium. It typically presents in large babies, born to diabetic mothers, is not related to meconium ileus. Hirschsprung's disease is the key differential diagnosis and can have similar radiological appearances. However, meconium is rarely passed following contrast examination and the given history of a diabetic mother is a leader to meconium plug syndrome.

Ref: Fundamentals of Diagnostic Radiology, 2nd Ed, p. 1287.

35 (e)
This is seen in over a quarter of cases. The remaining presentations are well-documented, but occur less commonly.

Ref: Clin Rad (2009); 64: 109–118.

36 (b)
Asymmetrical renal size may be the only US finding with a duplex system. The 'Weigert-Meyer' rule states that the lower pole ureter inserts in the normal position, the upper pole ureter inserts inferio-medially, tends to be stenotic and obstructed and is often associated with a ureterocoele. The lower ureter is prone to VUR. The renal pelvis will have a concave upper border due to inferior displacement by the obstructed upper pole, there is lateral displacement of the kidney and ureters and there are *decreased* calyces in comparison to the normal side, producing the 'drooping lily' sign.

Ref: Primer of Diagnostic Imaging, 4th Ed, p. 856–7 & Radiology Review Manual, 6th Ed, p. 985.

37 (a)
The normal thymus widens on expiration, and narrows/ elongates on inspiration. <5 yrs there are smooth biconvex lateral borders, with increasing age the lateral margins straighten or become concave. The anterio-lateral margins can be indented by anterior rib ends to give a scalloped 'wavy' appearance laterally, but not inferiorly. The right lobe often has a flattened inferior border near the horizontal fissure producing the 'sail sign'.

Ref: R-ITI 5_029 – Paediatric Mediastinum: Normal Anatomy and Appearances.

38 (d)
MCKD is normally unilateral (bilateral in 5–20%) and is thought to be caused by pelvi-infundibular atresia. US shows multiple cysts of variable size that are randomly arranged and are separated by little or no parenchyma; a renal pelvis cannot be seen. It is the 2nd most common cause of a neonatal abdominal mass (after hydronephrosis) and is the most common renal cystic disease in infants. Meckel-Gruber syndrome produces enlarged polycystic (2-10 mm cysts) kidneys *in utero*, and typically causes oligohydramnios and pulmonary hypoplasia. MLCN is characterised by large (> 10 cm) cystic spaces, which will compress or displace the parenchyma.

Ref: Primer of Diagnostic Imaging, 4th Ed, p. 861-2 & Radiology Review Manual, 6th Ed, p. 937-8.

39 (d)
Cervical spine injuries in children are usually located between the occiput and C2–C3, because the spine is hypermobile (ligament laxity), there is incomplete ossification of the odontoid process, a relatively large head, and weak neck muscles. The other options are normal variants, others include absent cervical lordosis, intervertebral widening, and pseudospread of the atlas on the 'Peg' view (pseudo–Jefferson fracture). Pseudo-widening of the prevertebral soft tissues can be normal, related to expiration.

Ref: Radiographics (2003); 23:539–560.

40 (a)
The presence of a posterior fat pad is always abnormal, an anterior fat pad can be normal. Fat pad elevation signifies a joint effusion and in the context of trauma this implies a fracture, even if occult by radiography. The fat pads will not be elevated if the fracture is extracapsular, or if the capsule ruptures. The elbow centres ossify in the sequence C-R-I-T-O-L (Capitellum, Radial head, Internal (medial) epicondyle, Trochlea, Olecranon, Lateral epicondyle). Although (rarely) this sequence varies, 'I' *always* comes before 'T', thus if the trochlea is present, the medial condyle has to be present - its absence implies an avulsion #. The medial epicondyle is extracapsular there is typically no fat pad elevation, however, there will be if the capsule is torn, in such cases there is a risk the medial epicondyle will be displaced into the elbow joint, thus cannot be seen on the initial radiographs (as implied in the scenario given).

Ref: Accident & Emergency Radiology, 2nd Ed, p. 100-6.

41 (d)
Neonatal causes include dehydration (vomiting, diarrhoea), sepsis, birth trauma and prematurity. Glycosuria in infants of diabetic mothers is another cause, and there is an association with increased maternal age. Left adrenal haemorrhage is a cause of RVT; the left adrenal vein drains to the left renal vein, the right adrenal drains directly to the IVC.

Ref: Radiology Review Manual, 6th Ed, p. 968.

42 (e)
The types of skeletal dysplasia include rhizomelic dysplasia: shortened proximal limb (*e.g.* humerus) relative to distal limb (*e.g.* radius), mesomelic: shortened distal relative to proximal, micromelic: shortened proximal and distal, and acromelic: distal extremity shortening (*e.g.* hand). The rhizomelic dysplasia described (femur lower limit of normal at 20 weeks) is most likely to be achondroplasia.

Ref: Primer of Diagnostic Imaging, 4th Ed, p. 883.

43 (b)
Meconium is the first stool passed, it is sterile and composed of epithelial cells, mucus, amniotic fluid, bile and water. Aspiration occurs if the meconium is expelled into the amniotic fluid prior to birth, or during labour. It is more common in post-mature births, if there is prolonged labour, and where foetal distress occurs during labour. Post-maturity is also associated with birth trauma and its sequelae, *e.g.* DDH. The other conditions are associated with prematurity.

44 (a)
Caffey's disease is idiopathic, presents at <6 months and results in asymmetric cortical periostitis of tubular bone diaphyses (epiphyses spared). Typical sites affected are mandible (80%), clavicle, ulna, tibia. Patients present with irritability, fever, and failure to thrive (if mandible affected). Post-treatment rickets can cause hyperostosis, scurvy occurs after 4 months, hypervitaminosis A occurs after 1 year. NAI is possible, but no other suspicious findings are apparent, and the sites are typical for Caffey's disease.

Ref: Radiology Review Manual, 6th Ed, p. 108.

45 (d)
If there is asymmetric transradiancy and the lungs are abnormal, there are 3 factors to consider: differences in aeration, vascularity and size. If there is different vascularity, the side with the decreased vascularity is abnormal. If there are differences in aeration, the side which changes least on expiration is usually abnormal. In this case the lungs are normal and the increased translucency must be due to another cause. Poland's syndrome has underdevelopment or absence of the pectoral muscle unilaterally (typically right); there may be associated webbing of the fingers.

Ref: R-ITI 5_014 – Unilateral Hyperlucent Hemithorax.

46 (c)
The small size of the neonatal heart and vessels is a challenge, which requires high resolution scans using a small FOV and small surface coils to maximise SNR. Neonates/ infants are typically anaesthetised and intubated, this stops spontaneous movement and allows breath-holding sequences to be performed. Some targeted studies may be as short as 10 minutes. Neonates have a fast heart rate, which necessitates high temporal resolution for accurate assessment of ventricular volume and flow.

Ref: Radiographics (2007); 27(1): 5–18.

47 (d)
Rickets is osteomalacia resulting from vitamin D deficiency that occurs during enchondral bone growth and can be primary or secondary (GI, renal, hepatic causes). There is failure of osteoid mineralisation; increased osteoid production elevates the periosteum and widens the epiphyseal plates. There is 'softening' of the diaphysis, resulting in bowing deformity of the long bones. The metaphyses are classically flayed (irregular), splayed (widened) and cupped. Blount disease presents > 6 years and may have bowing of the legs secondary to AVN of the medial tibial condyle.

Ref: Radiology Review Manual, 6th Ed, p. 156–7.

48 (a)
Gadolinium is not used because it crosses the placenta and is potentially teratogenic at high doses. After 13 weeks CRL is unreliable and biparietal diameter/ femur length are used. MRI can be used to assess specific foetal anomalies identified at US. It offers better visualization of the brain (not limited by the skull) and better soft tissue contrast. MRI is performed after 18 weeks to avoid exposure at times of peak organogenesis.

Ref: Primer of Diagnostic Imaging, 4th Ed, p. 801 & 814.

49 (d)
PVL is more common in preterm children, is secondary to ischaemia and usually occurs in the watershed areas. Initially there will be hyperechoic changes which gradually become cystic (>2 wks); the cysts are never septated and usually resolve over time. Porencephaly can be developmental or due to a vascular or infectious process which destroys brain tissue; it is almost always asymmetrical, rarely disappears over time and is often seen as an extension of the ventricle or sub-arachnoid space. If secondary to ischaemia it can also be in a watershed distribution.

Ref: Primer of Diagnostic Imaging, 4th Ed, p. 891 & Radiology Review Manual, 6th Ed, p. 313–4 & 324.

50 (a)
Malrotation is the abnormal position of the bowel due to a narrow mesenteric attachment following arrest of rotation and fixation *in utero*. The normal DJJ is at the ligament of Treitz, to the left of the vertebral (usually L1) pedicle at a level above or equal with the duodenal bulb on a true AP film. In malrotation, the mesentery is short, thus the DJJ does not reach the ligament of Treitz.

Ref: Radiology Review Manual, 6th Ed, p. 853

51 (a)
'Tetralogy of Fallot' consists of the 4 features listed in answers (b) – (e). Variations on the condition include 'Trilogy of Fallot' (PA stenosis, RVH and patent foramen ovale) and 'pink Tetralogy' (VSD with mild PS). The presence of ASD with the other features makes the diagnosis one of 'Pentalogy of Fallot'.

Ref: Primer of Diagnostic Imaging, 4th Ed, p. 128-9.

52 (a)
The 'double bubble' sign is described and implies obstruction at the level of the duodenum. Duodenal atresia (not stenosis) is the commonest cause (30%) and is associated with Down's. Annular pancreas is second commonest cause, others include: duodenal web/ diaphragm, pre-duodenal vein, midgut volvulus, and SMA syndrome.

Ref: Primer of Diagnostic Imaging, 4th Ed, p. 898.

53 (c)
Rhabdomyosarcoma represents 4–8% of cancers in children and is the 4th commonest after CNS tumours, neuroblastoma and Wilm's and is the commonest soft tissue sarcoma in children. The sites affected are: head and neck (28%), extremities (24%), genitourinary system, trunk (11%), orbits (7%), and retroperitoneum (6%); other sites in <3%.

Ref: Radiology Review Manual, 6th Ed, p. 971–2 & Clin Rad (1999); 54(1): 2-10.

54 (a)
DMSA is used for static renal imaging (scarring); MAG-3 and DTPA are dynamic renal tracers and can give split function. Pertechnatate can be used for testicular torsion, although is a secondary investigation following US and is rarely used now. The other combinations are commonly used.

Ref: Primer of Diagnostic Imaging, 4th Ed, p. 934–5 & p. 939–45.

55 (c)
Rebound hyperplasia is seen during recovery from illness, after chemotherapy or radiotherapy or following treatment for Cushing's disease. Hypoplasia or aplasia of the thymus is seen in DiGeorge syndrome. In infancy a prominent thymus is almost always normal and can occasionally extend as far as the diaphragm.

Ref: R-ITI 5_029 – Paediatric Mediastinum: Normal Anatomy and Appearances.

56 (c)
NHL is more common (55%) than HD (45%) in children. EBV infection is a risk factor; EBV genetic material can sometimes be detected in the Reed-Sternberg cells. The pathological diagnosis of HD is based on the presence of Reed-Sternberg cells. The nodular sclerosing type is commonest in children (50%). Females are at increased risk of breast cancer following treatment with mantle radiotherapy.

Ref: Primer of Diagnostic Imaging, 4th Ed, p. 78.

57 (e)
The US features described are those of agenesis of the corpus callosum. Other associations include: alobar and semi-lobar forms of holoprosencephaly, midline intracerebral lipoma, polymicrogyria, grey matter heterotopia and porencephaly.

Ref: Radiology Review Manual, 6th Ed, p. 264. & Primer of Diagnostic Imaging, 4th Ed, p. 572–4.

58 (a)
Congenital infections include HIV and TORCH (TOxoplasmosis, Rubella, CMV, and Herpes simplex). The findings described are classic for CMV (CT is adequate for diagnosis in up to 70% cases). There may be associated polymicrogyria. Toxoplasmosis and rubella calcification is distributed around the basal ganglia and in the parenchyma. HIV produces diffuse atrophy. Basal ganglia calcification may appear at 1 year.

Ref: Radiology Review Manual, 6th Ed, p. 232 & Primer of Diagnostic Imaging, 4th Ed, p. 568.

59 (b)
Chiari II malformation comprises a small posterior fossa, herniation of the tonsils and vermis through the foramen magnum, myelomeningocoele (90%), obstructive hydrocephalus (90%), agenesis of the corpus callosum, syringohydromyelia (50%) and abnormal cortical gyration. Chiari III is rare, has the features of Chiari II, but with an associated encephalocoele. Chiari I is associated with Klippel-Feil anomaly.

Ref: Primer of Diagnostic Imaging, 4th Ed, p. 571–2.

60 (a)
Aqueduct stenosis accounts for 43% of congenital hydrocephus. US assessment is difficult <20 wks because the ventricles normally occupy a large percentage of the cranial vault. The most sensitive modality for determining the cause (not presence) of hydrocephalus is MRI. Grade III germinal matrix haemorrhage has hydrocephalus, but in 2/3 this is stable and requires no treatment. Intracranial anomalies are associated in 37% (*e.g.* agenesis corpus callosum), extracranial anomalies in 63% (*e.g.* VSD, spina bifida).

Ref: R-ITI 5_029 – Paediatric Mediastinum: Normal Anatomy and Appearances.

61 (d)
TTN is the commonest cause of respiratory distress in the newborn. Risk factors include C-section, breech, or fast deliveries (thus fluid is not 'squeezed' from the lungs through the birth canal). Onset is typically within the first 6 hours (peak 1 day). The CXR findings given are typical and although there can be overlap, the history/ risk factors and subsequent resolution make TTN the most likely diagnosis.

Ref: Radiology Review Manual, 6th Ed, p. 528.

62 (c)
SUFE presents aged 10-15 years (typically overweight patients), and is bilateral in 15-25%. Early signs include widened growth plate and reduced height of epiphysis on the AP view (slips posteriorly), the 'frogleg' lateral is more accurate for showing a medial slip. Perthes disease (avascular necrosis) presents at 5–10 years, is bilateral in 15%, early features include widened joint space and subchondral fissure fracture; later features include fragmented epiphyses, subchondral cysts, increased density, and OA.

Ref: Primer of Diagnostic Imaging, 4th Ed, p. 878–9.

63 (a)
Brodie abscess is a subacute pyogenic osteomyelitis, most commonly caused by *Staphylococcus aureus*. It is a metaphyseal lesion, but may cross to the epiphysis before growth plate fusion; the proximal or distal tibia location is typical. The finding of a lucent channel extending to the physis ('serpentine' sign) is pathognomonic for Brodie abscess.

Ref: Radiology Review Manual, 6th Ed, p. 139–40.

64 (b)
In DDH there is an abnormally lax joint capsule +/- acetabular dysplasia ('shallow' acetabulum). Risk factors include girls, family history (12% if parent affected, 36% for subsequent siblings), breech delivery, and oligohydramnios (due to restricted space *in utero*). Duodenal atresia is a cause of polyhydramnios.

Ref: Radiology Review Manual, 6th Ed, p. 65–6.

65 (a)
Meconium ileus is the initial presentation in 10–15% of CF neonates, but over 90% of infants presenting with meconium ileus have CF (atresia of the pancreas or pancreatic duct are other causes). The 'soap bubble' appearance may be seen in the RIF and represents gas mixed with meconium. A water soluble contrast enema aids diagnosis (shows an unused 'micro' colon) and treatment (if unsuccessful, surgery is required).

Ref: R-ITI 5_026 - Cystic Fibrosis.

66 (c)
The features described are those of 'celery stalking', present in 50% of babies with congenital rubella. Growth retardation will not initially be apparent if contracted later in pregnancy. The absence of periosteal reaction distinguishes it from syphilis, scurvy does not develop before 4 months due to presence of maternal vitamin C.

Ref: Radiology Review Manual, 6th Ed, p. 159.

67 (d)
Tc-99m pertechnetate is the radiotracer used; cimetidine, pentagastrin and glucagon have been shown to improve the sensitivity of the test. Pentagastrin enhances tracer uptake in gastric mucosa, cimetidine 'traps' pertechnetate within the Meckel's, and glucagon reduces peristalsis, thus inhibits tracer washout. Potassium perchlorate given orally after the study protects the thyroid gland from accumulation of pertechnetate, however, if used prior to scanning it will block tracer uptake by gastric mucosa.

Ref: Clin Rad (2009); 64(2): 109–18.

68 (d)
PIE is typically due to positive-pressure ventilation leading to air leaks from the bronchi to the interstitium. PIE makes the lungs 'stiff' and more difficult to ventilate and leads to overinflated lungs, with the potential for pneumothorax or pneumo-mediastinum. BPD is diagnosed clinically as oxygen dependency at 28 days of age or 36 corrected weeks of gestation.

Ref: R-ITI 5_011 – Neonatal Respiratory Distress Medical Conditions.

69 (a)
All are causes of RAS, other causes include polyarteritis nodosa, post-renal transplantation and post-radiotherapy. FMD is the most common, the other conditions are rare. In adults, the majority of cases of RAS is secondary to atherosclerosis.

Ref: Primer of Diagnostic Imaging, 4th Ed, p. 871.

70 (a)
TS presents at 5-10 years and is the commonest cause of a non-traumatic limp in this age group. US is performed with the child supine and the hip in the neutral position, or in slight external rotation. US typically shows an effusion (capsular distension ≥ 2 mm), without synovial thickening. It is a diagnosis of exclusion, radiographs may help differentiate Perthe's disease; fluid aspiration helps exclude septic arthritis.

Ref: Radiology (1999); 210:499-507.

71 (d)
Vascular flow is a good sign - ischaemia is unlikely. A left-sided lesion is more difficult to treat, but the majority are ileocolic (75–95%) or ileo-ileocolic (9%); colocolic lesions are very rare. A short history (< 24 hours) suggests there will be less oedema and the intussusception is less likely to have passed through to the left colon. An older age (> 12 months) suggests a pathological lead point may be the aetiology. Intussusception is idiopathic in 95% of paediatric cases.

Ref: R-ITI 5_047 – Paediatric Intussusception.

72 (b)
A bone-in-bone appearance is often best seen in the vertebrae. It may be a normal appearance (particularly in the thoracic and lumbar vertebrae in infants). Secondary causes include Caffey's, SCD, thalassaemia, congenital syphilis, osteopetrosis, oxalosis, radiation, acromegaly, paget's disease (older population), rickets, TB, scurvy, hypoparathyroidism, hypothyroidism, lead poisoning and gaucher's disease.

Ref: R-ITI 5_138 – Bone Within a Bone Appearance.

73 (e)
All are causes of a generalised increase in bone density. Pyknodysostosis is also associated with dwarfism, mental retardation, widened hands and feet, brachycephaly, platybasia, widened sutures, and hypoplastic tapered terminal phalangeal tufts. It is possibly a variant of cleidocranial dysostosis, but this latter condition lacks the features of dense bones, phalangeal hypoplasia and short stature.

Ref: R-ITI 5_136 – Generalised Increased Bone Density.

74 (a)
Although less-specific for NAI, diaphyseal fractures are 4x more frequent than the more NAI-characteristic metaphyseal fractures. A key diagnostic feature of NAI is the presence of multiple fractures of differing ages. Other fractures that occur frequently but have less specificity are mid-clavicular fractures and simple linear skull fractures. Fractures of the scapula, spinous processes and sternum (the '3 Ss') and depressed fractures of the occiput are also considered specific for NAI, but rare.

Ref: Clin Rad (1999); 54(1):11-24.

75 (a)
Hirschsprung's disease presents in neonates with abdominal distension and failure to pass meconium. Proximal obstruction +/- perforation can be seen on AXR. The rectum is always involved, but the proximal extent of disease varies. The normal colon will be dilated. If the transition point lies near the recto-sigmoid junction, the rectum: sigmoid diameter ratio will be less than 1 (normal is > 1:1). Retention of contrast medium on a delayed 24 hours film is a classical feature, but definitive diagnosis is by biopsy.

Ref: Radiology Review Manual, 6th Ed, p. 856.

Central Nervous System and Head & Neck Mock Paper Questions

1 **A young man presents with a thunderclap headache. A CT examination is performed. Sub-arachnoid blood is seen with a localised clot which has a maximum thickness of 2 mm. No intraventricular nor parenchymal blood is seen.**

What is the Fisher Grade?
(a) Grade 0
(b) Grade I
(c) Grade II
(d) Grade III
(e) Grade IV

2 **A middle aged man with progressive lower-extremity weakness undergoes an MRI examination of the spine. T2W images demonstrate multiple small vessel flow voids on the cord pial surface, but no flow voids within the cord. The cord is enlarged, with oedema sparing the periphery.**

Which type of spinal cord arteriovenous malformation does this represent?
(a) Type I
(b) Type II
(c) Type III
(d) Type IV
(e) Type V

3 **A neonate presents with unilateral leukocoria and microphthalmia. An US reveals a hyperechoic band within the globe. CT demonstrates a hyperdense vitreous, fluid-fluid levels and an absence of calcification. No focal mass is seen.**

What is the most likely diagnosis?
(a) Coat's disease
(b) Persistent hyperplastic primary vitreous
(c) Retinal dysplasia
(d) Retinoblastoma
(e) Toxocariasis

4 **A 30 year old man presents with a progressive neurological deficit. A CT head demonstrates strongly enhancing, serpiginous structures. Catheter angiography subsequently visualises the lesion.**

What is the most likely diagnosis?

(a) Brain arteriovenous malformation
(b) Dural arteriovenous fistula
(c) Cavernous angioma
(d) Venous angioma
(e) Telangiectasia

5 **Which of the following is not a standard radiographic projection of the skull?**

(a) 30 degree fronto-occipital
(b) 20 degree occipito-frontal
(c) Occipito-mental
(d) 20 degree occipito-mental
(e) Posterior-anterior

6 **A patient presents with an enlarged, palpable cervical lymph node. Thyroid carcinoma is suspected, and an US is performed.**

What imaging feature would make a malignant node more likely?

(a) Short axis to long axis ratio (S/L) of 0.25
(b) Echogenic hilum
(c) Punctate calcification
(d) Central hilar flow pattern on colour doppler imaging
(e) Absence of visible subcapsular flow on colour doppler imaging

7 **A 30 year old man with learning difficulties presents to A&E after suffering facial injuries. An orthopantomogram is performed and demonstrates a multi-locular radio-lucent lesion in the angle of the mandible. He suffered from multiple carcinomatous lesions of the skin in childhood.**

What is the most likely diagnosis?
(a) Odontogenic keratocyst
(b) Dentigerous cyst
(c) Inflammatory odontogenic cyst
(d) Ameloblastoma
(e) Multiple myeloma

8 **A neck lump is found on clinical examination. Axial MR images of the neck demonstrate a mass displacing the parapharyngeal space posteromedially and the styloid musculature posteriorly.**

In which fascial space is the mass most likely to be located?
(a) Masticator space
(b) Carotid space
(c) Pharyngeal mucosal space
(d) Parotid space
(e) Retropharyngeal space

9 **A plain radiograph is performed on a male child. Unilateral, premature fusion of both the coronal and lambdoid sutures is evident.**

What is the most appropriate description?
(a) Scaphocephaly
(b) Brachycephaly
(c) Plagiocephaly
(d) Trigonocephaly
(e) Oxycephaly

10 A skull radiograph is performed on a patient who presented with a possible head injury. There is a solitary skull vault lucency, with a surrounding area of sclerosis.

What is the most likely diagnosis?

(a) Pacchionian granulation
(b) Multiple myeloma
(c) Hyperparathyroidism
(d) Langerhans cell histiocytosis
(e) Osteoporosis

11 A patient presents with sensorineural hearing loss. A cerebellopontine angle mass is demonstrated on MR imaging.

Which of the following features support a diagnosis of schwannoma over menigioma?

(a) High signal intensity relative to grey matter on T2W imaging
(b) Enhancement with *i.v.* gadolinium
(c) Calcification
(d) Unilateral lesion
(e) Durally based lesion

12 A patient develops dissociated anaesthesia of the legs. An MRI brain demonstrates herniation of the cerebellar tonsils.

Which of the following is not associated with Chiari type I malformation?

(a) Hydrocephalus
(b) Syringohydromelia
(c) Platyblasia
(d) Incomplete ossification of the C1 ring
(e) Myelomenigocoele

13 A middle-aged man presents with an acute onset facial nerve palsy and has MR imaging with the *i.v.* administration of gadolinium.

Which of the following features would support the diagnosis of a Bell's palsy?

(a) Enhancement of the tympanic portion of the facial nerve
(b) Enhancement of the intracanalicular portion of the facial nerve
(c) Enhancement of the mastoid portion of the facial nerve
(d) Continuing symptoms at 9 months
(e) Demineralisation of the petrous apex

14 Which of the following structures does not typically calcify in normal individuals?

(a) Parasellar ligaments
(b) Dentate nucleus
(c) Pineal gland
(d) Choroid plexus
(e) Perimesencephalic grey matter

15 A patient presents with multiple relapsing focal neurological deficits.

Which MR imaging feature would be unusual in multiple sclerosis?

(a) Cortical central atrophy
(b) Atrophy of the corpus callosum
(c) Hypointense thalamus on T2W
(d) Hypointense plaques on T2W
(e) Spinal cord involvement

16 A patient with a known intracerebral neoplasm suddenly deteriorates. A CT head demonstrates enlargement of left the CPA cistern and new areas of high attenuation in the anterior midbrain.

Which type of cerebral herniation is most likely?

(a) Subfalcine
(b) Transtentorial
(c) Transcalvarial
(d) Tonsillar
(e) Transalar

17 A patient presents with a lump thought to be arising from the thyroid gland. An US is arranged for further evaluation which confirms the solid lesion is thyroid in origin.

Which imaging feature would be most suggestive of a malignant lesion?

(a) Cystic nature
(b) Complete low-echogenicity halo
(c) Comet tail artefact
(d) Coarse calcification
(e) Hypoechoic

18 A young patient presents with dissociated sensory loss. MRI demonstrates spinal cord enlargement with an intra-medullary lesion.

Which of the following features would favour the diagnosis of astrocytoma, rather than ependymoma?

(a) Syrinx
(b) Haemorrhage
(c) Adult patient
(d) Ill-defined enhancement
(e) Bone remodelling

19 A patient is seen in the neurology clinic, referred by his GP with a chronic headache.

Which of the following features would not be an indication for imaging?

(a) Increasingly severe headache
(b) Recurrent episodes of headache in the early morning
(c) Constant headache for 2 years
(d) Blurring of vision for 1 month
(e) Early papilloedema

20 A patient presents with gradual onset of sensory symptoms affecting the right hand. CT reveals a superficial mass within the fronto-parietal region.

Which imaging feature would not support the diagnosis of menigioma?

(a) Inward bulging of the grey-white junction
(b) Surrounding oedema
(c) Hyperdense on unenhanced images
(d) Enhancement with intravenous contrast medium
(e) Intralesional haemorrhage

21 A 45 year old female presents with facial pain and abnormal eye movements. A cerebellopontine angle lesion is identified on MR imaging.

Which feature would not be consistent with an epidermoid tumour?

(a) Iso-intense to CSF on T1W Imaging
(b) Low signal on DWI
(c) Heterogeneous signal on FLAIR
(d) Lack of enhancement
(e) Low signal on balanced sequence/ true FISP

22 A young man suffers a subarachnoid haemorrhage. A CT angiogram fails to demonstrate an aneurysm, and a cerebral angiogram is performed.

Which of the following is not a recognised complication of cerebral angiography?

(a) Hydrocephalus
(b) Stroke
(c) Migraine
(d) Memory loss
(e) Contrast neurotoxicity

23 A man referred from the memory clinic has a ^{99m}Tc-HMPAO cerebral SPECT. Temporo-parietal hypoperfusion is found.

What is the most likely diagnosis?

(a) Pick's disease
(b) Chronic alcoholism
(c) Aids-related dementia
(d) Lewy-body disease
(e) Multi-infarct dementia

24 An MR reveals a lesion within the globus pallidus.

Which of the following is incorrect?

(a) The lesion is within the corpus striatum
(b) The lesion is within the lentiform nucleus
(c) The lesion is within the diencephalon
(d) The lesion is within the striatum
(e) The lesion is within the lenticular nucleus

25 A 30 year old pregnant patient is found unconscious and neurological examination reveals bilateral Babinski's sign. CT and MR imaging is suggestive of cerebral infarction.

Which of the following imaging features would support an arterial rather than a venous infarct?

(a) A hyperdense superior sagittal sinus on unenhanced CT imaging
(b) Bilateral areas of increased T2W signal
(c) Prominent haemorrhage
(d) Maximal brain swelling at 4 days
(e) Intense dural enhancement

26 A female patient is seen in the endocrine clinic and a pituitary microadenoma is suspected.

Regarding the imaging of the pituitary gland, which of the following is an abnormal appearance?

(a) High signal in the posterior pituitary on T1W
(b) Intermediate signal intensity in the posterior pituitary on T2W
(c) Enhancement of the posterior pituitary on T1W after gadolinium administration
(d) Convex superior margin of the pituitary gland in pregnant subjects
(e) High signal in the anterior pituitary on T2W

27 A patient with known HIV develops neurological symptoms and a CT head examination is performed. Multiple ring-enhancing lesions are seen.

What imaging features would support the diagnosis of toxoplasmosis rather than lymphoma?

(a) Hyperdense on unenhanced CT imaging
(b) Eccentric enhancing nodule
(c) Callosal involvement
(d) Subependymal spread
(e) Periventricular location

28 Thickening of the extra-ocular muscles is seen on MR imaging.

What features would support the diagnosis of pseudotumour rather than thyroid ophthalmopathy?

(a) Bilaterality
(b) Ocular muscle tendon involvement
(c) Atrophy of the lacrimal gland
(d) Minimal response to steroids
(e) Painless proptosis

29 An MRI brain is performed and a lesion is seen in the suprasellar region.

Which of the following imaging characteristics is not typical?

(a) Craniopharyngioma – calcification and nodular enhancement
(b) Epidermoid – isointense to CSF on T1W and T2W
(c) Tuber cinerum – isointense to grey matter on T1W
(d) Schwannoma – T1W hypointensity and marked enhancement with *i.v.* gadolinium
(e) Rathke's cleft cyst – T1W hypointensity and lack of enhancement with *i.v.* gadolinium

30 A teenager presents with a small midline neck lump. On examination, the lump is noted to move superiorly upon protrusion of the tongue.

Which of the following statements is incorrect regarding such lesions?

(a) They are characteristically suprahyoid
(b) Presentation with a painless midline mass is common
(c) Can appear anechoic by US imaging
(d) Can appear uniformly echogenic by US imaging
(e) Can appear heterogeneous by US imaging

31 An adolescent undergoes MR imaging and an incidental suprasellar mass is found.

What feature would suggest a diagnosis of craniopharyngioma rather than a Rathke cleft cyst?

(a) Absence of calcification
(b) Predominantly high signal on T1W imaging
(c) Smooth contour
(d) Homogeneous signal intensity
(e) Nodular enhancement

32 An elderly gentleman has an episode of amaurosis fugax and undergoes Doppler ultrasound assessment of his carotid arteries.

Which of the following features is not an indication of either internal carotid artery or common carotid artery stenosis?

(a) Peak systolic velocity of 160 cm/s
(b) Significant quantities of visible plaque
(c) End diastolic velocity of 120 cm/s
(d) Spectral broadening
(e) ICA/ CCA peak systolic velocity ratio of 1.5

33 An elderly gentleman presents with a hemiplegia. Both MR diffusion and perfusion-weighted imaging are performed.

Which of the following would suggest the presence of an ischaemic penumbra?

(a) A lesion which appears the same size on diffusion and perfusion weighted imaging
(b) A lesion which appears larger on perfusion-weighted than diffusion weighted imaging
(c) Visualisation of a lesion on perfusion-weighted imaging
(d) Changes in the perfusion parameters over time
(e) A lesion which appears larger on diffusion-weighted than perfusion weighted imaging

34 A 55 year old patient presents with head trauma. A CT head is performed and bilateral calcification of his basal ganglia is noted.

Which of the following is not a recognised cause?

(a) Sturge-Weber-Dimitri syndrome
(b) Fahr's disease
(c) Hypoparathyroidism
(d) Pseudo-pseudohypoparathyroidism
(e) Hypoxia

35 An elderly, hypertensive man is found collapsed. MR imaging demonstrates a large intracerebral haematoma, with intermediate signal intensity on T1W and high signal intensity on T2W.

How old is the haematoma likely to be?

(a) 0–12 hours
(b) 12–72 hours
(c) 4–7 days
(d) 8–30 days
(e) More than 1 month

36 An elderly lady has an MRI brain examination as part of a research study. A number of lesions are noted in the basal ganglia, most prominently around the atria. They are hypointense to brain parenchyma on T1W, hyperintense to brain parenchyma on T2W and isointense to CSF on FLAIR.

What is the most likely diagnosis?

(a) Lacunar infarction
(b) Virchow-Robin spaces
(c) Lyme disease
(d) Periventricular leukomalacia
(e) Multiple sclerosis

37 A lateral skull x-ray in a short male child demonstrates multiple wormian bones and a small, receding jaw, with an obtuse angle to the mandible.

What syndrome could explain these findings?

(a) Menke's (Kinky hair) syndrome
(b) Crouzon syndrome
(c) Down's syndrome
(d) Clediocranial dysostosis
(e) Pyknodysostosis

38 An elderly, hypertensive man was found collapsed. MR imaging reveals a large infarct, with low signal intensity on T1W, high signal intensity on T2W, high signal on DWI and low signal on the ADC map.

How old is the infarct likely to be?

(a) 0–6 hours
(b) 6 hours to 4 days
(c) 4–14 days
(d) 14–30 days
(e) More than 1 month

39 A young man suffers a severe head injury and a CT head identifies a significant haematoma.

Which feature would be more suggestive of an extra-dural, rather than sub-dural haematoma?

(a) High attenuation
(b) Absence of skull fracture
(c) Peripheral enhancement
(d) Mixed density
(e) Crosses the tentorium cerebelli

40 MR imaging demonstrates bilateral acoustic neuromas.

Which of the following is not a recognised association?

(a) Optic pathway gliomas
(b) Parasagittal meningomas
(c) Paraspinal neurofibromas
(d) Facial nerve schwannomas
(e) Meningiomatosis

41 A neonate presents with a soft, painless mass in the posterior triangle of the neck. MR imaging demonstrates a multi-loculated, insinuating mass of intermediate signal on T1W and high signal on T2W.

What is the most likely diagnosis?

(a) Epidermoid cyst
(b) Dermoid cyst
(c) Lipoma
(d) Cystic hygroma
(e) Laryngocoele

42 Which two optic nerves are most commonly affected by skull base injury?

(a) I and II
(b) III and IV
(c) V and VI
(d) VII and VIII
(e) IX and X

43 Which of the following imaging features would not support the diagnosis of diffuse axonal injury?

(a) Multiple ovoid lesions ranging in size from 5–15 mm
(b) Involvement at the grey-white interface
(c) Lesions seen more prominently on CT than MR imaging
(d) On CT imaging, lesions demonstrate a low attenuation margin
(e) Sparing of grey matter

44 A male adolescent suffers from recurrent epistaxis and the subsequent imaging investigations reveal a likely juvenile angiofibroma.

Regarding this condition, which of the following statements is incorrect?

(a) The majority extend within the sphenoid sinus
(b) The majority extend within the pterygopalatine fossa
(c) Embolisation may be undertaken *via* the maxillary artery
(d) Biopsy should be performed prior to therapy to confirm the diagnosis
(e) The lesion may recur following treatment

45 A smoker suffers from a hoarse voice and is found to have a glottic laryngeal carcinoma. The tumour is seen to have supra-glottic extension and fixes the cords.

What is the tumour stage?

(a) T1
(b) T2
(c) T3
(d) T4
(e) T5

46 A 61 year old, known hypertensive man has an episode of expressive dysphasia which lasts a total of 90 minutes and resolves spontaneously in the A&E department. He is currently asymptomatic with no focal neurology.

What is the most appropriate management step?

(a) Carotid imaging within 48 hours, with a view to endarterectomy within 1 week
(b) Discharge with routine GP follow-up
(c) Give 300 mg Aspirin
(d) Urgent CT (with CT angiogram/ perfusion if available)
(e) Urgent MRI, including DWI

47 A 40 year old man presents with a seizure and a CT head reveals an intracranial lesion. An oligodendroglioma is suspected.

Which feature would be least expected with this diagnosis?

(a) Ill-defined enhancement
(b) Cystic degeneration
(c) Absence of oedema
(d) Calcification
(e) Hyperdense on unenhanced imaging

48 Which of the following is not involved in a Le Fort type II fracture?

(a) Pterygoid plates
(b) Orbital floor
(c) Anterior wall of the maxillary sinus
(d) Posterio-lateral wall of the maxillary sinus
(e) Medial wall of the maxillary sinus

49 A young man is involved in an RTA and arrives in hospital with a markedly reduced GCS. CT imaging reveals a fracture of the temporal bone.

Which of the following features would be more typical of a transverse, rather than longitudinal fracture of the temporal bone?

(a) Facial nerve palsy
(b) Involvement of the ossicles
(c) Bleeding from the external auditory canal
(d) Sparing of the labyrinth
(e) Involvement of the tympanic membrane

50 A neonate is noted to have cataracts, microcephaly, basal ganglia calcification and a patent ductus arterious.

Which of the following *in utero* infections could explain all of these features?

(a) Toxoplasmosis
(b) Rubella
(c) Cytomegalovirus
(d) Herpes simplex
(e) HIV

51 MR imaging of a neonatal brain reveals an absent septum pellucidum, corpus callosum, third ventricle, and interhemispheric fissure. The thalami are fused.

Which variant of holoprosencephaly does this most likely represent?

(a) Alobar
(b) Bilobar
(c) Septo-optic dysplasia
(d) Lobar
(e) Semilobar

52 After review of a CT head examination, *i.v.* contrast medium is administered. The enhancement follows the gyral/ sulcal pattern and involves the meninges around the basal cisterns.

Which of the following conditions can give rise to this enhancement pattern?

(a) CSF leak
(b) Pachymeningitis
(c) Spontaneous intracranial hypotension
(d) An intraventricular shunt
(e) Sarcoid

53 A patient has a glioma resected and the post-surgical tumour bed is examined by CT imaging. Images are acquired both before and after the administration of *i.v.* contrast medium.

Which of the following features would lead one to suspect that there is residual tumour?

(a) Linear enhancement around the pre-operative tumour bed
(b) Enhancement within the pre-operative tumour bed, 1 day after surgery
(c) Enhancement within the pre-operative tumour bed, 4 days after surgery
(d) Evidence of haemorrhage
(e) Dural enhancement

54 An adolescent undergoes MR imaging after having a number of seizures. A mass is demonstrated within the periphery of the right temporal lobe. The lesion contains a number of cysts. There is no surrounding oedema and the mass does not enhance after the adminstration of *i.v.* gadolinium.

Which of the following is the most likely diagnosis?

(a) Desmoplastic infantile ganglioglioma
(b) Tanycytic ependymoma
(c) Oligodendroglioma
(d) High grade astrocytoma
(e) Dysembroplastic neuroepithelial tumour

55 A patient presents with a focal neurological deficit. CT imaging reveals multiple haemorrhagic foci.

Which of the following features would be more consistent with haemorrhagic metastases, rather than haemorrhagic cerebrovascular malformations?

(a) Incomplete haemosiderin ring
(b) Surrounding oedema within the first week from symptom onset
(c) Central enhancement
(d) Calcification
(e) Lack of enhancement with *i.v.* contrast medium

56 A patient presents with left sided proptosis. A CT reveals a low-density mass causing expansion of the frontal sinus. There is focal thinning of the bony walls, dehiscence of the orbital roof and mass effect on the globe. There is no enhancement with *i.v.* contrast medium.

What is the most likely diagnosis?

(a) Rhinosinusitis
(b) Allergic fungal sinusitis
(c) Sinonasal polyposis
(d) Mucocoele
(e) Nasopharyngeal carcinoma

57 A patient with chronic alcoholic liver disease is admitted with confusion. MR imaging of the brain is performed.

Which of the following imaging features is not associated with alcohol intake?

(a) Enlargement of the mammillary bodies
(b) Periventricular demyelination
(c) Hyperintense focii within the corpus callosum on T2W
(d) Atrophy of the corpus callosum
(e) Hyperintense lesions within the pons on T2W

58 A child with fever and otalgia has a CT examination performed. There is opacification of both the middle ear and mastoid. Fluid levels can be seen. There is bony resorption of the mastoid and haziness of the air cell walls.

What is the most appropriate description?

(a) Acute mastoiditis
(b) Coalescent mastoiditis
(c) Bezold's abscess
(d) Osteomyelitis
(e) Subperiosteal abscess

59 A patient presents with pulsatile tinnitus. CT reveals a mass in the left temporal bone and there is focal uptake with ^{111}In octreotide imaging.

Which of the following is least likely?

(a) Glomus tympanicum
(b) Meningioma
(c) Carcinoid metastasis
(d) Small cell cancer metastasis
(e) Metastasis of papillary carcinoma of the thyroid

60 A 5 year old child presents with headache, vomiting and ataxia. On CT imaging, a high attenuation posterior fossa mass is seen to arise from the midline of the roof of the 4th ventricle.

Given the most likely diagnosis, which of the following is incorrect?

(a) There is hydrocephalus in the majority
(b) The mass tends to be hyperintense on T1W
(c) There is an association between enhancing pial nodules and seizures
(d) In children older than 3 years, the mass tends to be resected
(e) Recurrence is common

61 You are reporting an MR of the nasal sinuses, and you notice a mass within the right maxillary sinus. The request card reads: '?squamous cell carcinoma ?mucocoele/secretions.'

Which of the following features would be more supportive of a diagnosis of benign disease, rather than squamous cell carcinoma?

(a) Bony destruction
(b) Low T2W signal
(c) Peripheral enhancement
(d) Heterogeneous MR signal intensity
(e) Occupational exposure to nickel

62 A 50 year old patient presents with headache and visual disturbances. MR imaging is performed, and a mass is seen within the clivus. A chordoma is suspected.

Which of the following features would be unusual for this diagnosis?

(a) Isointense to brain parenchyma on T1W
(b) Calcification
(c) Lack of tracer uptake on a ^{99m}Tc-MDP bone scintigram
(d) Lack of enhancement with *i.v.* gadolinium
(e) Some regions of low signal on T1W

63 A patient presents with seizures. An MR of the brain reveals an apparent area of linear meningeal thickening adjacent to an intracranial tumour.

Which of the following would make the description of this thickening as a 'dural tail' less appropriate?

(a) The adjacent tumour is an extra-axial
(b) The area of thickening does not enhance
(c) The thickening is only present on two contiguous 5 mm sections
(d) The adjacent tumour is intra-axial
(e) There is adjacent hyperostosis

64 A patient presents with a cranial nerve palsy, and a CT head reveals a mass in the region of the jugular foramen.

Given this location, which of the following structures is least likely to be involved?

(a) The spinal accessory nerve
(b) The vagus nerve
(c) The middle meningeal artery
(d) The inferior pertrosal sinus
(e) The glossopharyngeal nerve

65 A middle aged man has acute, profound loss of a visual hemi-field. MR imaging reveals an acute infarct of the left occipital pole and inferior temporal lobe.

To which arterial territory does this correspond?

(a) Anterior cerebral artery
(b) Middle cerebral artery
(c) Posterior cerebral artery
(d) Posterior inferior cerebellar artery
(e) Superior cerebellar artery

66 An immuno-compromised patient presents with symptoms of encephalitis. MR imaging is performed and primary CNS lymphoma is considered likely.

Which of the following features would be unusual for this diagnosis?

(a) Supratentorial location
(b) A large, discrete solitary lesion
(c) Ring enhancement with *i.v.* gadolinium
(d) A peripheral rim of high signal on T2WI
(e) Decreased uptake of thallium-201 on SPECT imaging

67 A patient presents with a neurocutaneous disorder.

Which of the following is not a recognised association?

(a) Neurofibromatosis-1 and plexiform neurofibromas
(b) Osler-Weber-Rendu syndrome and cavernomas
(c) Von Hippel Lindau disease and pheochromocytomas
(d) Tuberous sclerosis and pial enhancement
(e) Sturge-Weber syndrome and cerebral atrophy

68 A patient presents with a sudden onset headache and a CT head is performed. No intravenous contrast medium was administered. An arbitrary region of interest is drawn, and the attenuation is found to be 25 HU.

What tissue type is this likely to represent?

(a) Bone
(b) Congealed blood
(c) Grey matter
(d) White matter
(e) Cerebrospinal fluid

69 A child undergoes MR imaging of their spine. A review of the lower lumbar levels reveals that the dorsal dura is incomplete and the subarachnoid space lies ventral to a neural placode, which is directly continuous with the skin. The ventral subarachnoid space does not appear to be dilated.

What would be the most appropriate term to describe this spinal dysraphism?

(a) Myelocoele
(b) Myelomeningocoele
(c) Lipomyelocoele
(d) Lipomyelomeningocoele
(e) Spinal lipoma

70 A middle aged man has an acute onset headache and subarachnoid blood is seen on a CT head. An MR angiogram is considered.

Regarding cerebral MRA, which of the following is incorrect?

(a) MRA should be avoided following the endovascular 'coiling' of aneurysms
(b) Giant aneurysms are better visualised on CT angiography rather than 3D time of flight MRA
(c) Aneurysms smaller than 3 mm are more difficult to detect by MRA imaging
(d) Recent subarachnoid haemorrhage may degrade time of flight MRA imaging
(e) MRA may show aneurysms missed on a digital subtraction angiogram

71 A child presents with a lump in the neck, and a branchial cleft cyst is suspected.

Which of the following features would be unusual for this diagnosis?

(a) Attenuation of 10 HU on unenhanced CT
(b) High signal on T2W MR imaging
(c) Located deep to a sternomastoid muscle
(d) Lack of rim enhancement on CT
(e) Present in the posterior triangle of the neck

72 A 42 year old woman presents with weakness in her hands. On examination she is noted to have wasting of the small muscles of the hand, burns and cuts to her fingers. There are reduced biceps reflexes, increased tone in the legs and upgoing plantars. An MRI brain and spine are requested.

What is the most likely unifying diagnosis?

(a) Cervical spondylosis
(b) Chiari II malformation
(c) Motor neurone disease
(d) Multiple sclerosis
(e) Rheumatoid arthritis

73 You are shown a set of paediatric MR and CT head images in a teaching session. There is a well defined, lobulated mass within a dilated left lateral ventricle. There is hydrocephalus. It is hyperdense on CT and returns moderately high signal on T2W. There is intense contrast enhancement.

What is the most likely diagnosis?

(a) Colloid cyst
(b) Meningioma
(c) Chorid plexus papilloma
(d) Ependymoma
(e) Giant cell astrocytoma

74 You are reporting plain radiographs. You note a suture line posterior and inferior to the occipitomastoid suture on a lateral skull radiograph of an infant.

What is this suture most likely to be?

(a) Innominate
(b) Mendosal
(c) Squamosal
(d) Coronal
(e) Sagittal

75 You are asked to review an MRI brain, and note that there is a focal abnormality of the left globe. There is a localised outpouching of the vitreous near the site of the optic nerve attachment.

What is the most likely diagnosis?

(a) Normal variant
(b) Phthisis Bulbi
(c) Buphthalmos
(d) Staphyloma
(e) Coloboma

Central Nervous System and Head & Neck Mock Paper Answers

1 (d)
The Fisher scale is useful in communicating the description of SAH. Grade 1: no haemorrhage evident, grade 2: SAH < 1 mm, grade 3: SAH > 1 mm, grade 4: associated intra-ventricular haemorrhage or parenchymal extension.

Ref: RITI 6b_093 SAH: Acute investigation, treatment and prevention.

2 (a)
This is a spinal dural AV fistula (type I), the fistula is present within the dura, producing distended draining veins on the pial surface and cord oedema secondary to venous hypertension.

Ref: RITI 6b_105 Spinal Vascular Anomalies.

3 (b)
Persistent hyperplastic primary vitreous is caused by the persistence of the embryonic hyaloid vascular system. Its features are microphthalmia, a vitreous body remnant of the hyaloid artery, retinal detachment and leukocoria, a hyperdense vitreous from previous haemorrhage, fluid-fluid levels from the degradation of haemorrhage, and an absence of calcification.

Ref: Aids to Radiological Differential Diagnosis, 4th Ed, p. 381.

4 (a)
Brain AVMs are the most common symptomatic vascular malformation. They typically present in 20-40 year olds with ictus from intracranial haemorrhage, progressive neurological deficit or headaches. Imaging features include: at CT: serpiginous, densely enhancing vessels without mass effect or oedema; at MR: a nidus of flow voids on T2W and PD sequences, at catheter angiography: grossly dilated vessels like a 'bag of worms'. CT imaging of a dural AVM is typically normal unless haemorrhage has occurred. Catheter angiography of a cavernous angioma is either normal or demonstrates only a faint vascular stain. Venous angiomata and telangiectasia are typically asymptomatic.

Ref: Aids to Radiological Differential Diagnosis, 4th Ed, p. 408–410.

5 (d)

Ref: RITI 6b_008 Plain Skull Radiography.

6 (c)
A number of features are suggestive of nodal metastases: a round, rather than elliptical shape (S/L axis ratio > 0.5), the absence of an echogenic hilum, a cystic area suggestive of necrosis, an ill-defined border, peripheral colour flow with regions of relative avascularity and subcapsular vessels, and punctate calcification (seen in metastases from papillary thyroid carcinoma).

Ref: RITI 6a_058 Ultrasound of the Thyroid and Parathyroid Glands.

7 (a)
This patient suffers from Gorlin-Goltz/ basal cell naevus syndrome, associated with multiple cutaneous basal cell carcinomas during childhood, odontogenic keratocysts, ectopic calcifications, and multiple skeletal anomalies. Mental retardation is another recognised association. All of the above answers above can present as cystic lesions of the jaw.

Ref: RITI 6b_048 Dental Pathology.

8 (a)
The displacement of the parapharyngeal space and styloid musculature can help localise neck lesions:

Fascial space	Displacement of parapharyngeal space	Displacement of styloid musculature
Masticator space	Posteromedial	Posterior
Carotid space	Anterior	Anterior
Pharyngeal mucosal space	Posterolateral	Posterior
Parotid space	Anteromedial	Posterior
Retropharyngeal space	Anterolateral	Anterior

Ref: RITI 6b_053 Imaging Neck Masses in Adults & Neuroradiology: the requisites, 2nd Ed, p. 698.

9 (c)
The common craniosynostoses include:

Craniosynostosis type	**Sutures prematurely fused**
Scaphocephaly	Sagittal
Brachycephaly	Coronal or lambdoid (but not both; can be bilateral)
Plagiocephaly	Coronal and lambdoid
Trigonocephaly	Metopic
Oxycephaly	Sagittal, coronal and lambdoid
Cloverleaf	Multiple paired sutures to produce a 'trilobar skull'

Ref: Radiology Review Manuel, 6th Ed, p. 178 & Aids to Radiological Differential Diagnosis, 4th Ed, p. 487.

10 (d)
Although all the above conditions can result in skull vault lucencies, LCH is the only one that is also associated with surrounding sclerosis. In this case, the sclerotic border indicates the healing phase of LCH. Other conditions that can produce a lucency with sclerosis include: epidermoid, encephalocoele, haemangioma, chronic osteomyelitis, and frontal sinus mucocoele.

Ref: Aids to Radiological Differential Diagnosis, 4th Ed, p. 481.

11 (a)
Schwannomas are the most common CPA mass. The epicentre of the lesion is typically in the epicentre of the internal auditory canal, typically causing a >2 mm difference in canal diameter on the effected side. Extension into the CPA causes an 'ice cream cone' appearance. On MR imaging, the lesion is iso-intense on T1W, hyper-intense on T2W and has dense enhancement (however, meningiomas also typically enhance). Calcification is not typical.

Ref: Primer of Diagnostic Imaging, 4th Ed, p. 544.

12 (e)
Chiari I is herniation of the cerebellar tonsils below a line connecting the basion and opisthion. Unlike Chiari II, III and IV, Chiari I is not associated with myelomeningocoeles. Indeed, the condition is frequently isolated without supratentorial anomalies. As well as the listed associations, Chiari I occurs with: basiliar impression, cranio-vertebral fusion, and Klippel-Feil anomaly.

Ref: Radiology Review Manuel, 6th Ed, p. 275.

13 (b)
Although non-specific, enhancement of the intracanalicular and labyrinthine portion occurs in Bell's palsy (other inflammatory and neoplastic conditions should also be considered). Enhancement of the tympanic and mastoid portions of the facial nerve is a normal variant. Demineralisation does not occur.

Ref: Primer of Diagnostic Imaging, 4th Ed, p. 612.

14 (e)

Ref: Aids to Radiological Differential Diagnosis, 4th Ed, p. 428.

15 (d)
MS plaques are typically of high-signal intensity on T2W and Proton density imaging. The hypointense thalamus (and putamen) are due to increased ferritin.

Ref: Radiology Review Manuel, 6th Ed, p. 311.

16 (b)
Descending transtentorial (or uncal) herniation is associated with: effacement of the ipsilateral suprasellar cistern, enlargement of the ipsilateral CPA cistern, Duret haemorrhages in the midbrain (which would feature as regions of high attenuation), and PCA ischemia.

Ref: Primer of Diagnostic Imaging, 4th Ed, p. 531.

17 (e)
A number of features are suggestive of a benign, rather than malignant, lesion. Cystic lesions are usually benign; a comet tail artefact usually indicates a (benign) colloid cyst; a complete low-echogenicity 'halo' increases the odds of a benign lesion 12 times. The overall echogenicity is another indicator: 96% of hyperechoic lesions are benign, compared to 74% of isoechoic and 39% of hypoechoic lesions.

Ref: RITI 6b_058 Ultrasound of the Thyroid and Parathyroid Glands.

18 (d)

	Ependymoma	**Astrocytoma**
Age	Adult	Children
Bone remodelling	More common	Less common
T1W signal	Low	Low/intermediate
Enhancement	Well defined, strong	Ill defined
Syrinx	More common	Less common
Haemorrhage	More common	Less common

Ref: RITI 6b_123 Primary tumours of the spinal cord.

19 (c)
'Red flags' for potentially serious headache include: precipitation with valsalva manoeuvre, age over 50, new abnormal neurological signs, progressive headache, onset in early morning, associated fever or systemic symptoms, change in character of headache.

Ref: RITI 6b_160 Acute and Chronic headaches.

20 (e)
Only 1% of meningiomas are associated with internal haemorrhage. Regarding the other characteristics: the inward bulging of the grey-white junction is suggestive of an extra-axial lesion, such as a meningioma; 60% of meningiomas are associated with oedema; meningiomas are typically hyperdense on unenhanced CT imaging and are seen to enhance with *i.v.* contrast medium.

Ref: RITI 6b_116 Characteristic appearances and differential diagnosis of meningiomas.

21 (b)
Epidermoid tumours are typically iso-intense to CSF on T1 and T2W imaging, with high signal on diffusion weighted sequences and heterogeneous signal on FLAIR imaging. They do not typically enhance.

Ref: RITI 6b_118 Acoustic Schwannomas.

22 (a)
In older patients with significant atheroma, there is a 1–2% risk of neurological deficit. This is reduced to < 0.5% in younger patients.

Ref: RITI 6b_034 Intra-arterial cerebral angiography: implications, technique and complications.

23 (d)
Temporo-parietal hypoperfusion is typically caused by Alzheimer's type dementia or Lewy body disease. Two other patterns to consider include: firstly fronto-temporal hypoperfusion, caused by Pick's disease, fronto-temporal dementia, chronic alcoholism and schizophrenia; and secondly patchy/ multiple perfusion defects, caused by AIDS-related dementia, schizophrenia and multi-infarct dementia.

Ref: RITI 7n_005 HMPAO 2.

24 (d)
The striatum comprises the caudate nucleus and putamen; the corpus striatum also includes the globus pallidus.

Ref: Primer of Diagnostic Imaging, 4th Ed, p. 500.

25 (d)
Venous occlusion progresses to infarction in approximately 50% of cases. These infarcts do not conform to arterial territories: occlusion of the midline veins may result in bilateral infarction (low attenuation on CT and increased T2W signal on MRI). Acute thrombus is hyperdense on pre-contrast CT imaging; however, *i.v.* contrast medium results in more intense enhancement of the walls of the sinuses than of their contents (the 'delta sign'). Haemorrhage is common. Brain swelling is prominent early in the clinical course; this is in contradistinction to arterial infarcts, where swelling is maximal at 3–5 days.

Ref: Aids to Radiological Differential Diagnosis, 4th Ed, p. 400.

26 (e)
On T1W imaging, the anterior pituitary is typically iso-intense and the posterior pituitary hyperintense; on T2W imaging, both the anterior and posterior pituitary are typically iso-intense. The gland is normally flat or concave superiorly, but may be convex in pregnancy.

Ref: Primer of Diagnostic Imaging, 4th Ed, p. 580.

27 (b)
An eccentric enhancing nodule may be seen in cases of toxoplasmosis, but is rare in lymphoma. Callosal involvement, ependymal spread and high attenuation on unenhanced CT imaging are typical features of lymphoma.

Ref: Primer of Diagnostic Imaging, 4th Ed, p. 549.

28 (b)
Orbital pseudotumour tends to: be unilateral (85%), involve the tendons, cause stranding of the intra-orbital fat, enlarge the lacrimal gland, be painful, and have a good response to steroids.

Ref: Primer of Diagnostic Imaging, 4th Ed, p. 624.

29 (e)
A Rathke's cleft cyst is typically hyperintense on T1W, and has smooth peripheral enhancement with intravenous contrast medium.

Ref: Diagnostic Radiology, 5th Ed, p. 564.

30 (a)
A thyroglossal duct cyst is described. Many are infrahyoid (25-60%), the US appearances can be extremely variable.

Ref: Clin Rad (2008); 63:613-622.

31 (e)
A craniopharyngioma would typically be seen as a cyst with a mural nodule. Calcification is present in 90% of cases in the younger age group. Both craniopharyngiomas and Rathke cleft cysts have variable signal intensities on MR imaging, but most commonly craniopharyngiomas have a low signal on T1W imaging. The enhancement pattern is typically ‘solid’ or ‘nodular’, as opposed to the ‘rim-like’ pattern seen in Rathke cleft cysts.

Ref: Neuroradiology: the requisites, 2nd Ed, p. 542–547.

32 (e)
A consensus panel has recently defined the US criteria for gauging carotid artery stenosis. Quantitative criteria include:

		Stenosis			
	Normal	**< 50%**	**50–69%**	**> 70%**	**Total occlusion**
ICA PSV (cm/s)	< 125	< 125	125 –130	> 230	undetectable
ICA/CCA PSV ratio	< 2.0	< 2.0	2.0 - 4.0	> 4.0	N/A
ICA EDV (cm/s)	< 40	< 40	40 - 100	> 100	N/A

Ref: Radiology (2003); 229:340–346.

33 (b)
A region that shows both diffusion and perfusion abnormalities represents irreversibly infarcted tissue, while a region that shows only perfusion abnormalities and has normal diffusion represents viable but ischaemic tissue: a ‘penumbra’.

Ref: Radiographics (2006); 26:S75–95.

34 (a)
Sturge-Weber syndrome is associated with calcification of the cortical gyri, rather than the basal ganglia. The cause of basal ganglia calcification can be divided into: physiologic, endocrine, (*e.g.* hypothyroidism, hypoparathyroidism, pseudo- and pseudo-pseudohypoparathyroidism), metabolic (*e.g.* Fahr's disease and mitochondrial cytopathies), congenital/ developmental (*e.g.* Cockayne's syndrome), infection (*e.g.* TORCH, cystercercosis, tuberculosis), toxic (*e.g.* CO poisoning, hypoxia, lead), and chemotherapy/ radiotherapy.

Ref: Aids to Radiological Differential Diagnosis, 4th Ed, p. 430.

35 (a)

Time	T1WI Signal	T2WI Signal
0–12 hours (hyperacute)	Intermediate	High
12–72 hours (acute)	Intermediate	Low
4–7 days (early subacute)	High	Low
8–30 days (late subacute)	High	High
more than 1 month	Low	Low

Ref: Aids to Radiological Differential Diagnosis, 4th Ed, p. 404.

36 (b)
Virchow-Robin spaces are invaginations of the sub-arachnoid space into the brain parenchyma. They are seen with increasing frequency with age. The signal intensity is identical to CSF: in the case above, none of the other causes would appear isointense to CSF on FLAIR imaging.

Ref: Radiographics (2007); 27:1071–81.

37 (e)
Pycnodyostosis is an autosomal recessive inherited disease featuring dwarfism, learning difficulties, nail dystrophy, receding jaw, wide cranial sutures, and multiple wormian bones.

Ref: Aids to Radiological Differential Diagnosis, 4th Ed, p. 486.

38 (b)

Time	T1WI Signal	T2WI Signal	DWI	ADC
0–6 hours (hyperacute)	Isointense	Isointense	High	Low
6 hours to 4 days (acute)	Low	High	High	Low
4–14 days (subacute)	Low	High	T2 shine through	Pseudonormalization
more than 14 days (chronic)	Low (encephalomalacia)	High through	T2 shine	High

Ref: Neuroradiology: the requisites, 2nd Ed, p. 194.

39 (e)
The ability to cross dural reflections, such as the falx and tentorium cerebelli, places the haematoma in the extra-dural, rather than sub-dural space.

Ref: Neuroradiology: the requisites, 2nd Ed, p. 247.

40 (a)
The patient fulfils the diagnostic criteria for Neurofibromatosis type 2. Unlike NF-1, there is no association with Lisch nodules, skeletal dysplasia, optic pathway gliomas or vascular dysplasia.

Ref: Radiology Review Manual, 6th Ed, p. 319.

41 (d)
The commonest ‘soft’ neck masses in infants and children are lipomas, haemangiomas and cystic hygromas. The latter have low-to-intermediate signal intensity on T1W and high signal on T2W.

Ref: Aids to Radiological Differential Diagnosis, 4th Ed, p. 394.

42 (a)
The olfactory (I) and optic (II) nerves are most often affected by skull base injury.

Ref: RITI 6b_062 Brain Complications of Injury.

43 (c)
The typical lesions of diffuse axonal injury are seen more prominently on MR than CT imaging.

Ref: RITI 6b_060 Diffuse Brain Injury.

44 (d)
The vascular nature of the tumour contraindicates biopsy.

Ref: Radiology Review Manual, 6th Ed, p. 387.

45 (c)
The staging is: T1: tumour confined to vocal cord. T2: supra/ subglottic extension with or without impaired mobility. T3: fixation of true vocal cord. T4: destruction of thyroid cartilage/ extension outside larynx. There is no T5.

Ref: Radiology Review Manual, 6th Ed, p. 387.

46 (c)
The patient has had a transient ischaemic attack (TIA). The Rothwell classification counts a score of ≥4 counts as a high risk TIA; the risk of a stroke within 4 weeks is up to 20%. 1 point is scored for each of: age (≥ 60), hypertension (≥140/90), diabetes, symptom duration of 10-60 minutes and speech disturbance alone; 2 points for symptoms of >60 minutes or a unilateral weakness. The described patient scores 5 and is therefore high risk, however, recent NICE guidelines state the following management plan for high risk TIAs: 300 mg aspirin should be started immediately, specialist assessment and investigation should be undertaken *within 24 hours* of onset of symptoms (7 days for low risk patients), and that measures for secondary prevention should be introduced. MR imaging (with DWI) should only be performed if there is uncertainty over the diagnosis or the vascular territory involved. The guidelines also advocate carotid imaging within 7 days with a view to endarterectomy (if appropriate) within 2 weeks.

Ref: Lancet (2005); 366: 29–36 & NICE guideline CG068 (published July 2008).

47 (e)
Oligodendrogliomas are slowly growing gliomas, most commonly located in the frontal lobes. Large nodular calcification is present in approximately 90% of cases. Cystic degeneration, ill-defined enhancement and a lack of oedema are all common. Over 80% are either hypo- or iso- dense on unenhanced CT imaging.

Ref: RITI 6_108 Primary tumours Gliomas – astros, oligos.

48 (e)
The medial wall of the maxillary sinus is spared in a type II fracture. The pterygoid plates are involved in all Le Fort fractures.

Ref: RITI 6a_024 Trauma of the face, orbit and mandible.

49 (a)
Longitudinal fractures are parallel to the axis of the petrous pyramid and predominantly affect the middle ear (including the ossicles and tympanic membrane). Transverse fractures are perpendicular to the axis of the petrous pyramid and affect the labyrinth. Facial nerve palsy occurs in 50% of transverse fractures, but only 20% of longitudinal fractures.

Ref: Radiology Review Manual, 6th Ed, p. 208.

50 (b)
In addition, rubella is associated with hearing loss, autism, pigmentary retinopathy, vasculopathy, pulmonic stenosis, and hepatosplenomegaly.

Ref: Neuroradiology: the requisites, 2nd Ed, p. 443.

51 (a)
This is the most profound form of holoprosencephaly, where there is almost no separation of the cerebral hemispheres or ventricles. There is a 'horseshoe' configuration of neural tissue with a single crescent-shaped ventricle. There is no 'bilobar' form of holoprosencephaly. Septo-optic dysplasia can be considered part of the holoprosencephaly spectrum.

Ref: Neuroradiology: the requisites, 2nd Ed, p. 421.

52 (e)
This is a leptomeningeal pattern of enhancement. This can be seen in acute stroke, leptomeningeal meningitis, inflammatory diseases such as sarcoid, and metastasis.

Ref: Neuroradiology: the requisites, 2nd Ed, p. 281.

53 (b)
Within the first 2 days, enhancement within the pre-operative tumour bed should be regarded as suspicious of incomplete resection. After this time, it is common for enhancing granulation tissue to develop. Dural enhancement is a normal post-operative finding.

Ref: Neuroradiology: the requisites, 2nd Ed, p. 167.

54 (e)
DNETs are benign tumours arising from cortical gray matter, most commonly found in the temporal lobes. They are characterised by the presence of multiple cysts and a lack of surrounding oedema. Desmoplastic infantile gangliogliomas typically occur before the 2nd birthday; Oligodendrogliomas typically occur in 30–60 year olds.

Ref: Neuroradiology: the requisites, 2nd Ed, p. 167.

55 (a)
Haemorrhagic metastases typically have an incomplete or absent haemosiderin ring. Calcification is rare. Most commonly, there is either nodular, eccentric or ring enhancement. This contrasts with haemorrhagic cerebrovascular malformations, which typically show minimal or central enhancement. Surrounding oedema is present in both the acute/ subacute phase.

Ref: Neuroradiology: the requisites, 2nd Ed, p. 135.

56 (d)
A mucocoele is the accumulation of mucous secretions behind an obstructed ostium. This causes expansion of the sinus cavity and bone remodelling. Differentiation from carcinoma can be difficult.

Ref: Diagnostic Imaging: Head and Neck, 1st Ed, p. II-2-57.

57 (a)
Wernicke's encephalopathy is associated with necrosis of the mammillary bodies and periventricular demyelination. Marchifava-Bignami disease is associated with hyperintense foci within the corpus callosum on T2W; pontine myelinosis is associated with hyperintense lesions within the pons. Atrophy of the corpus callosum is a recognised feature.

58 (b)
This is a description of coalescent mastoiditis. A Bezold's abscess represents extension of infection down into the tissues of the neck.

Ref: RITI 6a_017b Petrous temporal bone: infection, cholesteatoma and glomus tumour.

59 (e)
Octreotide is a somatostatin analogue, and uptake is seen where somatostain receptors are expressed, such as neuroendrocine tumours (*e.g.*, glomus tympanicum), and other malignancies (*e.g.*, small cell lung cancer, lymphoma, and breast cancer). There is also uptake in a few tumours that do not express the receptor (*e.g.*, meningioma, astrocytoma).

Ref: Nuclear Medicine –The Requisites, 2nd Ed, p. 223-5.

60 (b)
The mass is most likely a medulloblastoma. These tend to be iso-to-hypo intense on T1W. Leptomeningeal metastases, seen as enhancing nodules, can cause seizures. Hydrocephalus is present in 90% of cases.

Ref: RITI 6b_110 Medulloblastoma.

61 (c)
Squamous cell carcinoma is usually of heterogeneous, low T2W signal, with a solid enhancement pattern. Bony destruction is seen in approximately 80% of sinonasal SCCs at first presentation. Occupational exposure to nickel, chrome pigment and the use of Bantu snuff are recognised risk factors.

Ref: Neuroradiology: the requisites, 2nd Ed, p. 634.

62 (d)
Chordomas originate from the remnants of the embryonic notochord, and may occur at any point along the neural axis. The clivus is the second most frequently affected site. The tumour is locally aggressive, calcified in approximately 50% (giving rise to areas of low T1W signal) and enhances. They are typically isointense to brain parenchyma on T1W.

Ref: Neuroradiology: the requisites, 2nd Ed, p. 560.

63 (b)
The 3 main criteria for the definition of a dural tail are: presence on at least two contiguous 5 mm sections through the tumour (although now sections tend to be less than 5 mm thick); the greatest thickness being adjacent to the tumour; and enhancement being greater than the tumour itself. Dural tails have classically been described in association with meningiomas, but can occur with other extra-axial and even intra-axial tumours.

Ref: Clin Rad (2005); 60:171-188.

64 (c)
The contents of the jugular foramen include: cranial nerves IX, X and XI, the inferior petrosal sinus, the internal jugular vein, and the posterior meningeal artery. The middle meningeal artery runs within the foramen spinosum.

Ref: Netter's Concise Neuroanatomy, 1st Ed, p. 13.

65 (c)
The posterior cerebral artery supplies the mesial inferior temporal pole, occipital lobe, and perforators to the thalamus and midbrain.

Ref: Netter's Concise Neuroanatomy, 1st Ed, p. 65.

66 (e)
CNS lymphoma has increased uptake of thallium-201 on SPECT imaging.

Ref: Radiology Review Manual, 6th Ed, p. 304.

67 (d)
Tuberosis sclerosis is associated with, amongst other features: cortical tubers, subependymal nodules, giant cell astrocytomas, white matter lesions, retinal phakomas and vascular abnormalities.

Ref: Aids to Radiological Differential Diagnosis, 4th Ed, p. 450.

68 (d)
The typical attenuation values for commonly encountered tissue types are: bone, 400-1000 HU; congealed blood, 56-76 HU; grey matter, 36-46 HU; white matter, 22-32 HU; water (CSF), 0.

Ref: A Textbook of Radiology and Imaging, 5th Ed, p. 1724.

69 (a)
In the case above, if the ventral subarachnoid space were dilated, this would be more appropriately termed a myelomeningocoele. If the dorsal placode were continuous with a lipoma, continuous with the subcutaneous tissues, this would represent a lipomyelocoele.

Ref: Fundamentals of Diagnostic Radiology, 2nd Ed, p. 312.

70 (a)
MRA is often used to follow 'coiled' aneurysms. Giant aneurysms are rarely visualised to their full extent on 3D time-of-flight MRA because of flow in their nidus. Time-of-flight MRA images may be degraded by the T1-effects of blood degradation products.

Ref: Diagnostic Radiology, 5th Ed, p. 1313.

71 (e)
Branchial cleft cysts are derived from the 1st or (more commonly) the 2nd cervical pouch. These are usually anterior triangle lesions and of water CT attenuation (< 20 HU). Rim enhancement is seen in infected cysts.

Ref: Diagnostic Radiology, 5th Ed, p. 1455.

72 (b)
The patient has lower motor neurone signs in the upper limbs and upper motor neurone signs in the lower limbs. The most likely diagnosis is a syrinx (syringohydromyelia) within the cervical cord. A Chiari II malformation is usually accompanied by a myelomeningocele, abnormal development of the cerebellar vermis and hydrocephalus. The herniated cerebellum blocks CSF circulation and leads to the formation of a syrinx within the spinal cord.

73 (c)
The imaging characteristics are those of a choroid plexus papilloma. Meningiomas are rarely intraventricular and most frequently occur in middle aged women. Colloid cysts occur within the third ventricle. Ependymomas typically arise from the floor of the fourth ventricle.

Ref: Clinical Imaging: An Atlas of Differential Diagnosis, 4th Ed, p. 1124.

74 (a)
The innominate suture is present in all neonates and can be seen posterior to the occipitomental suture. It rarely persists in adulthood.

Ref: Accident and Emergency Radiology, 2nd Ed, p. 37.

75 (e)
A coloboma represents incomplete closure of the foetal choroidal fissure, affecting the eyelid, retina, choroid and iris. It can be associated with microphthalmos and the morning glory anomaly (where the optic disk is enlarged and elevated). It is commonly bilateral.

Ref: Radiology Review Manual, 6th Ed, p. 620.

Bibliography

Adam A, Dixon AK, Grainger RG, Allison DJ (eds.) 2008. Diagnostic Radiology. 5th Ed. New York: Churchill-Livingstone

Albrecht T, Thorelius L, Solbiati L, Cova L, Frauscher F (eds.) 2005. Contrast-Enhanced Ultrasound in Clinical Practice. 1st Ed. Springer

Brant WE, Helms CA (eds.) 1999. Fundamentals of Diagnostic Radiology. 2nd Ed. Philadelphia: Lippincott Williams & Wilkins

Case SM, Swanson DB (eds) 2008. Constructing Written Test Questions for the Basic and Clinical sciences. 3rd Ed. Publisher: National Board of Medical Examiners, Philadelphia

Chapman S, Nakielny R (eds.) 2003. Aids to Radiological Differential Diagnosis. 4th Ed. Philadelphia: Saunders Ltd

Dahnert W (ed.) 2007. Radiology Review Manual. 6th Ed. Philadelphia: Lippincott Williams & Wilkins

De Lacey G, Morley S, Berman LH (eds.) 2007. The Chest X-Ray: A survival Guide. 1st Ed. Elsevier, Saunders

Eisenberg RL (ed.) 2003. Clinical Imaging: An Atlas of Differential Diagnosis. 4th Ed. Philadelphia: Lippincott Williams & Wilkins

Guglielmi G, van Kuijk C, Genant H (eds.) 2001. Fundamentals of Hand and Wrist Imaging. 1st Ed. Berlin: Springer-Verlag

Graham R, Gallagher FA (eds.) 2009. Emergencies in Clinical Radiology. 1st Ed. Oxford University press

Grossman RI, Yousem DM (eds.) 2003. Neuroradiology: the requisites. 2nd Ed. Philadelphia: Mosby

Hansell DM, Armstrong P, Lynch DA, McAdams HP (eds.) 2005. Imaging of Diseases of the Chest. 4th Ed. Philadelphia: Mosby

Harnsberger HR, Hudgins PA, Wiggins RH, Davidson HC (eds.) 2004. Diagnostic Imaging: Head and Neck. 1st Ed. Elsevier

Hathout GM (ed.) 2009. Clinical Neuroradiology: A Case-Based Approach. 1st Ed. Cambridge University Press

Helms CA (ed.) 2004. Fundamentals of Skeletal Radiology. 3rd Ed. Elsevier, Saunders

Kessel, Robertson (eds.) 2005. Interventional Radiology: A survival guide. 2nd Ed. Elsevier, Churchill-Livingstone

Kovacs GT, Norman (eds.) 2007. Polycystic ovary syndrome. 2nd Ed. Cambridge University Press

Making the Best Use of Clinical Radiology Services: Referral Guidelines (2007). 6th Ed. London: Royal College of Radiologists

Manaster BJ, May DA, Disler DG (eds.) 2006. Musculoskeletal Imaging: The requisites. 3rd Ed. Philadelphia: Mosby

Middleton WD, Kurtz AB (eds.) 2003. Ultrasound: The Requisites. 2nd Ed. Philadelphia: Mosby

Moore KL, Dalley AF (eds.) 2005. Clinically Oriented Anatomy. 5th Ed. Philadelphia: Lippincott Williams and Wilkins

Raby N, Berman LH, De Lacey G (eds.) 2005. Accident & Emergency Radiology. 2nd Ed. Elsevier, Saunders

Radiology Integrated Training Initiative. Website: http://www.e-lfh.org.uk/projects/radiology. The Royal College of Radiologists, London

Rubin M, Safdieh JE (eds.) 2007. Netter's Concise Neuroanatomy. 1st Ed. Saunders

Sidhu PS, Baxter GM (eds.) 2002. Ultrasound of Abdominal Transplantation. 1st Ed. Stuttgart: Thieme

Sutton D (ed.) 1992. A Textbook of Radiology and Imaging. 5th Ed. Churchill Livingstone

Thrall JH, Zeissman HA (eds.) 2000. Nuclear Medicine -The Requisites. 2nd Ed. Philadelphia: Mosby

Weissleder R, Wittenberg J, Harisinghani MG, Chen JW (eds.) 2007. Primer of Diagnostic Imaging. 4th Ed. Philadelphia: Mosby

Wittekind C, Sobin LH, Greene FL, Hutter R, Klimpfinger M (eds.) 2005. TNM atlas. 5th Ed. Wiley